The Psychology of
Pleasantness *and* Unpleasantness

By

J. G. BEEBE-CENTER

NEW YORK / RUSSELL & RUSSELL

1965

The Psychology of
Pleasantness *and* Unpleasantness

To
OUISTITI

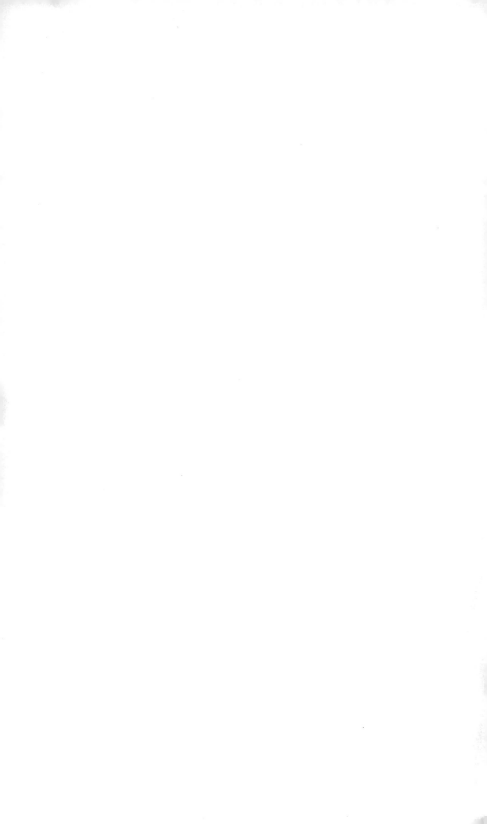

Introduction

The psychology of pleasantness and unpleasantness is at present a potential body of knowledge rather than an actual one. This is not due to any dearth of facts. Appropriate psychophysical methods were provided as early as 1871 by G. T. Fechner, and their application has yielded a considerable mass of information concerning the relation of pleasantness and unpleasantness to external stimuli and to motivating factors. In the 'nineties, the Wundtian school began the study of the vaso-motor and respiratory concomitants of pleasantness and unpleasantness, and this work, although it failed to live up to Wundt's expectations, yielded a further increment of useful information. Since 1910, finally, with the work of Head and Holmes, we have valuable data concerning the relation of pleasantness and unpleasantness to processes in the brain. These facts, however, lie scattered through the journals of many different nationalities and of many different periods. No attempt has been made to bring them together into a concrete systematic unit.[1]

This circumstance is doubly unfortunate. An adequate understanding of the conditions of pleasantness and unpleasantness would constitute not merely an advance of psychology, but a contribution to human welfare. However diverse they may be, all systems of ethics agree that some form of well-being should be the lot of mankind. Religions, for instance, promise beatitude, if not on this earth, at least in heaven,[2] and even for Kant the complete good must needs involve happiness.[3] True, mere knowledge of the conditions of pleasantness and unpleasantness would be far from sufficient to bring about universal well-being. Pleasantness is in all likelihood but one aspect of well-being. Besides, there would always remain the problem of application. Acquisition of this knowledge, however, would undoubtedly constitute a definite step toward the achievement of such an end.

The purpose of the present volume is to remedy the ghost-like state of the psychology of pleasantness and unpleasantness by bringing its facts together into a single orderly structure. The first chapter defines a systematic variable, hedonic tone, whose positive and negative values correspond respectively to pleasantness and unpleasantness. The second chapter discusses experimental methods. Chapters three to ten deal with the relation of hedonic tone to stimuli, to motivating factors, to memory, to muscular responses and to the nervous system. A final chapter is devoted to the theory of hedonic tone. The effort throughout has been to state the facts with a minimum of interpretation. Conclusions are separated from the results which underlie them, and the results themselves are placed in their experimental settings. Whatever value the work may have should thus prove relatively independent of personal systematic bias.

FOOTNOTES AND REFERENCES

[1] The nearest approach to such an integration is A. Lehmann's Hauptgesetze des Menschlichen Gefühlslebens, published originally in 1892 and in revised form in 1914. Excellent though it is in many ways, Lehmann's book is less an organized exposition of facts than a detailed formulation of theory with factual illustrations.

[2] Cf. J. RIBET. L'ascétique chrétienne, 7th edit., Paris, 1920, 225; Mahomet, Le Koran, translated in French by M. Savary, Paris, 1920, 12.

[3] I. KANT. Kritik der praktischen Vernunft, Erster Teil, Zweites Buch, Zweites Hauptstück (Sämtliche Werke, Vorländer edit., Vol. II, Leipzig, 1915, 142).

ACKNOWLEDGMENTS

I am indebted to a large number of authors and publishers for permission to reproduce passages, tables and figures. The indebtedness to authors is acknowledged by means of detailed references. However, these references do not always make apparent the indebtedness to publishers. In consequence I wish here to thank Harcourt, Brace and Company for permission to reproduce two tables from "The Effects of Music," edited by M. Schoen; Longmans, Green and Company for permission to quote a paragraph from William James' "Varieties of Religious Experience"; The Macmillan Company for permission to reproduce two figures from E. B. Titchener's "Experimental Psychology" and two paragraphs from the same author's "Textbook of Psychology"; and D. Van Nostrand Company, Inc., for permission to reproduce a table and a figure from M. Luckiesh's "Color and Its Application," and also several passages from L. T. Troland's "Fundamentals of Human Motivation."

In addition, I wish to thank the editors of the *American Journal of Psychology,* the *Journal of Experimental Psychology* and the *Psychological Review* for allowing me to reproduce the major portion of several of my own articles.

J. G. Beebe-Center

CONTENTS

vii

Chapter I

Definition of Pleasantness and Unpleasantness and of Hedonic Tone

It is well, before starting an investigation, to have clearly in mind that which one is to investigate. Strictly speaking, pleasantness and unpleasantness are mere words. The investigation of words, however, is a matter for the philologist. Our concern is not with the words themselves but with that which they represent. What is the meaning of the terms pleasantness and unpleasantness?

Let us first consider the colloquial meaning of these terms. Both involve the suffix -ness. According to Webster's dictionary, this suffix is "used primarily to form abstract nouns denoting in general *quality* or *state*." The implications of this definition are well borne out by everyday observation. When confronted with actual objects people rarely use the terms pleasantness and unpleasantness. Instead, they use the corresponding adjectives: "this perfume is very pleasant"; "this wet weather is unpleasant." As for children, the terms pleasantness and unpleasantness do not appear in their vocabulary until long after they have been accustomed to characterize objects as good or bad, pleasant or unpleasant. It seems clear that in colloquial usage the words pleasantness and unpleasantness are what logicians call *abstract* terms, as opposed to *concrete,* i.e., terms which refer to *attributes* and not to *things.*

The technical meaning of these terms is similar to their colloquial meaning. In the great majority of experiments upon pleasantness and unpleasantness the observers do not use the terms at all. Their reports are of the type: "x is pleasant," "y is unpleasant," "x is more pleasant than y." Pleasantness and unpleasantness do not appear until the ex-

1

perimenter begins to systematize the reports of his observers. It is obvious that in such cases pleasantness and unpleasantness do not denote actual data, items or constituents of the experience of the observers, but concepts, entities constructed by the psychologist to describe the actual data.

The concepts denoted by the words pleasantness and unpleasantness are quantitative ones. When an observer is asked to make judgments of pleasantness, for instance, he is able to state which of two objects is the *more* pleasant, and whether a single object is only *slightly* pleasant, *moderately* pleasant, or *very* pleasant. The experimenter can consequently arrange objects into a series, each member of which is related to its neighbors by being more pleasant than the preceding one and less pleasant than the following one. Such series are generally transitive, i.e. given any three members a, b and c, if a > b and b > c, then a > c. Difference in position in such series is considered to represent difference in amount of pleasantness. The concept pleasantness thus becomes a variable. But experimentation yields more than mere rank orders of pleasantness. By means of proper psychophysical technique it is possible to construct series of objects in which each member (other than the first) is just noticeably more pleasant than the preceding one. In accordance with custom in sensory psychophysics, just noticeable difference with respect to pleasantness is conceived to represent a difference of one unit in amount of pleasantness. The concept pleasantness thus becomes a truly quantitative variable. As a rule it is represented by a vector, relative position on the vector indicating relative amount of pleasantness. The same is true, naturally, of unpleasantness.

To say that the concepts pleasantness and unpleasantness are quantitative variables is not to say that experience itself is quantitative. These concepts are wholly distinct from the experience which they characterize. They are quantitative because the psychologist makes them so. Whether or not the experience to which they refer is likewise quantitative is a problem that I do not have to discuss, as I shall deal in this volume only with pleasantness and unpleasantness. It is a problem which I should not care to discuss, for I consider it to be not psychological but metaphysical. From the linguistic point of view pleasantness and unpleasantness are opposites. This has led a good many psychologists to consider the variables which they represent as positive and negative phases of a single more general variable. L. T. Troland, for instance, writes: " . . . Pleasantness can be treated as positive affection of a certain intensity, and unpleasantness as negative affection having a definite negative value. If we use this method of conception we do not have to distinguish constantly between pleasantness and unpleasantness, but may speak generally of affection or affective intensity—the measure of affection at any instant—which may have either positive, negative or zero values." [1] Such a view, however, has not met with universal acceptance. Thus in an article published in 1925, C. A. Ruckmick raises the query: "May pleasantness and unpleasantness be qualities of different orders?" [2] and concludes that "the opposition between these qualities is probably logical and not psychological." [3]

What are the facts concerning the relation of the variables pleasantness and unpleasantness? Experiments dealing with this question have been carried out by E. B. Titchener,[4] S. P. Hayes,[5] S. Fernberger[6] and W. S. Foster and K. Roese.[7] All four experiments agree with each other, so that it will suffice to describe only the most striking of them, that by Fernberger. This experimenter worked with the method of paired comparisons in which each stimulus of a group was compared with every other stimulus in the group with respect either to pleasantness or to unpleasantness, and the frequency of preference was taken as an index of the degree of pleasantness or unpleasantness.[8] The stimuli were 21 Milton-Bradley colors. There were 15 observers. The experiment involved two distinct series. In the first series the observers were instructed to judge in the case of each pair of stimuli which was the more pleasant. In the second series, they were instructed to judge in the case of each pair of stimuli (the same pairs as in the first series) which was the more unpleasant. The results are shown in Fig. 1, reproduced from Fernberger's article. The continuous line indicates for each stimulus (abscissae) the average of the frequencies with which it was judged *more pleasant* than the other stimuli by the 15 observers (ordinates). The broken line indicates for each stimulus

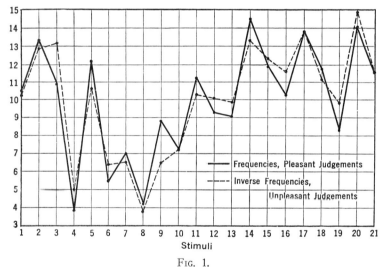

Fig. 1.

(After Fernberger)

the difference between the maximal frequency with which it could have been judged *more unpleasant* than the other stimuli, and the average of the frequencies with which it actually was so judged. Thus the continuous line indicates *relative pleasantness*, the broken one *relative lack of unpleasantness*. The high degree of correspondence between the two lines clearly shows that these two conceptions are equivalent.

The relationship, then, of the variables pleasantness and unpleasantness is such that a change towards the maximum of the one is equivalent to a change away from the maximum of the other. This relationship can be expressed in very simple fashion by making these two variables positive and negative phases of a single more general algebraic variable. As pointed out by Troland, such a convention obviates the necessity of distinguishing constantly between pleasantness and unpleasantness. We shall adopt this convention and shall henceforth consider pleasantness and unpleasantness to be respectively the positive and negative values of a single algebraic variable. In so doing, however, we shall not be maintaining that experience characterized by a negative value of the variable lacks some feature which is present in experience characterized by a positive value. Our convention applies solely to the concepts pleasantness and unpleasantness, not to the experience characterized by these concepts.

What name shall we give to this general algebraic variable? In his "Fundamentals of Human Motivation," Troland uses the term *affection* for this purpose.[9] This conflicts, however, with the widespread use of the term affection to represent an element having pleasantness and unpleasantness for its qualities.[10] This latter circumstance led Troland to avoid the term in his "Mystery of Mind" and to use *feeling* instead.[11] Here, however, we have a worse conflict. The term feeling has been used extensively by psychologists whose systems involved elements to represent combinations of affections (in the sense of elements) with sensations.[12] I myself have used the term *affectivity* to represent the general algebraic variable defined above,[13] but experience has shown this to be too radical a departure from custom. Either *feeling-tone* or *affective tone* would be good terms—they have been used in this sense by many well-known psychologists including Stout[14]—but their adoption would conflict with Wundt's use of feeling to indicate any "subjective" experience.[15] It seems to me at present that the best term is *hedonic tone*. The term has never to my knowledge been used in any other sense, and its use in the sense proposed is advocated by Baldwin's Dictionary of

Philosophy and Psychology.[16] In the present volume, then, the general algebraic variable, whose positive values correspond to pleasantness and whose negative values correspond to unpleasantness, will be called hedonic tone.

If the positive values of our general algebraic variable represent pleasantness, and its negative values, unpleasantness, what does its zero-value represent? Does it represent merely an ideal boundary between pleasantness and unpleasantness or a definite concept? Experimentation seems at first sight to support the latter alternative. If a set of very similar objects be presented to an observer with instructions to judge their pleasantness or unpleasantnes, he will usually judge several of them to be indifferent, and state that they are more pleasant than unpleasant objects but less pleasant than pleasant objects. It would seem, then, that there is a definite concept called indifference which refers to contents of experience different from those referred to by the concepts pleasantness and unpleasantness, and that it is this concept which is represented by hedonic tone of zero value.

In my opinion, however, this inference is erroneous. In an experiment upon habituation I had occasion to make my observers judge pairs of stimuli both relatively and absolutely. The observers were instructed to state, in the case of each pair, not only which stimulus was the more pleasant, but whether each was pleasant, indifferent or unpleasant. One observer astounded me by giving a considerable number of reports in which one stimulus was judged more pleasant than the other although both were judged to be indifferent. Upon being questioned, this observer explained that his procedure in arriving at a judgment was to represent the two stimuli in visual terms by two points on a vertical scale. Pleasantness was represented by the upper part of the scale, unpleasantness by the lower part, and indifference—this is the crux in the present connection—was represented not by a point in the centre of the scale, but by a range extending an appreciable distance above and below the centre. Thus if two stimuli were represented on the scale as shown below, the observer would naturally report that the first was the more pleasant, though both were indifferent. For the purpose of my experiment it was necessary to secure fine discrimination in terms of absolute judgments. I consequently instructed this observer to keep his range of indifference as narrow as possible. Within a few trials he ceased to give reports of the type mentioned above, and such reports did not recur during the remainder of the experiment.

This case clearly proves that indifference is equivocal insofar as it is a concept referring to a class of contents of experience. The contents to which it refers are not always the same. The case further indicates that such a concept overlaps the concepts pleasantness and unpleasantness, and consequently that it corresponds not to zero of hedonic tone, but to a range of values of hedonic tone centered upon zero. It follows that zero value of hedonic tone represents not a definite concept distinct from pleasantness and unpleasantness, but rather an ideal boundary between the latter.

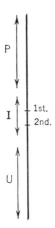

Fig. 2

Is this to state that the concept indifference is super-fluous? If, as I have sought to show, this concept represents merely a small and indeterminate range of hedonic tone around zero, and if such a range is covered by the concepts pleasantness and unpleasantness, it is clear that the concept is logically superfluous. It is superfluous, however, only in the logical sense. It remains a useful, albeit rough, means of referring to values of hedonic tone in the neighborhood of zero.

We are now in position to answer in detail the question asked at the beginning of the chapter. Pleasantness and unpleasantness are concepts characterizing experience. They are quantitative variables so related to each other that they may be represented respectively by the positive and negative values of a single algebraic variable. This single variable we shall call hedonic tone. The problem which we undertook to investigate in the introductory chapter thus becomes the problem of establ:shing the conditions of hedonic tone.

REFERENCES

[1] L. T. TROLAND. The Fundamentals of Human Motivation, New York, 1928, 282.

[2] C. A. RUCKMICK. The Psychology of Pleasantness, *Psychol. Rev.*, 32, 1925, 370.

[3] *Ibid*, 380.

[4] E. B. TITCHENER. Ein Versuch die Methode der paarweisen Vergleichung auf die verschiedenen Gefühlsrichtungen anzuwenden, *Philos. Stud.*, 20, 1902, 382.

[5] S. P. HAYES. A Study of the Affective Qualities, I. The Tridimensional Theory of Feeling, *Amer. J. Psychol.*, 17, 1906, 358.

[6] S. FERNBERGER. Note on the Affective Values of Colors, *Amer. J. Psychol.*, 25, 1914, 448.

[7] W. S. FOSTER and K. ROESE. The Tridimensional Theory of Feeling from the Standpoint of Typical Experiences, *Amer. J. Psychol.*, 27, 1916, 157.

[8] For a much more complete exposition of the method of Paired Comparisons, vide infra the chapter entitled "Methods."

[9] L. T. TROLAND. The Fundamentals of Human Motivation, New York, 1928, 266 seq.

[10] E. B. TITCHENER. A Textbook of Psychology, New York, 1909, 227.

[11] L. T. TROLAND. The Mystery of Mind, New York, 1926, 132.

[12] E. B. TITCHENER, *Op cit.*, 228.

[13] J. G. BEEBE-CENTER. The Relation Between Affectivity and Specific Processes in Sense-Organs, *Psychol. Rev.*, 37, 1930, 327.

[14] G. F. STOUT. A Manual of Psychology, 3rd Edit., London, 1924, 310 seq.

[15] W. WUNDT. Outlines of Psychology, translated by C. H. Judd, Leipzig, 1902, 33.

[16] J. M. BALDWIN. Dictionary of Philosophy and Psychology, New York, 1901, Vol. 1, 453.

Chapter II

Methods of Experimentation

INTRODUCTION

Experimental results constitute the backbone of psychology. In order to understand these results it is necessary to understand thoroughly the methods by which they have been secured. Before discussing data concerning hedonic tone we shall therefore deal with the methods of experimenting upon this variable.

In a paper read before the 6th International Congress of Psychology in 1910, Külpe suggested that these methods be classified not as units, but according to the various partial procedures of which they consist: "If ohe wishes to make a systematically complete and at the same time logically satisfactory survey of the methods used in the psychology of feeling, it is necessary to classify separately the *elementary* procedures involved in every one of the methods which are actually in use." [1] The classification which he proposed was as follows:

"A. *Methods of interpretation,* which are applied to expressions of feeling separated from the individual in whom they originate, e.g. to works of art, autobiographies, scientific performances. In the case of these methods it is sometimes necessary to institute a preliminary investigation concerning the genuineness, credibility and completeness of the evidence. The methods of interpretation are closely allied to the methods developed by the science of history.

"B. *Methods of observation,* which may be distinguished as follows:

1. Free and limited observation.
2. Casual and systematic observation.

3. Single observations and series of observations.
4. Simultaneous observation and retrospective observation.
5. Observation with full knowledge of the problem, with partial knowledge, and with no knowledge.
6. Noticing, perceiving, comparing, as particular forms of the observational relationship.
7. Observation while fully awake and while partially awake.

"C. *Methods of expression.* These divide into methods of verbal expression and methods involving other motor expressions.
1. *Methods of verbal expression,* or of report.
   (a) Free and limited reports; in the latter case the observer is instructed to use specific forms of report.
   (b) Terminologically *definite* and *indefinite* reports. The latter cannot always be avoided, and in certain cases the necessity of limiting himself to certain terms may constitute a disturbing obligation for the observer. One has to reckon with the possibility that reality is richer than our concepts.
   (c) Absolute and relative reports.
   (d) Direct and indirect reports. In the case of the latter one utilizes circumlocution or metaphors.
   (e) Description, explication, interpretation, explanation.
   (f) Reports of perceptions, recollections and conjectures.
   (g) Varying degrees of certainty of reports.
   (h) Spontaneous reports and answers to questions.

2. *Methods of motor expression.*
   (a) Of mimicry; (b) of gesture; (c) of movements of the entire body.

"D. *Methods of producing impressions,* of experimental procedure in the narrower sense:
1. Presentation, production and suggestion.
2. Production of constant and variable impressions.
3. Regular and irregular alternation of impressions.
4. Single impressions, paired impressions, serial impressions.
5. Direct and indirect production of impressions.

"E. *Methods of registering reactions.*
1. Writing down reports or phonographic reading of them.
2. Measurement of time.
3. Photographic and cinematographic recording of mimicry, gestures, movements of the entire body.
4, 5, 6. Sphygmography, pneumography, plethysmography.
7. Measurement of blood pressure (sphygmomanometry).
8. Determination of the number of blood corpuscles.
9. Measurement of temperature.
10. Determination of rates of metabolism and of conversion of energy.
11. Determination of muscular strength (dynamometry, ergography).
12. Determination of the psycho-galvanic phenomenon.
13. Determination of absolute sensitivity and of sensitivity to differences.
14. Determination of ideational processes and of thought processes.

"F. *Methods of treating data.*
1. Arrangement into categories.
2. Computation, statistical treatment, presentation in tabular and graphical form.
3. Separation of essential matter from the unessential.
4. Separation of typical cases from individual ones.

5. Derivation of laws, correlations.
6. Theoretical systematization and explanation." [2]

There is no question but that this classification constitutes the most thorough available analysis of the methods of studying hedonic tone. Were logical adequacy identical with meaningfulness, we should adopt it without question. But no such identity exists, and in following Külpe's analytic approach, we should run a great risk of learning much concerning relatively unimportant details of procedure but little concerning the concrete methods themselves. We shall consequently refrain from following Külpe, and adopt a form of classification which, whatever its logical weakness, will enable us to deal with the various methods as units.

It has long been customary to divide experimental methods dealing with hedonic tone into two groups, according to whether they emphasize the relation of hedonic tone to stimuli or its relation to responses of the organism. Methods emphasizing relation to stimuli are called *methods of impression.* Methods emphasizing relation to responses are called *methods of expression.* We shall deal with these two methods successively, beginning with the methods of impression.

METHODS OF IMPRESSION

Like the psychophysical methods used in the study of sensory and perceptual variables, the methods of impression have their origin in the work of G. T. Fechner. In an article entitled "Concerning Experimental Æsthetics," published in 1871,[3] Fechner proposed three methods involving what he called an "extensive measure" of hedonic tone— a measure determined by the *number of individuals* expressing preference, rather than by the *degree of preference* of a given individual.[4] These methods are:

1. The method of choice: this method is described by Fechner as follows for the particular case of a set of rectangles differing in the proportion of base to height: "One

presents to a large number of persons the proportions which are to be judged in respect to their relative pleasingness. The proportions should be arranged in as simple a fashion as possible. If the question is one of direct pleasingness, one instructs the observers explicitly to refrain from thinking of any particular use, and asks them to designate the proportion which according to its own nature seems the most pleasing, and that which is the least pleasing. One then records each preference in the appropriate column of a preference-table, and each dislike in the appropriate column of a table of dislikes, entering a 1 when the preference or dislike refers to a single proportion, and entering the fractions 1/2 or 1/3 when there is hesitation between two or three proportions. Finally one adds the figures in each column of the two tables, and compares the totals. With this procedure the less important judgments of dislike (often disregarded by me) can serve as a kind of check, for the proportions most rarely chosen must be at the same time rejected the most frequently if the method is to be consistent." [5]

2. The method of production: Fechner describes this method as follows (again in its application to rectangles differing in the proportion of base to height) : "A large number of persons, instead of being asked to choose the most pleasing among a number of proportions, are asked to *produce* the most pleasing proportion in as simple form as possible. One then ascertains the proportion corresponding to the greatest number of productions, or that around which the greatest clustering takes place. Lesser degrees of pleasingness are measured according to the lesser number of productions corresponding to any particular proportion." [6]

3. The method of use: with this method, according to Fechner, the following procedure takes place: "One measures the dimensions or subdivisions of the simplest objects which one finds in use or in commerce, in short, in everyday life. These objects, however, must be such that the form is determined directly by considerations of pleasingness

(provided that this pleasingness be inherent) rather than by considerations of the end for which they are used or of their meaning or of their harmony with other objects. They must not, furthermore, allow any arbitrariness in the mode of application of the measure. According to this method the relative measure of pleasingness is again determined by the relative frequency of the occurrence of this or that proportion." [7]

The two latter methods have been little used since the time of Fechner and have consequently undergone but little change. The method of choice, however, besides undergoing minor variations, has been developed in three different directions to give rise to the methods of order of merit, of paired comparison, and of single exposure,—the three classical quantitative methods of impression.

Minor Variations of the Method of Choice.—The most important minor variation of the method of choice is that described in 1905 by L. J. Martin under the name "method of gradual variation." This method is practically identical with the method of limits of general psychophysics. An object is changed *continuously* with respect to some one dimension (length for instance), and the observer judges what state is optimal. L. J. Martin applied this method to the investigation of the comic. She used an extensible picture of a dachshund to determine what length of the animal was the most comical. The method is obviously applicable to studies of hedonic tone whenever it is desired to determine optima.[8]

Development of the Method of Order of Merit.—In 1893, Witmer suggested the following improvements in Fechner's method of choice, calling his new method the "method of regular arrangement of figures." [9]

1. The use of a complete and regularly spaced series of stimuli,—i.e. of a series in which the aspect to be judged varies in regular steps from a value of $1/\infty$ to a value of ∞.[10]

2. The simultaneous presentation of the entire series of stimuli arranged in order of increasing (or decreasing)

magnitude of the aspect upon which judgments are made.[11]

3. The determination by the observers, not merely of the most agreeable and most disagreeable stimuli, but of the stimuli representing other important points on the curve of hedonic tone theoretically correlated with the series of stimuli.[12]

In his "Outlines of Psychology," published in 1893, Oswald Külpe spoke in very general terms of a method of studying hedonic tone, which he called the "serial method." [13] Not, however, until 1906 in a paper before the 2nd Congress of Experimental Psychology did he give a definite description of the method.[14] Its chief characteristic lay in making the observers not merely indicate the most pleasing and least pleasing objects of the set under investigation, but rather arrange *all* of these objects into an hedonic series. Külpe writes as follows concerning this method: "Its essential characteristic consists in having observers change a series of objects arranged according to mathematical or physical aspects into an hedonic series. Judging from the experiences which I gathered together previously and again recently in conjunction with Mr. Legowski, the most practical procedure is first of all to secure a rough ordering of groups and from these to work out then the finer divisions. Objects of equivalent æsthetic value are included in one group. The intervals between such groups are of different sizes and can also be judged by the observers. In the case of simple figures, the establishment of such series according to relative pleasingness took about three minutes on the average. Still another practical procedure with the serial method is to have the observer choose first of all the relatively most pleasing members of the series, and then again from those which remain the relatively most pleasing ones, and so on to the last number. In this manner a series of simple choices is first secured and afterwards the entire hedonic series may be considered and tested as a whole." [15] This method has become one of the three classical methods of impression. It is known in English as the method of order of merit.

It will have been noticed that the method of order of merit measures hedonic tone by relative position, not by units of amount. True, Külpe states that observers may estimate the distances between various members of the series once the latter has been established, but on the whole Fechner's "measure of extensive pleasantness" is dropped without being replaced by any other measurement in terms of units. More recently Thorndike has suggested several means of transmuting measures by relative position into measures in units of amount, one of which involves a unit very similar to Fechner's "measure of extensive pleasantness."[16] Suppose that in the case of a series of objects a b c d e f g h, ranked in order for some definite trait by a large number of judges (or many times by a single judge), the percentages of times that one member has been ranked below the next higher member are:

$$
\begin{array}{lll}
\text{a below b} & 74\% \\
\text{b \quad`` \quad c} & 74\% \\
\text{c \quad`` \quad d} & 74\% \\
\text{d \quad`` \quad e} & 70\% \\
\text{c \quad`` \quad f} & 80\% \\
\text{f \quad`` \quad g} & 60\% \\
\text{g \quad`` \quad h} & 90\%
\end{array}
$$

On the assumption that "equally often noticed" means "equal," "more often noticed" means "greater," and "less often noticed" means "less," we can consider that $(h - g) > (f - e) > (b - a) = (c - b) = (d - c) > (e - d) > (g - f)$. It is possible by making another assumption further to compute how much greater $h - g$ is than $f - e$, etc. This assumption is that given any two objects, a and b for instance, the frequency of the judgments $a > b$ will vary as a function of the difference between these objects with respect to a certain trait in accordance with a particular form of the mathematical function known as the phi function of gamma. Roughly speaking this means that when a is very much less than b, the frequency of the judgments $a > b$ will be very small, but never quite zero per cent (cf.

frequency for a — b = — 5 in the figure below) ; that as a increases by equal steps up to a = b, the frequency of judgments a > b will increase not by equal steps, but by increasing steps up to a value of 50% for a = b (cf. the frequencies

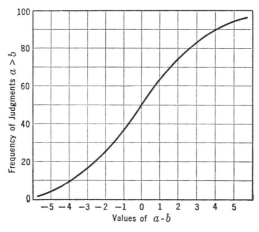

FIG. 3

for the values — 4, — 3, — 2, — 1, and 0 of the difference
a — b in the figure above) ; that beyond a = b, as a continues to increase by equal steps, the frequency of judgments
a > b will continue to increase, not by increasing steps, but
by decreasing steps (cf. the frequencies for the values 1, 2,
3 and 4 of the difference a — b in the figure above) ; and
finally that when a is very much larger than b, the frequency
of judgment a > b will be very large, though never 100%.
This assumption is essentially a complete generalization of
the so-called phi-gamma hypothesis of perceptual psychophysics, which has been borne out for the field of perception
by a great number of observations.

Thorndike gives a table for converting frequencies of
judgments a > b into amounts of difference a — b according
to what he terms the "probably best relation to assume"
between these variables. The table is reproduced in part
below. Amounts of difference are stated in terms (as mul-

tiples) of one particular amount of difference arbitrarily chosen as unit, namely that corresponding to a frequency of 75%. An excerpt from this table is given below. %r means "the percentage of judgments that x > y," $\dfrac{\Delta}{P.E.}$ means "x-y in multiples of the difference such that %r is 75."

TABLE I

%r	Δ/P.E.	%r	Δ/P.E.
50	.00	80	1.25
55	.19	85	1.54
60	.38	90	1.90
65	.57	95	2.44
70	.78		
75	1.00		

(*After Thorndike*)

A graphical representation of the relationship indicated by Thorndike's table is given below. As may be seen, it is

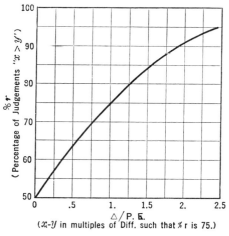

Fig. 4

one-half of the curve for a particular form of the phi function of gamma. It is only a half curve because the table deals only with frequencies of 50% and greater; and this circumstance in turn is due to the fact that frequencies of judgments a > b which are less than 50% may obviously be converted at once into frequencies of the converse judgment, namely b > a, which are greater than 50% (provided, naturally, that judgments "equal" have been ruled out by instruction or by mathematical treatment of the data before calculating the frequencies).

Thorndike's procedure for transmuting measures by relative position into measures of relative amounts has as yet received little application in the psychology of hedonic tone. This is very regrettable, for the high degree of specificity which it allows in the statement of functional relations is bound to be beneficial both in the verification of the relations and in their practical application. Consider, for instance, the work of Garth on changes in the color preferences of children with age.[16a] Using Thorndike's method, Garth ascertained for groups of children of various ages the hedonic value of seven colors relative to each other in terms of $\frac{\triangle}{P.\ E.}$, the ratio of difference to probable error of difference. He then constructed a scale, using as units a value of $\frac{\triangle}{P.\ E.}$ equal to .01, and computed the hedonic values of the colors according to this scale when white was arbitrarily assigned a value of zero. This procedure enabled him to describe the changes in color preferences of children with increasing age in the graphical form depicted below (abscissae represent school grades). Clearly the specificity of this description is far greater than could have been achieved by the mere use of rank orders. In the latter case, for instance, it would have been impossible to bring out the shift with increasing age of the hedonic value of red, green, orange, violet and yellow away from blue towards white.

Development of the Method of Paired Comparison. —Another development of Fechner's method of choice gave rise to what is known today as the method of paired comparison. This method was first suggested by Fechner himself. In the course of his experimentation he noticed in his observers a tendency to prefer the middle members of a series of objects irrespective of their nature.[17] In order to

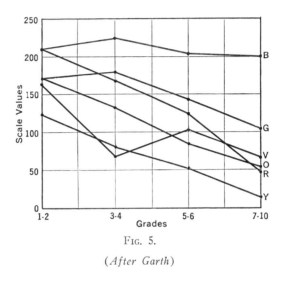

FIG. 5.

(*After Garth*)

eliminate this "influence of the mean," he advocated a modification of his original method of choice such that the objects to be judged would be presented to the observers not all simultaneously, but in successive pairs.[18] He himself, however, made but little use of this method and it was left to his successors to try the method out thoroughly and to formulate it with exactitude.

In 1894, Jonas Cohn gave a precise formulation of the method, suggesting at the same time that the pairs of stimuli be presented, not in haphazard order as with Fechner, but according to a definite sequence.[19] He wrote: "Assuming that there is a series of ten members to be tested in respect to each other for their relative pleasingness by means of the method of paired comparison, for instance ten colors from all parts of the color circle, $\dfrac{10 \times 9}{2} = 45$ comparisons are possible. If these are completely carried out each color will have been compared with all the nine others. The judgments possible are each time only "right the better," or "the same"; judgments such as "doubtful" are regarded as analogous to judgments of identity, but are recorded separately. The type of protocol is as follows: all colors with the exception of the last one (thus 1, 2, 3 . . . 9) are written in the horizontal line, and all with the exception of the first (thus 2, 3, 4 . . . 10) in the left vertical line. The lower half, marked off by a heavier line

Colors

		I	II	III	IV	V	VI	VII	VIII	IX
	II	1								
	III	2	3							
	IV	18	4	5						
	V	19	20	6	7					
Colors	VI	31	21	22	8	9				
	VII	32	33	23	24	10	11			
	VIII	40	34	35	25	26	12	13		
	IX	41	42	36	37	27	28	14	15	
	X	45	43	44	38	39	29	30	16	17

FIG. 6.

(*After J. Cohn*)

from the original rectangle contains in each of its fields one of the 45 comparisons. It now remains to establish the order of the presentations. It is advisable so to choose this order that the observer shall not remark its regularity lest his judgment be influenced. On the other hand it is desirable that the order be easily comprehensible and familiar to the experimenter in order that despite the large number of presentations speed and accuracy may remain assured. The order expressed by numbers in the attached diagram best satisfies these requirements. If then the total number of preference judgments for each color be counted (judgments of identity being reckoned as $\frac{1}{2}$), a measure is secured for the relative pleasingness of the individual colors."[20]

Cohn further suggests a simple means of avoiding the space error: "At the same time," he writes, "this order makes possible continual change of spatial position, as each color occurs twice in succession and thus can occupy once the right side, once the left."[21] This same procedure is obviously applicable for avoidance of the time error in successive comparisons.[22]

In 1904, Kowalewski[23] sought to establish an order of presentation which would secure the greatest possible spacing between any two occurrences of the same stimulus. In the case of an uneven number of stimuli 2 m+1, he points out that this condition would best be fulfilled if any m pairs of the series consisted of different stimuli.[24] Kowalewski does not supply any general formula for the generation of such a series. He merely describes his empirical procedure in the case of series of 5 members,[25] and states the order—without description of how it is established—in the case of series of 7 and 15 members.[26]

In 1906, yet another order of presentation was suggested by Külpe.[27] The first member of a series of stimuli is compared successively with each of the following members (e.g. the pairs are 1-2, 1-3, 1-4, . . . 1-n); the second is likewise compared with all the following members (e.g. 2-3, 2-4, . . . 2-n); and so on for each successive member until member n — 1, which can be compared only with member n. "This order," writes Külpe, "is not at all complicated and requires very little time. When it was repeated after four weeks in the case of fourteen members, it yielded practically the same values."[28]

Of these various modes of presentation, that advocated by Kowalewski is obviously the best. It is, however, very difficult to prepare except in the case of sets of 5, 7 or 15 stimuli for which one can use the series worked out by Kowalewski himself. In other cases it seems most expedient to arrange a sequence of pairs of stimuli in accordance with Cohn's procedure, thus precluding any influence of the time-error or of the space-error, and then to arrange the sequence by trial and error in such a fashion that no two successive pairs contain a common member.

In its usual application the method of paired comparison yields measures of hedonic tone by relative position, not in units of amount. It is true that it yields in the case of each stimulus a frequency of preference. Each pair of stimuli, however, is judged but once, and consequently this frequency of preference is not the frequency with which one of two objects is judged the more pleasant, but the frequency with which one object is judged more pleasant than any of a number of objects. Such a frequency of preference cannot be translated into amount of pleasantness by any known hypothesis.

This limitation of the method of paired comparison has recently been obviated by L. L. Thurstone.[29] His procedure involves in the first place a statistical application of the method of paired comparison in which every pair of a given set of stimuli is presented for comparison not once, but a large number of times. This may involve either the use of many observers making each comparison once, or the use of one observer making each comparison a large number of times. The consequence of this procedure is that the results involve in the case of each pair not merely the information that one member is "greater than" or "equal to" the other with respect to the characteristic under investigation, but the far more accurate information that one member is judged greater than the other with a certain specific frequency.

The second main feature of Thurstone's procedure is the acceptance of the assumption that the frequency of judgments a > b varies as a function of the difference between a and b in accordance with a particular form of the phi function of gamma. By means of this assumption Thurstone is able in the case of each particular pair of a set of stimuli to determine the difference between these stimuli with respect to some particular trait in terms of a unit of amount. This is done by consulting a table of the normal probability integral.

The third important step in Thurstone's procedure is the determination of the values corresponding to the various stimuli upon a single scale. This is done by averaging for each stimulus the differences between it and the other stimuli with which it has been paired. In view of the fact that

$$\frac{(a-b) + (a-c)}{2} = a - \frac{(b+c)}{2} ,$$ this computation is

equivalent to determining the difference between each stimulus and the average of all stimuli in the series and yields for all stimuli a value relative to the same standard, thus allowing the assignment to them of values upon a single scale.

In his most recent article upon this general procedure Thurstone suggests an improvement in this last step which involves weighting the differences between any one stimulus and all others before these differences are averaged. The equations required for this weighting are fairly complicated, however, and I must refer those wishing to study them to Thurstone's article.[30]

Just recently, J. P. Guilford has suggested two short-cuts in the application of Thurstone's general procedure.[31] The first is for use in cases where none of the frequencies is less than 15% nor greater than 85%. It obviates all calculation from tables by considering the total number of times one stimulus of a set is judged "greater than" any of the other stimuli in the set to be a measure of its value relative to these others with respect to the particular trait under investigation.[32] Guilford states that in the case of two sets of data used by Thurstone the results by means of this short-cut correlate with those by Thurstone's lengthy procedure to the extent of .985 and .994 by Pearson's formula. The second short-cut is for use when the occurrence of extreme frequencies precludes the use of the first short-cut. It involves, in the case of each stimulus, first the determination of the average of the frequencies with which it is judged greater than each of the other stimuli in the set (with respect to the trait under investigation), and only subsequently the determination of the scale-value corresponding to this average frequency in a table of the normal probability integral. This scale-value is then considered the final measure of the stimulus relative to the other stimuli of the set.

Development of the Method of Single Stimuli.—A third development of Fechner's method of choice gave rise to what is known as the method of single stimuli. This method was first formulated by D. R. Major[33] under the name "method of isolated exposure." It was considered by him to be a mere modification of Külpe's serial method. Major thought that the latter in its usual form was inapplicable to experimentation upon colors because of the effects of color-contrast. He consequently determined to present his stimuli not all together, but singly, asking the observers to state their judgments of each experience according to the following scale:

    1. Very pleasant.
    2. Moderately pleasant.
    3. Just pleasant.
    4. Without affective tone.
    5. Just unpleasant.
    6. Moderately unpleasant.
    7. Very unpleasant.

This method was used with a slight variation by J. Segal in a research published in 1906.[34] Segal, instead of having seven categories, had only four, namely "most pleasing," "moderately pleasing," "displeasing," and "indifferent." Most subsequent investigators have retained the seven-step scale, altering the numerical values to $-3, -2, -1, 0, 1, 2, 3$. Some, however, have used as few as three, and some as many as twenty.

Major did not claim that this method yielded absolute results. He believed the scale might vary considerably from one observer to the other, and that the steps of the scale might not be comparable even for a single observer. Concerning this latter point there have recently been secured a number of interesting experimental data. In 1923, E. S. Conklin published an investigation of the method of single stimuli[35] in which he had 1699 observers rate six propositions such as "to do ridiculous initiation stunts in public" according to the following scale:

1. Greatest possible pleasure.
2. Very, very great pleasure.
3. Very great pleasure.
4. Great pleasure.
5. More than a little pleasure.
6. Just the slightest pleasure.
7. Neutral, neither.
8. Just the slightest displeasure.
9. More than a little displeasure.
10. Great displeasure.
11. Very great displeasure.
12. Very, very great displeasure.
13. Greatest possible displeasure.

Plotting the frequencies with which the various members of the scale were used yielded the graph reproduced in Fig. 7. It is obvious from this graph that certain members are used with special predilection, and the fact that these members are 1, 4, 7, 10 and 13,—evenly spaced—indicates that this predilection is due to the scale and not to the stimuli.

In an attempt to obviate the occurrence of preferential members, Conklin repeated the experiment with a scale of nine members and a lesser number of observers. The results do not show such regularly spaced preferred members, and Conklin concludes that a scale of nine members is adequate. Inspection of the graph in Fig. 8, however, indicating the frequencies for the nine categories, shows that members 4 (moderate pleasure), 6 (moderate displeasure) and

7 (great displeasure), received a marked preponderance of votes, and suggests that even nine members involve an artificial emphasis upon certain categories irrespective of stimuli.

Conklin's findings have recently been confirmed by P. T.

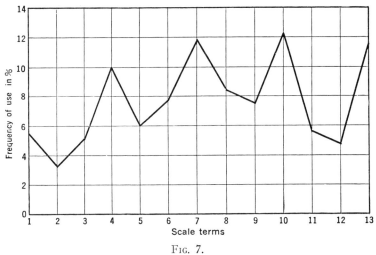

FIG. 7.

(*After Conklin*)

Young.[36] Using a scale of eleven members, he had 19 observers rate by this scale 43 common foods the names of which were read out aloud. The results showed a distinct predilection for the 3rd and 9th members, corresponding respectively to "pleasure" and "displeasure." Young points out that both his results and those of Conklin remind one of an investigation by Coover on mental habits in relation to judgment.[37] Young writes: "Bringing together available evidence from a wide variety of fields, Coover demonstrated a preference for round numbers. In the twelfth and thirteenth census reports, for example, the figures indicate that persons give their ages most frequently in multiples of 5 and 10. Also when students' grades are given on a percentile basis the figures indicate that the teachers have a distinct preference for multiples of 5 and 10. Coover found that judges, in giving a criminal sentence, have a marked preference for round numbers when the sentence is in years, and for quarters of a year when the sentence is

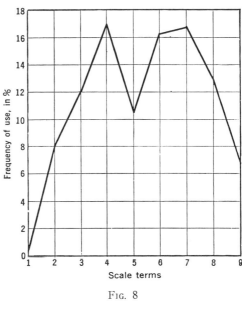

Fig. 8

(*After Conklin*)

in months. Further, in the estimation of star magnitudes a preference for round numbers is manifest. For example, one bit of evidence gives 1239 stars of the 6.5 magnitude, and only 159 of the 6.6. . ." [38]

This rapprochement by Young suggests that it might be the use of numbers in scales of value which determines the occurrence of preferential values. Recent experimentation by Mr. N. E. Cohen in this laboratory has shown this not to be the case. Mr. Cohen had his observers rate 10 odors according to the scale of eleven members used by Young, but the scale did not have any numerical designation of its members. The preferential nature of members

3 (pleasant), 6 (indifferent) and 9 (unpleasant) was nevertheless well-marked. (Fig. 9.)

It seems clear that scales of eleven or more members involve preferential values, and that this occurs whether or no the scales utilize numerical designation. It follows that such scales cannot yield accurate measures of hedonic tone. Whether the same is true of scales involving nine members or less is at present being investigated by Mr. Cohen. Until it is shown, however, that such is not the

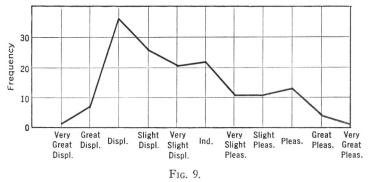

FIG. 9.

(*After N. Cohen*)

case the use of any scale involving gradations of pleasantness and unpleasantness must be fraught with the danger of inaccuracy.

The desire to obviate this difficulty has led me to adopt a form of the method of single stimuli in which measurement in terms of a scale is replaced by measurement in terms of frequency. Instead of judging a stimulus in terms of a scale, the observer judges it to be pleasant, indifferent or unpleasant. Each stimulus is presented to the observer a large number of times under identical conditions, and the proportion which the pleasant judgments plus one-half the indifferent judgments bear to the total number of judgments, expressed in percentage form, is considered to be an index of the hedonic value of the stimulus under the existing conditions. This index I have called percentage of pleasantness, and this method will henceforth be referred to as method of percentages of pleasantness. An illustration of its application is afforded by an experiment which I carried out in 1925-26 on habituation.[39] My purpose in this experiment was to study shifts in the hedonic tone of a set of stimuli due to repeated stimulation with some of its members. Fig. 10 shows the results in one part of the experiment for one observer. The curves indicate percentages of pleasantness (ordinates) for the different stimuli (abscissae) before and after repeated stimulation with certain

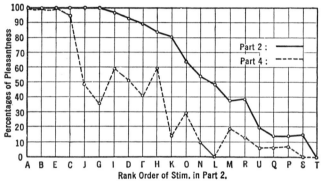

FIG. 10

of the stimuli. The curves are typical of those secured throughout the experiment. They show clearly the adequacy of the method of percentages of pleasantness in measuring the shifts determined in this particular experiment.

A very similar method was proposed in 1928 by R. Engel.[40] In an experiment upon the relation of hedonic tone to the intensity of the stimulus, he had his observers give judgments of pleasantness, unpleasantness and indifference upon stimuli of various intensities and then indicated graphically the number of judgments of each category which were made upon each stimulus. One of his figures is reproduced below. The maxima of the curves representing the various judgments were taken by him to indicate maxima and minima of pleasantness and unpleasantness.[41]

The development of the particular form of the method of single stimuli which I have called the method of percentages of pleasantness in such a fashion as to make it yield measures of hedonic tone in units of amount is a simple matter provided one accept the fundamental assumption made

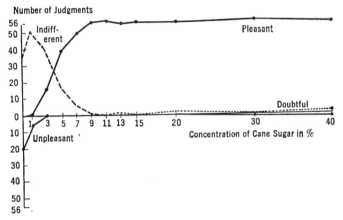

Fig. 11. Curve Representing the Hedonic Tone of Solutions of Cane Sugar for 10 Observers in 6 Sittings.

(After R. Engel)

by both Thorndike and Thurstone, namely that the frequency of the judgments a > b will vary as a function of the difference between these entities with respect to a certain trait in accordance with a particular mathematical function, namely the phi function of gamma. The judgment "pleasant" is obviously equivalent to the judgment "more pleasant than an indifferent object." Thus the percentage of pleasantness of an object may be considered to represent the frequency with which this object is considered greater with respect to pleasantness than a standard indifferent object. It follows that if one determine from a table of the probability integral the proportion of the standard deviation corresponding to the various percentages of pleasantness, these proportions may, on the basis of the assumption above, be taken to represent the relative amounts of hedonic tone of the stimuli yielding these percentages. The legitimacy of this assumption is indeed far greater in the case of the method of single stimuli than in the case of the two other methods of impression. It has been shown by E. G. Wever and K. E. Zener that if the ordinary psychophysical experiment upon weights is varied to the extent of presenting the variable weights singly and of asking the observer in each case to judge whether the weight is heavy, medium or light, the frequencies of the judgments "heavy" and "light" are found to be related to the physical heaviness of the weights by a function approximating closely to the phi function of gamma.[42]

Critical Examination of the Classical Methods of Impression.—We have seen that the method of choice of Fechner has been developed in three directions to give the methods of order of merit, of paired comparison and of single stimuli. These are the three classical methods of impression. Let us inquire into their relative value.

A first criterion is what I shall call *adequacy*. For a method to be adequate it must in no wise limit the occurrence of hedonic tone. On this score it would seem that the method of single stimuli is definitely superior to the two others. Indeed, Kaestner has criticized it on this very ground,[43] pointing out that its judgments are more affected by mood and "the feelings bound to the perceptual process as such" than are the comparative judgments of the two other methods. On the other hand, E. Bullough and C. W. Valentine prefer this method upon much the same grounds. According to Bullough, the method of comparison "destroys the preadaptation of the subject to æsthetic experiences, and thereby vitiates his whole mental attitude towards the object to be offered to his appreciation."[44] And Valentine, in discussing the results of an experiment upon musical intervals, writes: "The sound is, after all, such a simple thing and its æsthetic impression so fleeting that it cannot, as a rule, hold the emotional mood it has roused when another interval is presented with its appropriate æsthetic impression also struggling for existence. We either get an æsthetic impression due to the whole formed by both intervals (as was sometimes stated), and then there is no real comparison; or if this does not happen, there is a tendency for a purely critical attitude to be adopted, and especially for some one standard to be selected by which the two shall be judged, e.g., the degree of consonance." [45]   More recently, M. Yokoyama made a thorough investigation of the judgments involved in the method of paired comparisons.[46]   The frequency with which his observers reported pleasantness and unpleasantness not as "existential processes" but as "meanings," or "conscious attitudes," particularly towards the close of the experiment, made him feel "that the method of paired comparisons can no longer be taken as a typical laboratory setting for affections of process-nature, and that the experimental establishment of the process affection is therefore more than ever in need of an experimental method." [47]

A second criterion is *accuracy*. The comparative accuracy of the methods of order of merit and of paired comparison has been investigated experimentally by M. Barrett.[48]   Miss Barrett used three sets of stimuli, namely 15 weights, 15 specimens of handwriting and 15 propositions. The rank orders of the weights according to weight, of the specimens of handwriting according to excellence, and of the propositions according to belief, were established for 10 observers by both the method of order of merit and the method of paired comparisons. Miss Barrett found that the average correlation between the two methods for the three types of judgments was .987. "This indicates," she writes, "the absence of any basis of preference of one method over the other—with respect to the general results obtained." [49]   We may, I think, accept this conclusion.

The method of paired comparison has been compared experimentally to the method of single stimuli by two investigators, namely Valentine[50] and K. Danzfuss.[51] These investigators, both of whom used auditory stimuli, agree that there is considerable discrepancy between the results secured by the two methods for single individuals, but that collective results by the two methods are quite similar. Their experimental procedure, however, did not allow them to determine in the case of the discrepant individual results which method was the more accurate. The basis of judgment was hedonic tone and the series obtained by the two methods could consequently not be compared to any objective series.

The method of order of merit has also been compared to the method of single stimuli. E. S. Conklin and J. W. Sutherland[52] had 20 observers judge 40 jokes as to excellence in each of five successive trials. Ten of the observers were instructed to assign to each joke a degree of excellence from a scale involving ten degrees. It was found in the first place that the order of the jokes as determined by the two methods showed a coefficient of correlation of only .55. In the second place, it was found that the mean variation of a joke about its average position was greater in the case of the method of order of merit. In the third place, it was found that the correlations of the average positions of the jokes in the first and the four succeeding trials was higher for the method of order of merit. The experimenters believe that the relatively low correlation between the two methods is due to the fact that the one emphasizes feeling (as opposed to intellectual judgment) more than the other. Furthermore they believe that the lesser variability of the method of single stimuli shows that it is this method which emphasizes feeling to the greater extent.

The results of Conklin and Sutherland are much like those of Valentine and of Danzfuss. The results shed a certain amount of light on the relation of the method of single stimuli to the other two methods, but do not allow any definite conclusions on its relative accuracy. For such a conclusion to be possible it will be necessary to test the two methods using not hedonic judgments, but perceptual judgments,—judgments of weight, for instance, as in Miss Barrett's experiment. Certain other considerations suggest, however, that the discrepancy will be found due to inaccuracy of the method of single stimuli. E. G. Wever and K. E. Zener have compared results secured in experiments upon lifted weights by the method of single stimuli and the method of constant stimuli.[53] They found that the methods both yielded psychometric curves, that curves by the two methods were approximately of the phi function of gamma type, and that the measures of precision in the case of the two curves were practically the same. Indeed they concluded that the method of single stimuli is a practicable method for use in psychophysical investigation. We may infer, I think, that when a direct comparison is made with respect to accuracy between the particular form of the method of single stimuli which I have called the method of percentages of pleasantness and the two other methods of impression, the result will likely favor the former method.

A third criterion is *completeness*. All three of the classical methods yield relative information concerning the hedonic value of the processes under investigation. Two of them—that of order of merit and that of paired comparison, yield *only* relative information—they tell the experimenter nothing concerning the pleasantness, indifference, or unpleasantness of the various stimuli. Does the method of single stimuli yield more? Titchener has said no. In his Experimental Psychology, he called the method of single stimuli the "serial method" and pointed out that its results were no more absolute than those secured by the method of paired comparison.[54] Külpe, though leaning to the negative side, preferred to reserve his opinion on this matter.[55] Myers, finally, unequivocally said yes.[56] Whom shall we believe?

Titchener advanced the view that absolute judgments are generated from past relative judgments. It was his belief that an experience which has occurred repeatedly in connection with one or more experiences and has been followed by a judgment of relationship to these other experiences will subsequently, if occurring alone, be followed by a similar judgment formulated either in relative or absolute terms.[57] Let us for the sake of argument admit that absolute judgments are generated from relative judgments. Let us grant that any given absolute judgment is equivalent to a certain relative judgment in terms of some standard. With knowledge of the standard, we can derive the one from the other. Knowing, for instance, that chocolate is the standard of hedonic tone we can derive from the judgment "tea is less pleasant than chocolate" the equivalent judgment "tea is unpleasant." Without knowledge of the standard, however, the fact of equivalence is of no assistance. No matter how many relative judgments are available concerning tea, we cannot possibly determine its hedonic tone without knowledge of the hedonic standard. It is obvious, now, that we never know the hedonic standards of our observers and consequently that we can never actually measure hedonic tone by means of relative judgments. It follows that no matter what is the theoretical relationship between relative and absolute judgments, the former do not yield as much information concerning hedonic tone as do the latter, and consequently that in respect to completeness the method of single stimuli is superior to the two other methods of impression. Whether absolute judgments are logically absolute, i.e. independent of the previous experiences of the observer, is a very interesting question but one which has nothing to do with methodology. We shall see later that such independence does not obtain: that there is on the contrary a very definite relationship between the hedonic tone of any given object and that of similar objects preceding it.

A fourth criterion, finally, is *convenience*. It is clear that the method of paired comparison, involving for any set of n stimuli $\frac{n(n-1)}{2}$ judgments, is applicable only to restricted sets of stimuli. Use of this method for ranking a set of 50 stimuli would require $\dfrac{50(50-1)}{2} = 1225$ judg-

ments, — $24\frac{1}{2}$ hours with 50 judgments an hour—and for 100 stimuli, would require 4950 judgments,—99 hours, at 50 judgments per hour. As far as I know, it has never been used with sets of more than 25 members. Even for small sets of stimuli, it is more time-consuming than the method of order of merit.[58]

It has been pointed out that the method of order of merit can only be used with sets of stimuli subject to simultaneous presentation, and that this constitutes a grave limitation. The fact is correct, but the conclusion is not. The stimuli must indeed be subject to simultaneous presentation, but not necessarily to the sense-organs primarily involved in the judgment. Miss Barrett, for instance, used this method with much success upon 15 weights.[59]

As to the method of single stimuli, its convenience has never been questioned. It is obviously applicable to any set of stimuli, no matter what their nature and number.

Our inquiry concerning the relative merits of the three classical methods of impression shows that with respect to appropriateness, completeness, and convenience, the method of single stimuli is the best, and that with respect to accuracy it is probably at least on a par with the two other methods. We may conclude that the method of single stimuli is in general the best method. As to the relative merits of the two other methods, they have turned out to be equal except with respect to convenience. The method of order of merit turned out to be the more convenient whenever it could be used, and consequently, may in general be considered the next best method after the method of single stimuli.

METHODS OF EXPRESSION

The methods of expression may be said to have had their inception with Mosso's "Sulla circulatione del sangue nel cervello dell' uomo," published in 1880.[60] Mosso had occasion to make observations on a number of individuals with openings in their skulls, enabling him to record variations in pulse and volume of the brain cavity. For this purpose he used a pair of Marey tambours connected by an air-pipe. One tambour, which we may term the exploration tambour, was provided with a button and attached over the opening in the skull. The other tambour, the registering tambour, was provided with a hinged marker whose movements were recorded on the smoked roll of a kymograph. Mosso further recorded variations in the pulse of the arm (and sometimes of the leg) of his observers by means of what he called a hydrosphygmograph. This apparatus consisted essentially of a water-filled chamber enclosing the observer's forearm, this chamber being connected by an air-pipe to a Marey recording tambour. In addition to this air-pipe, the chamber was connected by a water pipe to an open water-filled vessel destined to compensate for volume changes.

With these two pieces of apparatus, Mosso recorded changes in the pulse and volume of the brain cavity and changes in the pulse of a limb during various mental states including ones characterized by hedonic tone. His interest lay primarily in establishing a relationship between circulatory changes and mental activity in general, and his work yields little information upon the circulatory correlates of hedonic tone. The fact, however, that he was able to demonstrate physiological correlates of mental states characterized by hedonic tone gives him the distinction of having originated the methods of expression in the study of this variable.

With the appearance in 1884 and 1885 of the theories of emotion of James[61] and Lange,[62] the investigation of the bodily concomitants of emotional variables, including hedonic tone, was given a strong impetus. But it was Wundt's appeal in 1899 to physiological concomitants in support of his tridimensional theory[63] which brought into prominence the methods of expression in their specific application to the study of hedonic tone. The work of Brahn[64] upon the vaso-motor concomitants of feelings, published in 1901, ushered in a long series of researches upon hedonic tone by the method of expression which, though it reached its maximum around 1906, continues even to this day. The methods of expression as applied to hedonic tone seek to correlate this variable with physiological processes and thus involve two distinct parts: (1) the determination of hedonic tone, and (2) the establishment of physiological processes.

The determination of hedonic tone has undergone a marked improvement since the early applications of the methods. Brahn, for instance, omitted introspection from his actual experiments, taking it for granted that stimuli which previously, in a totally different setting, had aroused pleasant or unpleasant experiences, would again arouse the same experiences during his actual experiment. The danger of this assumption was pointed out very forcibly in 1903 by Orth, and in 1907 by Alechsieff. The latter in his own experiments required introspections of his observers after each trial of the actual experiment, thus establishing beyond a doubt the particular hedonic tone correlated with any particular physiological change.[65] Alechsieff's insistence upon adequate introspection has been taken into account by most subsequent investigators.

The establishment of physiological processes has developed continuously since the earliest experiments by Mosso. This development has been almost wholly a matter of inventing new recording devices and has been carried out chiefly by physiologists.

It is impossible here to enumerate all the many devices which have been used in the study of hedonic tone by the method of expression. Those most commonly used are the following:

1. *The Plethysmograph.* This apparatus measures changes in the volume of a part of the body. It consists essentially "of a closed chamber in which part of the body, usually the forearm, comfortably rests. The chamber is connected with a distant tambour, so that any variations

of pressure due to increased or decreased volume of the arm are transmitted to a recording lever. In some types of the instrument the chamber enclosing the arm contains air, but more usually the air is replaced by lukewarm water." [66] Other parts of the body whose volume has been recorded plethysmographically are the ear and the finger. The movements of the lever are usually recorded on a kymograph, consisting essentially of a cylinder rotating at a constant speed. The cylinder is usually covered with smoked paper which can be removed after the experiment and which after being covered with shellac provides a permanent record of the results.

In connection with the plethysmograph it is well to mention a source of error which recurs in various forms in the case of practically all devices used in the method of expression. Changes in volume of a part of the body will indeed induce—provided the tambour is sufficiently sensitive— changes in the position of the lever. But a number of other circumstances will do the same. Gradual warming of the water in the direction of body-temperature will increase its volume and thus affect the lever. Movements of the arm, by increasing or decreasing the extent to which it is engaged in the plethysmograph, will likewise affect the lever. One must guard carefully against the introduction of such artifacts by making sure that all variables affecting the lever, with the exception of that under investigation, are held rigidly constant.

2. *The Sphygmograph.* This apparatus is used to record the frequency and the form of the pulse. The usual model involves a receiving drum which is placed over an artery in such a fashion that changes of arterial pressure can be transmitted to a recording drum by an air-pipe and thus registered upon a kymograph.[67]

3. *The Sphygmometer.* This instrument serves to measure the pressure of the blood in an artery. It is obvious, in view of the pump-like action of the heart, that blood-pressure in arteries is continuously varying. Corresponding to the end of one pulsation and the beginning of the next,

it is minimal. This is called the diastolic pressure. Corresponding to about the middle of a pulsation, it is maximal. This is called the systolic pressure.

The most obvious way to record blood-pressure is to connect the artery directly with a manometer—usually a U-shaped tube containing mercury, which has been calibrated in such a fashion that scale-readings indicate the pressures corresponding to the various positions of the column. This method is used extensively on animals,[68] but is obviously difficult of application to human beings. The most usual type of sphygmometer used upon human beings is the so-called cuff-sphygmometer. This apparatus involves essentially an air chamber in the form of a cuff, which is attached to the arm midway between arm-pit and elbow, a pump (usually a rubber bulb) and exhaust valve for regulating the air pressure in the cuff, and a manometer for recording this air pressure. By means either of a stethescope or of the fingers of his left hand the experimenter observes the pulse beats at the observer's wrist. With his right hand the experimenter increases the pressure in the cuff until the pulse at the observer's wrist is no longer perceptible. He then decreases the pressure very gradually by means of the valve until the pulse just begins again to become perceptible. At this point he reads the pressure recorded by the manometer. This is the systolic blood-pressure. The experimenter then further decreases the pressure in the cuff. The pulse gradually becomes stronger, passes through a maximum, and then decreases again. At the beginning of the latter phase the experimenter again reads the manometer. This is the diastolic pressure.[69]

In using this type of sphygmometer the usual procedure is to take records at intervals of at least a minute in order not to discommode the observer too much by protracted loss of blood-supply in the arm. Such a procedure is of little value in the study of hedonic tone. Experiment shows that changes in blood-pressure are extremely frequent and extremely marked even in the absence of any external stimulation. Within fifteen seconds, for instance, and in the absence of external stimulation, the writer found the systolic blood-pressure of an observer to change from a pressure of 104mm. of mercury to one of 122mm. Obviously readings at one-minute intervals may fall at the beginning or at the end of one of these rapid variations without enabling the experimenter to determine which. It follows that a variation in external stimulation correlated in general with a rise of blood-pressure may in a particular trial appear to correlate with a drop of blood-pressure, owing to the fact that the reading has taken place at the trough of a sudden change produced by internal stimulation. In many fields,—medicine, for instance—this difficulty may be overcome by repetition of observations. In the study of hedonic tone, however, repetition is frequently impossible except by the use of different observers, and this latter resort itself is sometimes of no avail. How, for instance, obtain a large number of blood-pressure readings correlated with success or failure in some important examination? An experimenter is lucky to obtain a very few records of this type from stoical friends or colleagues.

A procedure has been suggested by Bickel for securing a continuous record of blood-pressure by means of the cuff-sphygmometer. Observation and theoretical considerations both showed according to him that if the cuff is connected to a Marey tambour and the pressure in it is kept constant: (a) when the pressure in the cuff is between the diastolic and the systolic pressure, increase of blood-pressure corresponds to increase of the amplitude of movement of the lever on the tambour; (b) when the pressure in the cuff is below the diastolic pressure, increase in blood-pressure corresponds to decrease of the amplitude of movement of the lever.[70] Bickel consequently adopted amplitude of movement of the arm of the tambour under constant pressure in the cuff as an index of blood-pressure, increase in this amplitude indicating increase of blood-pressure with supra-diastolic pressures in the cuff, decrease of blood-pressure with infra-diastolic pressures in the cuff.[71]

Bickel's procedure requires high pressure in the cuff

because of the inertia of the Marey tambour. This in turn limits the length of the continuous record because of discomfort to the observer. The writer has found that if the Marey tambour be replaced by an alcohol bubble in a tube, one end of the tube being connected with the cuff and the other end with a fairly large sealed container, the oscillations of the bubble—corresponding to those of the lever on the tambour—have sufficient amplitude to give an excellent photographic record when the pressure in the cuff is as low as 50mm. of mercury—a pressure which arouses practically no discomfort in the observer. This "bubble-recorder" is illustrated below. During actual recording the

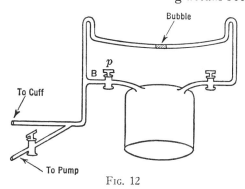

Fig. 12

petcock at p is closed, and consequently arm B of the system is out of use—or rather, acts as cul-de-sac. This arm, however, is essential in order that the bubble may retain a constant position while pressure is being raised in the cuff. When such adjustment is in progress petcock p is opened, with the result that the increase of pressure in the cuff increases the pressure on both sides of the bubble equally and does not move the bubble.

4. *The Pneumograph.* This instrument records the rate and extent of respiratory movements. In general it consists of an air-tight rubber tube, an inch or so in diameter, containing a coil-spring so attached as to keep the diameter of the tube constant and its length as small as possible. The tube is stretched across the chest by a chain attached at

both ends of the tube and going around the observer's back. The tube is further connected to a Marey tambour. As the observer breathes in, the tube is stretched, the coil-spring keeps its diameter constant and consequently the volume of the tube increases and there results a depression of the Marey tambour through suction. As the observer breathes out, the coil-spring shortens the tube, its volume decreases, and the Marey tambour comes back to its normal position.[72]

5. *The Dynamometer and Ergograph.* The dynamometer records the force exerted by a movement, usually by the flexion of some limb. This force is usually recorded in units of weight: pounds or kilograms. The best known dynamometers are the hand-dynamometer and the finger-dynamometer which record the force exerted in closing the hand or flexing the finger against a spring resistance.[73] The ergograph records the energy exerted by a series of movements, usually by the flexion of a member. It is essentially a recording dynamometer. The best-known type is that devised by Mosso, in which each flexion of the finger draws up a weight and the successive lifts carried out by a series of flexions are summated by means of a ratchet mechanism attached to a counter of revolutions. The energy is usually stated in foot-pounds or kilogrammeters.[74]

6. *The Automatograph.* This apparatus records involuntary movements, usually of the arm. In the case of the arm, the automatograph involves essentially a horizontal board hung from a support in such a way as to move freely in any direction in a horizontal plane. The board is suspended over a sheet of paper on which its movements are recorded by means of an attached pencil. The observer's arm is fastened to the board so that all of its movements in the horizontal plane move the board and thus record themselves on the paper.[75]

Very much more delicate automatographs have been devised for the recording of involuntary tremor, particularly of the fingers. Work on tremor appears to yield an excellent example of the danger of concluding from the movements of a recording lever to the response of the individual. For a long time it appeared that the normal tremor of the finger stretched motionless without support was around 10 per second.[76] The use of an electrical method of registration has recently yielded rates of 300 to 600 per second.[77] It seems likely that the type of apparatus yielding a frequency around 10 was recording not individual excursions but regular variations—the ebb and flow, as it were—in the length of these excursions.

7. *The Galvanometer.* This instrument records ex-

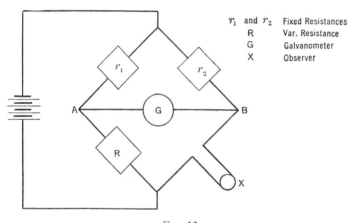

r_1 and r_2 Fixed Resistances
R   Var. Resistance
G   Galvanometer
X   Observer

Fig. 13

tremely minute flows of electro-motive force. It is used in both physiology and psychology to determine the electrical resistance of the body, and also occasionally to determine the electrical current generated in various parts of the body.

When used to measure resistance, it is as a rule mounted in a circuit of the type indicated above. In such a circuit no difference of potential exists across AB when $\dfrac{r_1}{R} = \dfrac{r_2}{X}$ Hence in such a case the galvanometer will register no deflection.

This fact makes possible two uses of this circuit. In the first place, one can determine the resistance of the observer.   As this resistance is usually around 50,000 ohms, and as the variable resistance V usually varies from 1 to 10,000 ohms, one usually selects r_1 and r_2 in the ratio of 1 to 10 (e.g. $r_1 = 1$, $r_2 = 10$). In this case, one has the equation

$$X = R \frac{r_2}{r_1}$$

$$X = R \frac{10}{1} = 10 \ R$$

With such a circuit one can determine resistances of X varying from $10 \times 1 = 10$ to $10 \times 10,000 = 100,000$ ohms.

In the second place—and this is the main use in psychology—one can readily determine variations in resistance. For this purpose one first "balances" the galvanometer, i.e. one fixes the variable at a value for which no deflection of the galvanometer results (in the circuit defined above, R would have the value $\frac{1}{10}$ X, but there is no need in this method to read the value of R). Any change in the resistance of the observer—e.g., the change following stimulation usually called the psycho-galvanic reflex—will thus occasion a deflection of the galvanometer.[78]

Is there any point in discussing the relative merits of the various methods of expression? I think not. The methods are not alternative ways of dealing with a single problem, but each is the *only* way of dealing with a particular problem. The only basis for comparing the methods with each other would be convenience in the sense of quickness and ease of application, and convenience is surely not—or at least should not be—important enough to dictate a choice of problems. As to the comparison of the different techniques which are possible in the case of each method—of various sphygmometric techniques, for instance,—this seems better left to physiologists.

APPENDIX: A STATISTICAL PITFALL

Experimentation upon hedonic tone frequently involves determination of gains or losses in hedonic tone as a function of some variable—number of repetitions, for instance, in investigation of habituation. In such cases the gross results are apt to be misleading. They must be corrected for the effect of chance-factors. If the measurements be independent of such factors, a stimulus ranking first according to one measurement will also rank first according to another measurement, provided conditions remain constant. If, however, the measurements, as is generally the case, depend upon chance-factors, a stimulus ranking first according to one measurement will in all likelihood rank lower than first according to another measurement, even though the known conditions of the two measurements remain identical. As Thorndike has written: "When the individuals in a varying group are measured twice in respect to any ability by an imperfect measure (that is, one whose self-correlation is below 1.00), the average difference between the two obtained scores will equal the average difference between the true scores that would have been obtained by perfect measures; but for any individual the difference between the two obtained scores will be affected by error. Individuals who are below the mean of the group in the first measurement will tend by error to be less far below it in the second, and individuals who are above the mean of the group in the first measurement will tend by the error to be less far above it in the second. The lower the self-correlation, the greater the error and its effects." [79]

The way in which chance-factors manifest themselves in gains or losses of hedonic rank is well illustrated by data which I secured some years ago in an investigation of habituation. The hedonic rank orders of 14 olfactory substances were determined for each of eight observers in each of three experimental series (series 1, 2 and 3). The conditions in all three experimental series were identical. The table below shows for each rank in series 1 (column a):

(α) the arithmetical average (average without regard to sign) of the differences between the ranks in series 1 and 2 of the stimuli which for each observer had the rank in question in series 1 (column b); (β) the arithmetical average of the differences between the ranks in series 1 and 3 of the stimuli which for each observer had the rank in question in series 1 (column c); (γ) the arithmetical average of the two averages defined in (α) and (β) above (column d).

TABLE II

(ARITHMETICAL AVERAGE)

a Rank in Ser. 1	b Diff. in Rank Ser. 1—Ser. 2	c Diff. in Rank Ser. 1—Ser. 3	d Average of Diffs. in Rank
1	.56	.17	.36
2	2.68	1.67	2.17
3	1.69	2.10	1.89
4	1.35	2.17	1.76
5	2.56	3.04	2.80
6	1.84	2.75	2.29
7	.65	2.21	1.43
8	2.15	2.02	2.08
9	2.81	2.29	3.05
10	1.31	2.28	1.79
11	1.89	2.74	2.31
12	2.03	2.29	2.16
13	1.25	1.29	1.27
14	.87	1.39	1.13

The figure below represents graphically the relationship between the values in column a of this table (abscissae) and those in column d (ordinates). It is clear that the arithmetical average of the rank differences for all observers is not the same for all ranks in series 1, but is minimal for ranks 1, 7 and 14, and maximal for ranks 5 and 9. It is consequently clear that given a set of stimuli arranged upon two successive occasions into hedonic rank orders, the difference between the rank of a stimulus on the first occasion and the rank of the same stimulus on the second occasion will not be the same for all stimuli in series 1, but will be minimal in the case of the first, median, and last

stimuli, and maximal in the case of stimuli lying near the
quartiles.

The table below indicates for each rank in series 1
(column a) : (α) the *algebraic* average of the differences
between the ranks in series 1 and series 2 of the stimuli

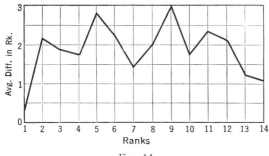

Fig. 14

which for each observer had the rank in question in series
1 (column b) ; (β) the algebraic average of the differences
between the ranks in series 1 and series 3 of the stimuli
which for each observer had the rank in question in series
1 (column c) ; (γ) the algebraic average of the two averages defined in (α) and (β) above (column d).

TABLE III

a Rank in Ser. 1	b Series 1 & 2	c Series 1 & 3	d Average
1	— .44	— .05	— .25
2	—2.07	—1.42	—1.74
3	— .14	—1.49	— .82
4	— .30	—1.70	—1.00
5	—1.52	—2.92	—2.22
6	.16	— .62	— .23
7	— .06	.67	.31
8	.62	1.70	1.16
9	1.15	1.60	1.37
10	— .53	—1.38	— .95
11	.73	1.92	1.32
12	1.77	1.93	1.85
13	.51	.50	.50
14	.62	1.33	.97

The figure below represents graphically the relationship between the values in column a of the table (abscissae) and those in column d (ordinates). Inspection of both table and figure shows clearly that for ranks 1-6 inclusive, the algebraic

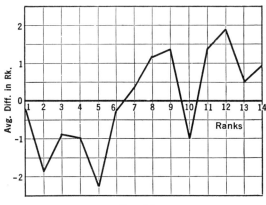

Fig. 15

value of rank differences is on the average negative, whereas for ranks 7-14 inclusive (with the single exception of rank 10), the algebraic value of rank differences is on the average positive. But the differences in rank were defined above as: difference in rank = rank in series 1—rank in series 2 (or series 3). It follows that a negative difference in rank indicates a change towards the low (unpleasant) end of the

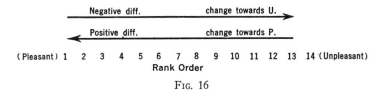

Fig. 16

rank order, and a positive difference, a change towards the high (pleasant) end. (Cf. Fig. above.) This clearly shows that, given a set of stimuli arranged upon two successive occasions in hedonic rank orders, the stimuli which occupied a high rank on the first occasion, will tend to occupy a lower rank on the second occasion, and those occupying a low rank on the first occasion will tend to occupy a higher rank on the second occasion. It should be clear from this illustration that when hedonic tone varies in a regular fashion from one occasion to another *with* variation of some condition c, it is by no means legitimate to infer that hedonic tone is varying as a *function* of condition c. It is imperative first to make sure that the regular variation observed is different from that to be expected from the operation of chance-factors.

FOOTNOTES AND REFERENCES

[1] O. Külpe. Zur Psychologie der Gefühle, *Rapport et C. R. du Vlme Congrès International de Psychologie,* Genève, 1910, 189.

[2] O. Külpe. *Op. cit.,* 189.

[3] G. T. Fechner. Zur Experimentellen Aesthetik, *Abh. d. Math.—Phys. Cl. d. k. Sächs. Ges. d. Wissensch.,* IX, Leipzig, 1871, 555-635.

[4] Fechner distinguishes "Mass der Extensiven Wohlgefälligkeit" from "Mass der Intensiven Wohlgefälligkeit." The latter he does not consider to be practical. "Direkt kann man den Grad der Wohlgefälligkeit oder Missfälligkeit, unter dem ein Verhältnis diesem oder jenem unter diesen oder jenen Umständen erscheint, nicht messen: dazu gälte es ein Mass der Einzel-Lust und Unlust zu haben, was wir noch nicht haben." (*Ibid.,* 598.)

In regard to the "Mass der Extensiven Wohlgefälligkeit," on the other hand, he writes: "Aber man kann das Mass andershin übertragen, indem man die Personen zählt, die dem einen und die dem andern Verhältnisse bei gleichzeitiger Vorlage derselben, oder überhaupt gleicher Möglichkeit der Wahl den Vorzug geben, und dasjenige Verhältnis für das wohlgefälligste zunächst für die Klasse von Personen, die man zu den Versuchen angezogen hat, erklärt, welches die meisten Vorzugsstimmen für sich vereinigt, oder, wenn es nicht mit vorliegt, ein solches, um welches sich die Vorzugsstimmen am dichtesten schaaren, überhaupt aber den Grad der relativen Wohlgefälligkeit eines gegebenen Verhältnisses für eine gegebene Menschenklasse nach der relativen Zahl der sich dafür vereinigenden Stimmen dieser Klasse beurtheilt. . . . Ich nenne . . . nicht nur etwas nach Massgabe wohlgefälliger, als es unter vergleichbaren Bedingungen mehr Vorzugsstimmen für sich vereinigt, sondern stelle auch ausdrücklich den Begriff grösserer oder geringerer Wohlgefälligkeit darauf . . . (*Ibid.,* 598.)

[5] *Ibid.,* 602.

[6] *Ibid.,* 602-603.

[7] *Ibid.,* 603.

[8] L. J. Martin. Psychology of Aesthetics, I, Experimental Prospecting in the Field of the Comic, *Amer. J. Psychol.,* 16, 1905, 73.

[9] L. Witmer. Zur Experimentellen Aesthetik einfacher Räumlicher

52 METHODS OF EXPERIMENTATION

Formverhältnisse, *Philos. Stud.,* IX, 1898, 122 seq. Witmer entitles the chapter in which he deals with these improvements, "A New Method of Choice."

[10] "Vorliegende Versuche sind in der Weise angestellt, dass die den Versuchspersonen zur aesthetischen Beurteilung vorgelegten Figuren nicht eine beschränkte Anzahl, sondern eine vollständige Reihe von Grossenverhältnissen in stetiger Abstufung bildeten. Für die Ausdehnung dieser Reihe, sowie für die Grösse des Zwischenintervalls je zweier benachbarter Glieder waren natürlich praktische Bedürfnisse Massgebend." (*Ibid.,* 122-123.)

[11]"Es ist ferner nicht ohne Bedeutung, in welcher Weise man die Figuren den Versuchspersonen vorlegt. Entweder kann man sie je 2 Figuren mit einander vergleichen lassen; oder man gibt ihnen die ganze Reihe auf einmal und zwar entweder in unregelmässiger Folge, oder so geordnet, dass die Grössenverhältnisse der Figuren stetig ab—resp. zunehmen. Von diesen drei Versuchsanordnungen ziehe ich die letzte vor denn dieselbe hilft nicht nur in der Ausschliessung störender Nebenassoziationen, sondern macht auch die Wahl bequemer und leichter und steigert endlich die Intensität des Gefühls selbst." (*Ibid.,* 125.)

[12] "Nach dieser Methods nun habe ich den Versuchspersonen eine Reihe von Figuren vorgelegt und sie aufgefordert, bei durchmusterung der einzelnen Verhältnisse genau auf die Intensitäts-schwankungen ihres Gefühls zu achten." (*Op. cit.,* 137.) . . . "Für die aesthetische Figurenreihe sind somit 7 Hauptpunkte ihrer Lage nach bestimmt und zwar: der Indifferenzpunkt, das Maximum, der Punkt der subjektiven Gleichheit nebst 2 aesthetisch gleichwerthigen Punkten rechts und links vom Curvenhöhepunkt und endlich das Minimum nebst seinem Aequivalenzpunkt." (*Ibid.,* 139.)

[13] O. KÜLPE. Gründriss der Psychologie, 1893, 239 seq. Cf. translation by E. B. Titchener under title "Outline of Psychology," N. Y., 1895, 233.

[14] O. KÜLPE. Der gegenwärtige Stand der experimentellen Aesthetik, *Ber. ub. d. II Kongr. f. exptl. Psychol.,* 1907, 11.

[15] *Ibid.,* 11.

[16] E. L. THORNDIKE. An Introduction to the Theory of Mental and Social Measurements, New York, 1913, 122-124.

[16a] T. R. GARTH. A Color Preference Scale for One Thousand White Children, *J. Exper. Psychol.,* 7, 1924, 233. Fcr detailed statement of procedure, cf. T. R. Garth, The Color Preference of Five Hundred and Fiftynine Full-blooded Indians, *J. Exper. Psychol.,* 5, 1922, 392-418.

[17] "Schon im gewöhnlichen Leben werden, abgesehen von manchen Personen, welche ausnahmsweise Extreme lieben, solche verworfen und sog. mittlere Verhältnisse im Urtheil wie in den Anwendungen bevorzugt, wonach sich nur fragt, welches darunter die meisten vorzugsstimmen für sich vereinigt, denn das an sich wohlgefälligste Verhältnis ist eben ein mittleres. Legt man nun eine beschränkte Zahl von Verhältnissen vor, so können dieselben entweder alle kleiner oder alle grösser sein als das vortheilhafteste Verhältnis, was als Definitivresultat aus allen Versuchen hervorgeht, oder können dasselbe zwischen sich fassen. Sind alle kleiner, só wird das grösste darunter dem Vortheilhaftesten Verhältnisse am nächsten liegen, und insofern Anlass sein, es zu bevorzugen; aber insofern es doch ein Extrem in der Reihe ist, die man gerade vor sich hat, wird das Urtheil

hiervon mitbestimmt, und man vielmehr geneigt sein, statt dessen ein mittleres Verhältnis *dieser Reihe* vorzuziehen, um so mehr, wenn die Reihe so nach der Grösse der Verhältnisse geordnet ist, dass das der Grösse nach mittlere Verhältnis zugleich der Lage nach ein mittleres ist . . . Ich nenne dies kurz den *Einfluss der Mitte* oder der *Abweichung von der Mitte*, je nach dem die Begünstigung des Verzugs durch die erstre oder die Benachteiligung durch die letzte in Betracht kommt." (Fechner, *op. cit.*, 629.)

[18] "Am sichersten schliesst man natürlich den Einfluss der Mitte nach Grösse und Lage aus, wenn man von den zu prüfenden Verhältnissen immer nur je zwei auf einmal dem Urtheil darbietet; und ich glaube in der That, dass sich hierauf überhaupt die an sich vortheilhafteste Anwendung der Methode der Wahl gründen lässt, habe auch Versuche danach eingeleitet, aber noch nicht weit genug durchgeführt, um über den Erfolg derselben schon sichere Angaben machen zu können." (Fechner, *Op. cit.*, 630).

[19] JONAS COHN. Experimentelle Untersuchungen über die Gefühlsbetönung der Farben, Helligkeiten und ihrer Combinationen, *Philos. Stud.*, 10, 1894, 562.

[20] *Ibid.*, 564-565.

[21] *Ibid.*, 565.

[22] For a discussion of the space and time errors, cf. section of Chapter IV, on hedonic tone as a function of position in space and time.

[23] A. KOWALEWSKI. Studien zur Psychologie des Pessimismus, *Grenzfragen des Nerven und Seelenlebens*, 1904, Heft 24.

[24] "Als das Erfordernis einer rationellen Ambenreihe erscheint mir, dass die Wiederholung jedes einzelnen Elements möglichst hinausgeschoben wird, d. h. also möglichst viele aufeinander folgende Amben lauter verschiedene Elemente enthalten. Bei einer ungeraden Zahl von Elementen $(2m + 1)$ wäre diese Forderung dann am vollkommensten erfüllt, wenn je m successive Amben sich aus lauter verschiedenen Elementen aufbauen. Greift man also irgend eine Ambe aus der Reihe heraus, so muss sie und die m— 1 folgenden amben (wenn es deren gibt) lauter verschiedene Elemente aufweisen." (*Ibid.*, 70.)

[25] "Bei 5 Elementen $(m = 2)$ gestaltet sich die Durchführung unserer Forderung folgendermassen. Als die beiden ersten Amben unserer Reihe wählen wir 1, 2, und 3, 4. Die nächste Ambe darf keines der Elemente 3, 4 enthalten, muss sich also aus den Elementen 1, 2, 5 aufbauen. Die Ambe 1, 2 ist bereits verbraucht. Es bleiben also nur die Amben 1, 5 und 2, 5 übrig. Da wir ohne Beschränkung 1 und 2 vertauschen dürfen, so können wir die drei ersten Glieder der gewünschten Reihe in folgender Weise festlegen : 1,2, 3,4, 1,5.

Durch ähnliche Ueberlegungen findet man, dass als nächstes Glied ohne Beschränkung 2,3 genommen werden kann. Beim darauffolgenden Schritt entsteht eine Gabelung, indem sowohl 1,4 als 4,5 die fünfte Stelle einnehmen kann. Die Verfolgung der Möglichkeit 1,4 führt aber zu Widersprüchen. Es bleibt also nur 4,5, und das folgende Glied muss dann, wie man leicht erkennt, 1,3 sein. Darauf tritt eine nochmalige Gabelung ein, und man findet schliesslich als Lösung unserer Aufgabe im Falle von fünf Elementen die beiden Ambenreihen :

| 1,2 | 3,4 | 1,5 | 2,3 | 4,5 | 1,3 | 2,4 | 3,5 | 1,4 | 2,5 |
| 1,2 | 3,4 | 1,5 | 2,3 | 4,5 | 1,3 | 2,5 | 1,4 | 3,5 | 2,4 |

Jede andere Ambenreihe die unserer oben aufgestellten Forderung genügt, muss sich, wie aus der Herleitung der beiden obigen Reihen unmittelbar hervorgeht, in eine derselben durch eine passende Vertauschung der Zahlen 1,2,3,4,5 überfuhren lassen. Die beiden Reihen selbst können aber direkt durch keine solche Permutation aufeinander reduziert werden. Schreibt man indessen die erste von ihnen umgekehrt.

2,5	1,4	3,5	2,4	1,3	4,5	2,3	1,5	3,4	1,2

so geht sie in die zweite über vermöge der Substitution (12345). Die beiden
(42531)
ausgezeichneten Ambenreihen, wie ich sie nennen möchte, sind also nicht wesentlich von einander verschieden. Jede ist die Umkehrung der anderen, abgesehen von einer Permutation der Ziffern 1 . . . 5.

Analoge Verhältnissen scheinen bei jeder ungeraden Zahl von Elementen zu bestehen, was ein ebenso neuer wie interessanter mathematischer Satz sein dürfte." (*Ibid.*, 71.)

[26] "Bei 7 Elementen lautet z. B. die eine der beiden Ausgezeichneten Ambenreihen:

1,2	3,4	5,6	1,7	2,3	4,5	6,7	1,3	2,5	4,7	1,6	3,5	2,7	4,6
1,5	3,7	2,6	1,4	5,7	3,6	2,4"	(*Ibid.*, 72).

In the case of 15 members, the order is:.

1,2	15,3	14,4	13,5	12,6	11,7	10,8	1,9	2,3	15,4	14,5	13,6	12,7	11,8	10,9
1,3	2,4	15,5	14,6	13,7	12,8	11,9	1,10	3,4	2,5	15,6	14,7	13,8	12,9	11,10
1,4	3,5	2,6	15,7	14,8	13,9	12,10	1,11	4,5	3,6	2,7	15,8	14,9	13,10	12,11
1,5	4,6	3,7	2,8	15,9	14,10	13,11	1,12	5,6	4,7	3,8	2,9	15,10	14,11	13,12
1,6	5,7	4,8	3,9	2,10	15,11	14,12	1,13	0,7	5,8	4,9	3,10	2,11	15,12	14,13
1,7	6,8	5,9	4,10	3,11	2,12	15,13	1,14	7,8	6,9	5,10	4,11	3,12	2,13	15,14
1,8	7,9	6,10	5,11	4,12	3,13	2,14	1,15	8,9	7,10	6,11	5,12	4,13	3,14	2,15

(*Ibid.*, 74).

[27]O. KÜLPE. Der Gegenwärtige Stand der experimentellen Aesthetik, *Ber. ub. d. II Kongr. f. exptl. Psychol.*, 1907, 1.

[28]*Ibid.*, 13.

[29] L. L. THURSTONE. Psychological Analysis, *Amer. J. Psychol.*, 1927, 38, 368-389; The Method of Paired Comparisons for Social Values, *J. Abn. Psychol.*, 1927, 21, 390; The Measurement of Opinion, *J. Abn. Psychol.*, 1928, 22, 415-430.

[30] L. L. THURSTONE. *J. Abn. Psychol.*, 1928, 22, 415-430.

[31] J. P. GUILFORD. The Method of Paired Comparisons as a Psychometric Method, *Psychol. Rev.*, 35, 1928, 494-506.

[32] It is obvious that the central portion of the curve representing the phi function of gamma roughly (very roughly!) approximates a straight line, and thus that this procedure is roughly legitimate.

[33] D. R. MAJOR. On the Affective Tone of Simple Sense Impressions, *Amer. J. Psychol.*, 7, 1895, 57.

[34] J SEGAL. Beiträge zur Experimentellen Aesthetik. I. Über die Wohlgefälligkeit einfacher räumlicher Formen, *Arch. f. d. ges. Psychol.*, 7, 1906, 53.

[35] E. S. CONKLIN. The Scale of Values Method for Studies in Genetic Psychology, *University of Oregon Publications,* Vol. 2, 1923, No. 1.

[36] P. T. Young. Studies in Affective Psychology, VIII. The Scale of Values Method, *Amer. J. Psychol.*, 42, 1930, 17.

[37] J. E. Coover. Experiments in Psychical Research, *Leland Stanford Junior University Publications, Psychical Research Monograph No. 1*, Stanford University, 1917, 230 seq.

[38] P. T. Young. *Op cit.*, 17.

[39] J. G. Beebe-Center. The Law of Affective Equilibrium, *Amer. J. Psychol.*, 41, 1929, 64.

[40] R. Engel. Experimentelle Untersuchungen über die Abhängigkeit der Lust und Unlust von der Reizstärke beim Geschmacksinn, *Arch. f. d. ges. Psychol.*, LXIV, 1928, 1-36.

[41] *Ibid.*, 10.

[42] E. G. Wever and K. E. Zener. The Method of Absolute Judgment in Psychophysics, *Psychol. Rev.*, 35, 1928, 466.

[43] G. Kaestner. Untersuchungen über den Gefühlseindruck unanalysierter Zweiklänge, *Psychol. Stud.*, 4, 1909, 475.

[44] E. Bullough. The "Perceptive Problem" in the Aesthetic Appreciation of Single Colors, *Brit. J. Psychol.*, II, 1908, 412.

[45] C. W. Valentine. The Method of Comparison in Experiments with Musical Intervals and the Effect of Practise on the Appreciation of Discords, *Brit. J. Psychol.*, VII, 1915, 126.

[46] M. Yokoyama. The Nature of the Affective Judgment in the Method of Paired Comparison, *Amer. J. Psychol.*, 32, 1921, 357-369.

[47] *Ibid.*, 369.

[48] M. Barrett. A Comparison of the Order of Merit Method and the Method of Paired Comparisons, *Psychol. Rev.*, 1914, 21, 278.

[49] *Ibid.*, 292.

[50] C. W. Valentine. The Method of Comparison in Experiment with Musical Intervals and the Effect of Practise on the Appreciation of Discords, *Brit. J. Psychol.*, VII, 1915, 118.

[51] K. Danzfuss. Die Gefühlsbetönung einiger unanalysierter Zweiklänge, Zweitonfolgen, Akkorde, und Akkordfolgen bei Erwachsenen und Kindern, *Philos. u. Psychol. Arbeiten,* 5, 1923, 875.

[52] E. S. Conklin and J. W. Sutherland. A Comparison of the Scale of Values Method with the Order-of-merit Method, *J. Exptl. Psychol.*, 6, 1923, 44.

[53] E. G. Wever and K. E. Zener. *Psychol Rev.*, 35, 1928, 484 seq.

[54] "If the method (Serial Method) is to be valid, O must keep in mind the serial nature of the impressions. . . . The affective curve in this case is no more absolute than are the curves of the preceding experiment (by the method of paired comparison). There is no guarantee, e.g., that 7 is as far below 4 as 1 is above it . . . and again, there is no guarantee that the figures as applied to colours mean the same thing as they would if applied, e.g. to smells. Indeed the contrary of this is pretty obvious: a 'very pleasant' smell is a great deal more pleasant than a 'very pleasant' colour." (E. B. Titchener, Experimental Psychology, Vol. 1, Part II, 157.)

[55] O. Külpe. *Bericht über den II Kongress für Experimentelle Psychologie*, 1907, 8.

[56] "In this method (i.e. of Single Stimuli) . . . the judgments of the subject are absolute instead of relative." (C. S. Myers, A Textbook of Experimental Psychology, Cambridge, 1911, 306.)

[57] E. B. TITCHENER. A Textbook of Psychology, New York, 1926, 312-313; 536-537. Cf. also C. S. Myers, A Textbook of Experimental Psychology, 2nd Edit., Cambridge, 1911, Part I, 256-260.

[58] L. WITMER. *Philos. Stud.*, IX, 1893, 128.

[59] M. BARRETT. *Psychol. Rev.*, 21, 1914, 278.

[60] A. MOSSO. Sulla circolatione del sangue nel cervelle dell' uomo; German edition, Uber den Kreislauf des Blutes im menschlichen Gehirn, Leipzig, 1881.

[61] W. JAMES. What is an Emotion? Mind, O. S., IX, 1884, 188.

[62] C. LANGE. Om Sindsbevaegelser, Kopenhagen, 1885. German translation by H. Kurella entitled "Über Gemüthsbewegungen," Leipzig, 1887.

[63] W. WUNDT. Bemerkungen zur Theorie der Gefühle, *Philos. Stud.*, 15, 1899, 149.

[64] MAX BRAHN. Experimentelle Beiträge zur Gefühlslehre, *Philos. Stud.*, 18, 1901, 127.

[65] N. ALECHSIEFF. Die Grundformen der Gefühle, *Psychol. Stud.*, 3, 1907, 169.

[66] C. S. MYERS. A Textbook of Experimental Psychology, 2nd Edit., Cambridge, 1911, Part II, 101. Extensive use of the plethysmograph has been made by Lehmann (A. Lehmann, Die körperliche Äusserungen psychischer Zustände, Leipzig, 1899). For a thorough discussion of various types of plethysmographs, cf. H. Bickel, Die wechselseitigen Beziehungen zwischen psychischem Geschehen und Blutkreislauf, Leipzig, 1916, 26-31.

[67] For a description of a very simple sphygmographic appliance involving merely a small glass funnel connected to a Marey tambour, cf. M. Verworn, Physiologisches Praktikum, 5th Edit., Jena., 1921, 120-121.

[68] W. H. HOWELL. A Textbook of Physiology, 10th Edit., Phila., 1929, 500.

[69] Cf. W. H. HOWELL. A Textbook of Physiology, 10th Edit., Phila., 1929, 505 seq. For an illustration of the use of the cuff-sphygmometer, cf. W. M. Marston, Blood-pressure Symptoms of Deception, *J. Exptl. Psychol.*, 2, 1917, 123.

[70] H. BICKEL. *Op. cit.*, 14 seq.

[71] E. WEBER has suggested an alternative method for the continuous registration of blood-pressure, in which a plethysmograph is used instead of a cuff. Cf. E. WEBER, *Arch f. Physiol.*, 1913, 205.

[72] For a discussion of pneumographic technique, cf. C. Landis and Gulette, *J. Comp. Psychol.*, 5, 1925, 221-253.

[73] For a description of a finger-dynamometer, cf. E. B. Titchener, Experimental psychology, Student's Manual, Qualitative, 100. For an application of the dynamometer to the patellar reflex, cf. Burtt and Tuttle, *Amer. J. Psychol.*, 1925, 36, 553.

[74] For a description of the ergograph after Kraepelin, cf. C. S. Myers, Textbook of Experimental Psychology, Part II, 59. For an application of this ergograph, cf. A. Ernst, *Archiv. f. d. ges. Psychol.*, 1926, 57, 445.

[75] For a description of the arm-automatograph, cf. E. B. Titchener, *Experimental Psychology*, Student's Manual, Qualitative, 95.

[76] Cf. W. A. BOUSFIELD. The Influence of Fatigue on Tremor, *J. Exptl. Psychol.*, 15, 1932, 104.

[77] L. E. TRAVIS and T. A. HUNTER, Muscular Rhythms and Action-Currents, *Amer. J. Physiol.*, 81, 1927, 355-359.

[78] For a most excellent and thorough discussion of the use of the galvanometer in psychological experimentation, cf. D. Wechsler, The Measurement of Emotional Reactions, *Arch. of Psychol.*, New York, 76, 1925.

[79] E. B. THORNDIKE. The Influence of Chance Imperfections on the Relation of Initial Score to Gain or Loss, *J. Exptl. Psychol.*, 7, 1924, 225.

[80] In view of the psychological complexity of this description I give a concrete illustration. Let us assume that two observers, Xa and Ya, have each arranged three stimuli, A, B, and C, into hedonic rank orders, series 1 and series 2, upon two successive occasions. (Cf. Table below.)

TABLE IV

	Obs. Xa.		Obs. Ya.	
Rank	Ser. 1	Ser. 2	Ser. 1	Ser. 2
1	A	B	C	A
2	B	A	B	B
3	C	C	A	C

The stimuli which for each observer have rank 1 in series 1 are: for observer Xa., stim. A; for observer Ya., stim. C. The difference between the ranks of those stimuli in series 1 and 2 will be for observer Xa., 1; for observer Ya., 2. The average defined above will consequently be for rank 1:

$$\frac{1+2}{2} = 1.5.$$

Chapter III

The Relation of Hedonic Tone to Mental Elements

INTRODUCTION

Towards the close of the XIXth century, when psychological laboratories first came into existence, the fundamental problem of experimental psychology was analysis into elements. As early as 1862 Wundt wrote in his "Beiträge": "There is no doubt that consciousness itself and everything occurring within it are already complicated phenomena. Here, as everywhere in nature, it is only the complicated events that offer themselves immediately to our observation, whereas simple events remain at first concealed. These simple events, to which we can attain only by dismemberment of the composite events, but which yield us the principles necessary for the exploration of these complex events, are in psychology the first stages both in the single conscious being and in the whole series of conscious creatures." [1] With the publication of the "Grundzüge," the fundamental importance of analysis into elements became explicit. He wrote: "The immediate contents of experience, which constitute the subject-matter of psychology, are invariably processes of a composite nature. . . . The perception of an external object, for instance, consists of the partial perception of its parts. . . . Faced with such a complicated state of affairs, scientific investigation must successively solve three different problems. The first problem involves the analysis of the composite processes, the second involves the establishment of the combinations into which may enter the elements discovered by analysis, the third involves the discovery of the laws which are operative in the establishment of such combinations." [2]

It is not surprising, therefore, that the first systematic issues to be raised in connection with hedonic tone were concerned with *its relation to mental elements.* The fundamental problem was conceived to be that of the nature of *affection,* by which term was meant the class of elements or of combinations of elements of which hedonic tone was an attribute. Two fundamental views were in conflict. One school of psychologists, led by Wundt and Titchener, believed hedonic tone to be an attribute of *special affective elements,* different from sensations. Another school, including Ziehen and Stumpf, denied the existence of special affective elements, believing hedonic tone to be an attribute of *sensations.*

These two basic views were in turn the starting point for further divergences. Those who agreed as to the existence of special affective elements disagreed as to their attributes. According to Titchener, for instance, the affective elements involved but one qualitative dimension, namely hedonic tone.[3] According to Wundt, they involved three qualitative dimensions, namely pleasantness-unpleasantness, strain-relaxation, excitement-depression.[4] Those who agreed to the sensory nature of affective elements were likewise at odds. Ziehen, for instance, considered hedonic tone to be an attribute of all sensations, though not a "necessary" attribute.[5] Stumpf, on the other hand, believed it to be an attribute of certain specific sensations, distinguished by him under the title "feeling-sensations."[6]

Experimental psychology around 1900 was essentially the psychology of Wundt and of his pupils. Little wonder then, that the first of these systematic issues to be dealt with experimentally was not the fundamental one of the existence of special affective elements, but a minor one, namely that concerning the number of qualities of the special affective elements. It is with reference to this minor issue that I shall begin my discussion of the relation of hedonic tone to mental elements, for emphasis in the present work is to be on experimental data rather than on the results of mere observation.

THE QUALITATIVE DIMENSIONS OF THE SPECIAL
AFFECTIVE ELEMENTS

The history of the problem of the qualitative dimensions of special affective elements is, from the point of view of the experimentalist, the history of Wundt's tridimensional theory of feeling. Lipps, it is true, maintained as early as 1903 that feelings involved, besides pleasantness-unpleasantness, a number of other qualitative dimensions.[7] But Lipps was an æsthetician and his views upon feelings were never subjected to experimental test by psychologists. Again, Royce advanced a two-dimensional theory of feeling,[8] but it was merely Wundt's theory divested of its third dimension, and Royce proclaimed himself ready to add this third dimension if future research demanded it.

It was in 1896, in the original edition of his "Grundriss der Psychologie," that Wundt first published his tridimensional theory of feeling.[9] According to this view, experience involves two kinds of psychical elements, sensations and feelings. The latter, distinguished from the former by their subjectivity, are almost infinite in variety. From the qualitative point of view they cannot be arranged into an uni-dimensional system, but only into a three-dimensional one. The three necessary dimensions are pleasantness-unpleasantness, excitement-depression, and strain-relaxation.[10]

In the latter part of the same year, O. Vogt[11] reported some observations upon a woman under hypnosis, which he believed to have bearing upon the tridimensional theory. The woman distinguished four qualities of feeling constituting two opposed pairs, namely pleasant-unpleasant, and elevating-depressing. She insisted, however, that the latter pair of qualities were very different from the former, indeed that she would not care to include them under the term "feeling." [12] They were characterized, she added, by a purely subjective character.[13] Vogt believed that these results supported the recently published Wundtian view, and they were later quoted in the same sense by Wundt himself.

In 1899, E. B. Titchener fired the opening gun of his long battle against the Wundtian view.[14] Besides purely theoretical criticisms, Titchener reported an experiment carried out upon a Cornell student with the purpose of securing evidence either for or against the view of Wundt. This young man was requested to introspect upon his occasional affective experiences and to write reports upon them. The result was "that except for pleasantness and unpleasantness, Mr. W. (the O in question) did not once find during the entire year an affective content that he could not localize accurately in some bodily organ, i.e. which did not show itself to be either a sensation or a complex of sensations." [15]

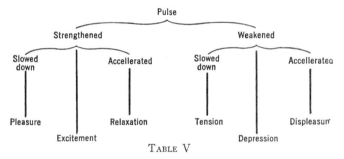

TABLE V

These results Titchener interprets as clearly against the Wundtian theory.

This attack called forth a prompt rejoinder from Wundt. In the same year he published a long defense of his tridimensional theory of feeling in which, besides calling upon the results of his own introspection and those of Vogt's hypnotized observer, he further sought evidence from the results of experiments upon the bodily concomitants of feelings.[16] The works of Mentz[17] and Lehmann[18] upon vaso-motor responses could be interpreted, he argued, as indicating characteristically different pulse-changes for his six different qualities. These changes he represented in the above schema.[19]

The problem of the physiological concomitants of pleasantness-unpleasantness, excitement-depression and strain-relaxation, thus raised by Wundt, led to a great deal of profitable research. We shall not, however, deal with this work here, for Wundt himself subsequently admitted its lack of evidential value with respect to the issue in which we are interested. "All these (objective) symptoms," he wrote, "have their psychological value solely in being objectively demonstrable events, which, insofar as they regularly accompany definite feeling processes, constitute in their differences indications of corresponding psychical differences. But it must never be forgotten that they are merely indications and not in the slightest degree proofs. Where introspection does not show univocally the existence of a definite feeling, such a feeling can naturally not be deduced from objective events, no matter how numerous they may be." [20]

In 1902,—peculiarly enough in a memorial volume in honor of Wundt—Titchener resumed his attack upon the Wundtian view.[21] Using two different sets of stimuli, the one involving 24 tones, the other 14 metronome-rates, he established for each set curves indicating the relative values (in terms of frequencies of "greater than" judgments) of the individual stimuli with respect to pleasantness, unpleasantness, excitement and depression. The results of this experiment are summarized by him as follows: "Observers of different degrees of training and of different intellectual capacities found it possible for different kinds of stimuli and both with and without knowledge of procedure, to react constantly with respect to Pleasantness and Unpleasantness. We have secured not a single univocal feeling curve which could not be considered identical with a Pleasantness-Unpleasantness curve. We have met with variability of feeling reaction and with hesitancy of judgment only outside of the Pleasantness-Unpleasantness dimension. With respect to Excitement, we found differences in curves which point unmistakably to a difference between the opposed pairs Pleasantness-Unpleasantness and Excitement-Depression, and consequently to the complexity of the emotional state called Excitement." [22]   These results are interpreted by Titchener as definitely against the Wundtian view.

Much of the research mentioned in the preceding pages had been carried out on the implicit assumption that there were definite observable criteria of feelings, and consequently that it was possible to determine experimentally whether a given process was or was not a feeling. This assumption was denied flatly in 1903 by Orth.[23] For Orth, feelings could be defined only as pleasure and displeasure, and consequently the tridimensional view of feeling could be proved only by proving that excitement, depression, strain and relaxation were processes similar to pleasure and displeasure. Experiments carried out by himself, however, showed in his mind that no such similarity existed, and consequently disproved the tridimensional view. He subjected four observers, including Marbe and Ach, to a variety of stimuli with the instruction to give a complete introspective report. They described strain, relaxation, excitement and depression in sensory terms. "It follows," writes Orth, "that these phenomena must have displayed themselves in the subjective experience in this fashion, and not required to be dealt with as feelings." [24]

In 1906, Hayes published the results of an experiment by the method of paired comparison patterned after that of Titchener reported above.[25] His data showed: (1) that judgments of pleasantness and unpleasantness were "easy, direct and natural";[26] (2) that judgments of strain were easy and direct, but further, that strain was described in muscular terms throughout and the curves of strain corresponded closely to the curves of unpleasantness; (3) that judgments of excitement and depression were less direct than judgments of pleasantness and unpleasantness, and that judgments of depression were often associatively motivated; (4) that judgments of relaxation, besides being sometimes associatively motivated, gave curves identical to those of either depression or pleasantness. He concluded that his evidence was opposed to the tridimensional theory.

The effect of Orth's criticism of previous investigations is very apparent in the work of Alechsieff, published in 1907.[27] Instead of taking for granted the existence of indubitable criteria of feeling, and attempting to judge the Wundtian view with reference to these criteria, he sought first to establish the characteristics of all six of the Wundtian fundamental types of feeling and then to judge the Wundtian view according to the relationship between these characteristics. His results showed that all six fundamental forms had the same characteristics. "Tension or excitement," he wrote, "can no more be localized or objectified than pleasure or displeasure. All these processes are independent of definite sense organs and forms of stimulation, but show a dependence on the condition of consciousness. None of these six processes could be subjected to a closer determination. They were reported to be indefinable and unanalyzable, and consequently classed as elementary psychical processes." [28]   He concludes: "The fundamental forms of feelings cannot be reduced to only two fundamental forms, pleasure and displeasure. They constitute a much greater variety and require for grouping, not one feeling-dimension, but three feeling-dimensions, characterized by the oppositions pleasure-unpleasure, strain-relaxation and excitement-depression." [29]

In 1916, Foster and Roese published the results of an experiment by the method of paired comparison similar to those already reported by Titchener and Hayes. [30]   Like the latter authors, Foster and Roese established curves of excitement, depression, strain, relaxation, pleasantness and unpleasantness for 24 tones. Instead, however, of leaving the interpretation of the terms excitement, depression, etc., to their observers, they gave these observers for use as standards, experiences which, according to Wundt, were typical of these six qualities. Thus standards of excitement and depression were provided by putting the observers in light and dark rooms respectively; for the experiences of strain and relaxation, the observers were forced to listen attentively to metronome clicks at intervals of 3 seconds, the impression of the waiting period being considered as representative of strain, and that during and immediately following each click as representative of relaxation; as a standard for pleasantness and for unpleasantness the observers were given syrup of sugar and a solution of sulphate of quinine. The main results were as follows:

1. The judgments of excitement, depression, strain and relaxation were as easy and direct, if not more so, than were those of pleasantness and unpleasantness.

2. Curves were plotted for the six qualities in the following fashion: a stimulus-scale was established by arranging the clangs in order of increasing frequency of vibration and representing neighboring members by equidistant positions along a line; along this scale there were plotted as ordinates the number of "more than" judgments for each stimulus. In the case of each pair of qualities the curves for the two qualities were opposites. The pairs of curves corresponding to the various pairs of qualities were of three main types, which the authors call the X, XO, and OX types. The pairs of curves for a single pair of qualities did not belong to the same type for all observers. Thus the excitement-depression curves were of the X type for three observers, but for a fourth belonged to the XO type. The strain-relaxation curves were of the X type for two observers, but of the OX type for two others. The pleasantness-unpleasantness curves were of the OX type for two observers, of the XO type for a third, and of the X type for a fourth.

3. The introspections of the observers upon the nature of the six processes and upon their judgments of these processes indicated that the judgments were being made not on affective values but upon sense-feeling values.

The authors argue that if the Wundtian theory were correct the observers should have had no difficulty in passing judgments upon the six qualities on the basis of the six standards given them; that they should have given typically different curves for the various qualities; and that they should have given curves identical in type with those of other observers for the same quality. The results show the opposite to have been the case. The authors conclude that their results do not support the Wundtian theory.

The research of Foster and Roese brings to an end the
list of experiments upon the tridimensional theory of feeling. This end, however, is a stalemate rather than a vic-
tory. In the last edition of the "Grundriss," in 1920, Wundt
was still arguing for the tridimensional theory.[31] In the
last edition of the Textbook, in 1926, Titchener was still
arguing against it.[32]

What may one conclude from these experiments? To
refresh the reader's memory the experiments are listed below in two columns according to whether or not they favor
the Wundtian view. If one study the table and if one remember that the experiments left both Wundt and Titchener with convictions unaltered, one must needs conclude
that the problem is unsolved. It seems to me, however,
that a further conclusion suggests itself, namely that special

TABLE VI

	Pro	Contra
1896	Vogt (elevating-depressing subjective like P & U).	
1899		Titchener (only P & U are non-localizable).
1899	Wundt (E-D & S-R have physiol. concomitant of same type as P-U).	
1902		Titchener (paired comp. judgments more difficult for E-D & S-R).
1903		Orth (S-R & E-D are sensory).
1906		Hayes (paired comp. judgments less direct for E-D and S-R).
1907	Alechsieff (E-D and S-R have same introsp. characteristics as P-U).	
1916		Foster & Roese (no typical curves for S-R, E-D or P-U).

affective elements are equivocal with respect to the number of their qualities—that they are three-dimensional in Leipzig but uni-dimensional at Cornell. This paradoxical statement is obviously in need of elucidation. I prefer, however, to postpone its discussion until the conclusion of the present chapter, for I believe that it can only be understood properly in the light of all the data on the relation of hedonic tone to mental elements.

THE EXISTENCE OF SPECIAL AFFECTIVE ELEMENTS

It is truly astonishing to what extent the psychology of Wundt, the great experimentalist, is based upon opinion rather than fact. A good illustration of this circumstance is afforded by his views upon the relation of hedonic tone to mental elements. It was in 1896 that he espoused the doctrine of special affective elements. It was not until 1907 that any of his pupils produced data apparently confirming the existence of such elements, and even then these data were secured with another end in view, namely that of supporting the tridimensional nature of the element.

In the preceding section it was pointed out that Alechsieff,[33] in order to test the tridimensional theory, sought to determine the characteristics of the six fundamental forms of feeling: pleasure, displeasure, strain, relaxation, excitement, depression, He found these processes to be non-localizable, non-objectifiable, independent of specific sense-organs, dependent upon the condition of consciousness, and non-describable. His major conclusion was in favor of the tridimensional theory because of the fact that these characteristics were common to all six forms of feeling. In addition, however, he pointed out that the nature of these characteristics indicates that feelings constitute a class of elements different from sensations.

The first experimental work to cast doubt upon the existence of special affective elements was that of Nakashima. In 1909, this investigator published two experiments upon the nature of affective judgments and of feeling itself.[34] In the first experiment, the method used was that of paired comparison. The stimuli were tones and colors. The observers were instructed to judge relative pleasantness and to "analyze their judgments introspectively, as fully and accurately as possible; especially they were to note the basis, motives, cues,—in short, the means by which these judgments were, or seemed to be, effected."[35] The results of this experiment are well illustrated by the following introspctive report of one of the observers at the close of the tonal series: " . . . I felt somewhat anxious about whether I had completely analyzed the situation or not. But when I look back I cannot find anything I left out, and I know now just as little as at the beginning why I like some tones better than others."[36]

In the second experiment, the method used was that of single stimuli. Various stimuli, such as sandpaper, ice water, carbolic acid, listerine, musk, were presented to the observers with the instruction "to take each (stimulus) as it came and to say what it did to consciousness—to give their immediate conscious reaction upon it, without making an effort to identify and analyze."[37] The results of this experiment were equivocal. "What we got," writes Nakashima, "was not any clear cut differentiation, on a positive basis, of affection and sensation, but rather a reflection of the theories and idiosyncrasies of our observers."[38]

Nakashima's experiments did not yield results contrary to the doctrine of special affective elements, they merely failed to support this doctrine. In 1914, however, Koch published an experiment whose results actually did conflict with the doctrine.[39] Koch's work was done for the purpose of testing Wundt's tridimensional theory. Its conclusions, however, bear wholly upon the problem of the existence of special affective elements, and that is why I am dealing with it here rather than in the preceding section. Koch felt that a prerequisite to the discussion of the tridimensional theory was the experimental determination of the criteria of pleasure and displeasure. Only then, by ascertaining whether strain, relaxation, excitement and depression conform to these criteria could one hope to learn whether these latter processes were likewise to be considered as feelings. In order to determine the criteria of pleasure and displeasure Koch established a list of 11 criteria proposed by psychologists at one time or another. He then aroused pleasant and unpleasant experiences in his observers by means of various stimuli, usually acoustic or visual, and had them report upon the applicability of these criteria to their pleasures and displeasures. The criteria the validity of which he thus sought to test were:

1. Arousal independent of specific sense organs.
2. Relative independence from outer stimuli.
3. Dependence upon "total consciousness."
4. Non arousal without cognitive concomitants.
5. Usually longer latent period than cognitive contents.
6. Non persistence after cessation of cognitive contents.
7. Always determine occurrence of attention. (i.e. cannot be "unnoticed.")
8. Weaken under attention.
9. Not objectivated but are experienced as states of a subject.
10. Not reproducible. (No affective imagery.)
11. Mutual exclusiveness and opposition of pleasure and displeasure.
12. Non localization of pleasure and displeasure.

Koch concludes against the validity of these criteria on the following grounds. (In the list below the number indicates the criterion similarly numbered in the list above.)

1. Observers invariably report organic sensations as concomitants of pleasure and displeasure.
2. True not only of pleasure and displeasure, but of organic sensations.
3. True not only of pleasure and displeasure, but of organic sensations.

4. Observers report that pleasure and displeasure may precede cognition.
5. Observers report simultaneity and sometimes precedence of pleasure and displeasure (especially when reproducing them in imagery).
6. Observers report cases where pleasure and displeasure persist after related cognitive content has vanished.
7. Observers report pleasure and displeasure are weakened by attention.
8. Observers report cases of increase of pleasure or displeasure under attention.
9. True of organic sensations.
10. Observers report imaginal pleasure or displeasure.
11. Observers report coexistence of pleasure and displeasure.
12. Observers report cases of localized pleasure or displeasure.

As none of these criteria is valid to distinguish pleasure and displeasure from sensations, Koch further concludes that the problem whether strain, relaxation, excitement and depression are to be classed with pleasure and displeasure or with sensations no longer exists—all of these processes must be classed as sensory.

In 1921, M. Yokoyama published an article upon the nature of the hedonic judgment in the method of paired comparison.[40] In an experiment carried out by this method with geometrical forms cut out of colored paper with a view to determining the manner in which judgments of pleasantness were dependent upon color and form, he secured a great many introspective reports upon the mental processes involved in these judgments. Examination showed that "P and U may be meanings for any observer; for B[41] and D always, for F consistently at one stage; for P occasionally. Organic sensory content is the *sine qua non* of P and U, except in advanced stages of degeneration; for B and D as carriers of the pleasant and unpleasant meanings; for F as concomitant or carrier; for P as con-

comitant." [42]   Yokoyama concluded: "(a) that P and U
(of the method of paired comparisons) are most univer-
sally and definitely statable as meanings; (b) that on the
side of process P and U are predominantly sensory; and
(c) that there exists a portion of the process-aspect of P
and U which is equivocal in its essential nature (i. e. it
is not certain whether it is sensory or non sensory) but
that this equivocal portion of the process-complex follows
a law of sensory decay." [43]   He added, however, that these
results need not be considered at all conclusive against the
existence of special affective elements, but might well indicate inadequacy of the method of paired comparison in the
investigation of affections of a process nature.

By this time it was clear that the doctrine of special
affective elements was anything but secure. As this doctrine
was a corner-stone of Titchener's psychology, its complete
establishment or complete disproval became a pressing
problem at Cornell. An intensive experiment was under-
taken upon this problem by J. P. Nafe, and its results published in 1924.[44] Using eight observers, Nafe presented a
great variety of visual, auditory, olfactory, gustatory and
tactual stimuli with the following instructions: "I shall give
you a stimulus which is intended to arouse a moderately
pleasant or a moderately unpleasant sensory experience.
You are to direct your attention as exclusively as possible to
the affective side of the experience. When you judge that the
feeling is at its maximum, break off your observation and
describe the feeling itself as accurately as you can." [45]

The most striking feature of the result is described by
Nafe as follows: "All of our Os, early in their reports,
make attempts to describe the qualities of P and U. From
first to last the reports are made in terms of touch. The O
may begin by saying the affective quality is like pressure but
isn't one,—yet reports in pressure terms continue. All Os
eventually describe P and U as 'sensory' pressures. They
are 'as much alike as if from the same matrix.' There are
many reports to the effect that there is no qualitative variation, and there is not one report that indicates any such

variation. P in quality is a bright pressure or a quality lying between bright pressure and tickle. It is described as bright; sparkling; brilliant; active; like effervescence; like tickle; dancing; shimmering; like points of light pressure; mild; misty; yielding; buoyant; vaporous; diffuse; light; airy; thin; fluffy; ethereal; smooth; soft; oily; welling; spreading; like the pressure component in warmth; like goose flesh, fur and glass; like muscle pressure in quality (not in density or localization), but brighter; like expansiveness of the body. The quality of the U is that of dull pressure or, according to some Os, of a pressure between dull pressure and neutral pressure or between dull pressure and strain. It is described as dull; drab; dead; rigid; less lively; somber; inert; stiff; gloomy; more dense; heavy; sinking; leaden; thick; cold; hard; rough; harsh; grating; insistent; condensed; like bodily contraction; like neutral pressure but duller; like dull strain. . . . It must be remembered that our Os were feeling for words; there is no reason at all to think that the various characterizations here listed refer to different modes of experience. Indeed, at the end of the experiment, all Os (except A and Br, to whom the question was not put) were ready to accept the designations 'bright pressure' and 'dull pressure.' " [46]

The general outcome of his inquiries is summarized by Nafe as follows. He insists, however, that each item of the summary must be qualified by the phrase "under the conditions of the present experiment."

"(1) Sensory experience may or may not also be affective; it may be characterized as P or U or neither. If sensory experience becomes P or U, it alters as a whole; something is added to it that is not present while it remains indifferent.

"(2) Qualitatively this increment, in the case of a P experience, is bright pressure or a touch-quality lying between bright pressure and tickle; in the case of an U experience, the increment is dull pressure or a quality lying near dull pressure.

"(3) The bright pressure is more extended than the

dull pressure of the same general intensity, and is usually greater in extensity than the accompanying sensory experience. Both P and U may vary in extensity. P is very voluminous, without limit or restraint. U is voluminous, but less so than P; it is without limit, but is somehow constrained or contracted. Neither P nor U has definite form, limit or boundary.

"(4) The affective increment is sometimes beaten up with the rest of the experience, and sometimes there is a quasi-spatial separation, which, however, is never complete.

"(5) P and U are both inherently weak, mild; but they may vary in intensity. The Os do not, at all times, report changes in the same variable as intensive changes. The 'intensity' of P may increase as the brightness increases, as the volume increases, with the increase of some variable in the nature of the chroma, or with the intensity of the stimulus. The 'intensity' of U may increase as the dullness increases, as volume decreases, as density increases, or again, with increase in the intensity of the stimulus.

"(6) There are patterns of density for both P and U. P shows streaks in a roughly radial direction, and is more dense, more intense, more prominent or more dominant somewhere out from the center, toward the periphery. U is more prominent at the center. Both dwindle at the extreme limits, though there are no definite limits in the sense of boundaries.

"(7) At a high degree of intensity affective experience becomes perceptive and, in the case of U, passes over into emotion. This passage was not reported for P.

"(8) The affective component of an experience goes on at the same time with the sensory component. It rises after the sensory component; P comes in gradually though quickly, while U comes in at full strength. Both P and U run a course, which may be either continuous or intermittent, and disappear with or before the sensory (or imaginal) component.

"(9) Affection is palpable; it stands up under observation.

"(10) The affective component is not definitely localized. Usually it is not localized at all. It may, however, be vaguely localized as within the body, or as projected out from the body; or it may be referred to some more or less well defined part of the body. There is some evidence to show that whenever affection is dominant for attention there is no localization.

"(11) Neither P nor U appears in isolation. The affective component ties up, under various aspects, to the sensory component of the total experience.

"(12) Affection is not simply a meaning carried by organic sensations. Nor is it a blend of organic sensations.

"(13) Experience from every sense department may take on the increment of bright or dull pressure, that is, may become affective experience. To arouse an observably affective experience the stimulus must be only mildly intensive, not so intense as to arouse a perceptive experience, and the O must maintain a psychological, non-perceptive attitude. The attitude may be active within these limits.

"(14) P and U are inherently alike, as if made from the same matrix. Their differences are of the sort that occur within one and the same modality.

"(15) There is no qualitative variety either of P or of U. Nor are there qualitative differences within the spread or volume of a given P or U.

"(16) P and U do not occur together; they may appear in rapid alternation." [47]

Are these conclusions in favor of affective elements or against them? In 1924, Nafe does not commit himself. He writes: "We do not, indeed, venture at this time upon any sort of systematic discussion of our results." [48] In two subsequent articles, however, he makes clear his systematic point of view. Pleasure and Unpleasure are for him *patterns of specific sensory experiences, namely bright and dull pressures:*[49] "Pleasantness, as a psychological experience, consists of discrete bright points of experience in the general nature of a thrill but usually much less intensive. It is vaguely localized in the upper part of the body and quickly adapts or fatigues. Unpleasantness is similar but characteristically duller, heavier, more of the pressure type of experience and is localized in the abdomen or in the lower part of the body." [50]

Since the publication of Nafe's work two attempts have been made to check up on his results. In 1927, P. T. Young published an experiment which was an exact duplicate of that of Nafe: the stimuli were the same, the instructions the same, and the total experimental situation the same insofar as possible.[51] Young used three observers, one of whom had been an observer in Nafe's experiment. Each observer was made to give 80 reports, 8 per day for 10 days. The observer who had worked for Nafe confirmed Nafe's results. Another observer "who had had a radically different type of psychological education, failed completely to confirm Nafe's results, but gave reports consistent with his theoretical views upon P and U." [52] The third observer likewise failed to confirm the results of Nafe. Young concludes that Nafe's results must be dependent upon a particular kind of training in his observers.

Young's experiment, whatever its interest in connection with the effects of training, was not a fair test of Nafe's work. Nafe specifically states that "to arouse an observably affective experience the stimulus must be only mildly intensive . . . and the O must maintain a psychological, nonperceptive attitude." [53] There is little doubt but that the two observers of Young who failed to duplicate Nafe's results were maintaining anything but a psychological attitude, for the one "was of the behaviourist's faith" [54] and the other was "a junior at the University of Illinois, a normal, competent individual who is quite innocent of theoretical views upon introspection, feeling and other psychological matters." [55]

The other attempt to check up on Nafe's results was made by W. A. Hunt in the Harvard laboratory.[56] The experiment was planned in such a way that it allowed for the dependence of "observably affective" experiences upon a "psychological" attitude, and at the same time avoided the influence of laboratory training emphasized by Young. In the main part of the experiment fifteen colored papers were shown singly to each of six observers on four different occasions separated by intervals of one week. On the first and third occasions the observers were instructed to judge whether the experience involved in looking at a color involved a bright pressure or a dull pressure. On the second and fourth occasion the observers were to judge whether the colors were pleasant, indifferent or unpleasant. Each color was shown three times in each sitting. Thus in the case of each observer the experiment yielded for each color six judgments of the brightness-dullness of pressure concomitants and six judgments of hedonic tone. From these judgments Hunt computed for each observer by means of numerical symbolization the average brightness of the pressure concomitants of each color and its average hedonic tone. This yielded data from which it was possible to determine the correlation between hedonic tone and brightness of concomitant pressures. The coefficients of correlation in the case of the six observers are given below:[57]

TABLE VII

Observer	r	P.E.
K	0.72	0.08
G	0.94	0.02
J	0.86	0.05
H	0.88	0.04
B	0.96	0.03
C	0.99	0.003

It is obvious that these coefficients confirm the general results of Nafe's work in that they show a connection on the one hand between pleasantness and bright pressure, on the other hand between unpleasantness and dull pressure. The exact nature of this connection, however, remains a matter of conjecture. Hunt himself favors the view that "affection is *accompanied* by bright and dull pressure." [58] He believes, however, that two other views are possible: (1) "Affection *is* bright and dull pressure" (Nafe's view) [59] and (2) "Affection and bright and dull pressure depend upon identical processes in proprioceptive end-organs, but upon different attitudes of report." [60]

In order to refresh the reader's memory I have listed. below the experiments discussed in the present section, together with their results.

TABLE VIII

Affection is

1907	Alechsieff	a special element
1909	Nakashima	experimentally equivocal
1914	Koch	a sensory experience
1921	Yokoyama	a meaning, at least in the case of judgments by paired comparison
1924	Nafe	a pattern of pressure
1927	Young	experimentally equivocal
1930	Hunt	accompanied by pressures

It is obvious what conclusion is implied by these results with respect to the particular doctrine at issue in the present section, namely that of special affective elements. Of seven experiments, but one supports this doctrine. We must conclude that the evidence is distinctly contrary to the existence of special affective elements.

It is also clear what conclusion is implied with respect to the general problem of the relation of hedonic tone to mental elements. The series of experiments started with the purpose of choosing between two alternatives: the view that hedonic tone is an attribute of special affective elements, and the view that it is an attribute of sensations. It ends with the quasi-elimination of one alternative, but not with the selection of the other. Instead, the series brings forth two new views, that of Nafe, according to which hedonic tone is an attribute of a pattern of particular sensory elements, and that of Yokoyama, according to which hedonic tone is an attribute of a meaning in Titchener's sense of the word, i.e. in the sense of a particular pattern of sensory elements. No one view, furthermore, is supported by more than a single experiment.[61] Indeed, the only two experiments whose results agree concerning the problem are those of Nakashima and Young, and these results indicate that the problem is experimentally equivocal. It would seem that it is this negative conclusion which best accords with all of the data of the series, and consequently that it is this conclusion which we must tentatively accept.

MIXED FEELINGS

The preceding sections have made it clear that interest in the relation of hedonic tone to mental elements led to considerable emphasis upon the *characteristics* of *affection* —upon the characteristics of the elements or groups of elements of which hedonic tone was considered an attribute. This emphasis was displayed not only in experiments on the characteristics in general, such as some of the experiments described above, but also in experiments on some one characteristic alone. It is my intention to adapt my exposition to this specialization and to turn now to a discussion of the data available concerning four particular characteristics,— or supposed characteristics—of affection, namely the co-occurrence of pleasant and unpleasant affections (the occurrence of so-called mixed feelings), the clearness of affection, its localization and its extensity. I shall begin with the data on mixed feelings.

Casual observation, as Titchener points out, yields evidence both for and against the occurrence of mixed feelings. "We go back to school after the holidays with mixed feelings; we visit our old home, after a long absence, with mixed feelings; there is, indeed, hardly anything that we may not look upon, or look back or forward to, with mixed feelings. Juliet tells us that parting is sweet sorrow, a pleasant unpleasantness; and Tennyson's Geraint watches the mowers, whose dinner he has just eaten, with humorous ruth (pity), that is, with a pleasantly unpleasant feeling. There is no pleasure we are told, without its alloy of pain; there is no despair so dark that it is not lightened by a ray of hope.

"On the other hand, we know that a single trifling annoyance may color our whole mood. When Othello behaves unkindly to Desdemona, she excuses him on the ground that he is worried by affairs of state; 'for let our finger ache,' she says, 'and it indues our other healthful members ev'n to that sense of pain.' We know, too, that if we are in a particularly good temper we take everything good-temperedly; we may even ask pardon of the man who has trodden on our corns. And there is really no proof that the pleasantness and unpleasantness of the mixed feelings are strictly coincident: Juliet may be alternately glad and sorry; sorry now to part from Romeo, but glad the next moment that he is there, as her lover, to be parted from, and glad a moment after in the thought of seeing him again. How quickly the pendulum of feeling may swing we see in the case of the child who is crying bitterly at its hurt and then, within a few seconds, is smiling over a lump of sugar." [62]

Little wonder, then, that psychologists have failed to agree upon this problem. In "Emotion and the Will," Bain considered the opposition of pleasantness and unpleasantness to imply their incompatibility. "Pleasure and Pain are opposites in the strongest form of Contrariety; like heat and cold, they destroy or neutralize each other." [63] This view gradually became subject to doubt. In 1893, Külpe wrote: "In our own view, mixed feelings are certainly less well authenticated than cancellation of feeling." He went on to add: "It is hardly possible in the present state of our knowledge to decide positively for or against the reality of these mixed feelings." [64] More recently, McDougall has categorically championed the opposite view. He writes: "I have no hesitation in rejecting this doctrine and in following Professor Stout, in recognizing states of feeling in which pleasure and pain are conjoined." [65]

As far as I know, the first experimental contribution to the problem of mixed feelings is to be found in an investigation by Orth, published in "Gefühl and Bewusstseinslage," in 1903.[66] In an attempt to test Wundt's theory of doubt, according to which doubt involved a "total feeling" generated by alternations of pleasure and displeasure, Orth presented to his observers groups of lines and of dots, instructing them in the case of the former to judge which line was the longer, and in the case of the latter, what was the number of dots. Orth further instructed his observers to give a complete report,—"of all experiences during the trials." [67] The results, insofar as they bear upon mixed feelings, were as follows. Out of 28 tests (each of 7 stimuli presented to each of 4 observers) pleasure was reported 5 times, displeasure 10 times, and the simultaneous occurrence of pleasure and displeasure not once. Furthermore, one observer reported in one and the same test a sequence of 4 hedonic states, first pleasure, then displeasure, then again pleasure, then again displeasure. Of this latter report, Orth writes: "This sequence seems to me to point to the non-occurrence of mixed feelings." [68]

In 1905-6, S. P. Hayes carried out some experiments upon mixed feelings, but never published the results. The data, however, were communicated to P. T. Young, who wrote of them as follows: "The work was done in the Cornell laboratory in 1905-06 with two subjects, but the unpublished article is based upon 134 reports of a single subject. Pairs of simultaneous stimuli were used, a stimulus to P with a stimulus to U; (1) taste solutions containing sugar and quinine in various percentages; (2) taste solutions (sugar and quinine) and sounds (chords or discords from forks); (3) sounds (chords or discords) and odors (valerianic acid, carbon bi-sulphate, essence of peppermint, cinnamon). The subjects were instructed to 'attend to the sensations aroused . . . and then to recall the experience and report on the sensations and affections experienced.' The result of the experiment was negative; it seems that we often have side by side in consciousness, sensations (or complexes of sensations) that when alone are distinctly P or U. Here then we might expect to find P and U side by side, but the observer confidently asserted that they never did coexist." [69]

In 1906, C. H. Johnstone published an extensive experiment upon the results of combining various pleasant and unpleasant impressions, seeking particularly to determine "whether it is really impossible that various feelings co-exist and remain distinguishable." [70] The procedure involved the simultaneous presentation of two stimuli affecting different sense organs—a color stimulus and a touch stimulus, for instance—under instructions to give an introspective report. There were seven observers, two women and five men. No introspections are given by the author, but we are told that "in this investigation, after considerable training, the subjects, with a single exception, were all convinced that both feeling tones, for tactual and visual impressions, could be present at once." [71] This is not by any means invariably the case, according to Johnstone, for "the various phenomena of fusion, summation, partial re-enforcement, merely simultaneous, independent co-existence, partial and total inhibition, of one by the other occur." [72]

The problem of mixed feelings was investigated by Alechsieff in his extensive research published in 1907 under the title "Die Grundformen der Gefühle." [73] Alechsieff subjected his observers simultaneously to two stimuli affecting different sense organs. The usual procedure was either to place a bottle of oil of rose under the observer's nose and to apply a quinine solution on his tongue, or to have him smell valerian and at the same time taste raspberry juice. The results were in accord with the conclusions of Orth, and contrary to those of Johnstone. Alechsieff's observers reported that pleasure and displeasure frequently alternated, but never occurred simultaneously.

In 1909, T. Nakashima published an experiment on the time relations of hedonic tone in which the instructions to the observers included the task of reporting upon mixed feelings.[74] The observers were shown pictures tachistoscopically, each trial involving the presentation of two pictures in quick succession. Nakashima stated: "There are a few cases of mixed feeling mentioned in the records of H, F, D and I." [75] He did not further discuss the matter.

In the same year, Nakashima published another experiment upon the nature of pleasure and displeasure in which he secured a few incidental data on mixed feelings.[76] Using the method of single stimuli, he presented to his observers cutaneous and olfactory stimuli with the instruction to "say what (the stimuli) did to consciousness." [77] Only one of four observers reported mixed feelings and this observer upon being asked to comment upon his report at the close of the experiment stated that he might well have reported as simultaneous processes which were not so in reality.[78]

In 1913, Koch published a research involving a subsidiary experiment directly upon the problem of the existence of mixed feelings.[79] Four observers were subjected to various acoustic stimuli including two pieces of music played in immediate succession. Three of them reported co-occurrences of pleasure and displeasure.

In an article published in 1915, C. E. Kellogg undertook a thorough examination of the problem.[80] This article begins with a very interesting historical sketch showing among other things that the problem was already a real one to Socrates. It then goes on to describe Kellogg's experimental work, which like that of Johnstone was done at Harvard. Kellogg's purpose was to produce pleasure and displeasure in such a manner as to lead to interference. To do this he selected a large number of pictures and exposed two of them, usually one pleasant and the other unpleasant, alternately in a slightly modified form of the Dodge tachistoscope. Fourteen observers took part in the experiment. The results indicate the occasional occurrence of mixed feelings. One observer, for instance, stimulated for 20 seconds with pictures alternating at the rate of 10 presentations per minute, reported: "One pleasant all the time, the other disgusting. Contrast made pleasantness stronger, and the pleasantness seemed to last and be contrasted with the disgust during exposure of '92.' " [81] Kellogg adds that "this was not true in the other direction. The pleasant feeling was pure." [82] And another observer, stimulated for 24 seconds with two other pictures alternating at the same rate (10 per min.) reported: "Pleasure overbalanced the displeasure. No surprise this time, sinking not noticed. Pleasant feeling begins the moment the picture appears, just the same as real scenes. Other just slightly unpleasant. Made a conscious effort to endure it. Less unpleasant than the black intervals in the case of the road alone. Pleasant feeling seemed to last during exposure of 3, but under a mist." [83]

Kellogg concludes that mixed feelings actually occur, though only under certain conditions. "When the two feeling-tendencies are of like intensity, if the total reactions, the apperceptive attitudes are widely dissimilar, the result is inhibition, whether the feeling-tendencies are of the same or of unlike sign. Inhibition diminishes with increasing similarity, until with some subjects, there is a tendency to parallelism, and, rarely fusion. . . . When the feelings are of unequal intensity, inhibition continues farther up the scale of similarity." [84]

In his well-known monograph upon olfaction, published in 1916,[85] Henning claims to have experienced definite mixed feelings under certain specific conditions. "If I smell oil of mustard localized in the right half of the nose, and oil of jasmin (or Khasana-perfume, etc.) localized in the left half, both partial experiences being experienced as a plurality and simultaneous, though disconnected, then it is only the oil of mustard which has a sensory unpleasantness, whereas I notice simultaneously a tone of pleasantness in the case of the odor of jasmin." [86] He does not, however, indicate whether this result has been found to obtain for other observers.

P. T. Young published in 1918 an extensive experiment on mixed feelings carried out in the psychological laboratory at Cornell.[87] His general method was "to establish a relatively permanent affective consciousness of moderate intensity, and then .by stimulation to superinduce a brief affection of opposite sign." [88] The experiment consisted of four main divisions. In the first, Young devised "natural" situations that would evoke a relatively permanent feeling-consciousness. For instance, he "asked the subject to omit breakfast; and when a hunger U had been obtained, (he) superinduced P by the smell and taste of food." [89] In the second division, Young used single stimuli, odors, tones and noises, taste complexes and tactual complexes. In the third division, he used simultaneous stimuli: "At first a stimulus to P was presented and when E thought it had exerted its full effect a stimulus to U was added, and conversely." [90] In the fourth division, he used alternate presentations of two stimuli, the stimuli being pictures. The instructions to the observers were as follows: "There will be two signals: 'Now . . . now.' After the second 'now' you will report the course of feeling during the interval between the signals." [91]

The frequency of mixed feelings for the different observers is shown in the table below, copied from Young.

TABLE IX

(From P. T. Young)

Subject	Positive Reports	Doubtful Reports	Positive by Questioning	Total 1, 2, 3	Total No. Reports	Percentage Mixed Feelings
B	0	0	0	0	193	0.
Da	0	1	0	1	275	0.36
Di	0	2	0	2	242	0.82
F	4	2	1	7	252	2.77
G	0	5	0	5	232	2.15
H	4	7	0	11	242	4.54
K	21	6	10	37	307	12.05
O	2	3	1	6	278	2.15
W	0	2	0	2	191	1.04
	31	28	12	71	2,212	3.21

Young's comments upon these figures are as follows: "Out of a grand total of 2212 reports, there are 71 or 3.21% mixed feelings. Of these 71 reports, 37 or 52% are reported by a single subject (K). If we eliminate doubtful reports, there are left 43 of almost 2% mixed feelings. If we limit our consideration to positive mixed feeling reports, we find 31 or 1.4% of which 21 or 67.7% are reported by subject K. Five subjects (B, Da, Di, G, W) report no positive mixed feelings. Coexisting P and U is at best a rare experience . . . Not only is mixed feeling a rare experience, but it is also a doubtful one. Of the 71 mixed feelings, 28 or 39.4% contain expressions of doubt and uncertainty." [92] Examination of the distribution of mixed feelings within the experiment showed that "mixed feelings are reported in sporadic groups throughout the course of a single experimental hour." [93]

Besides considering the quantitative side of his reports, Young subjected them to an extremely thorough analysis. He found that they could be classed into two main categories, which he terms "psychological reports of experience" and "common sense statements about the object of experience." The "psychological reports are characterized by clearness and definiteness of statement regarding the temporal relations and course of P and U during the interval reported. They contain no temporal ambiguity. *They are detailed accounts of the rise and fall,* the fluctuations and alternations of P and U." [94] An example of such a report is: "There was pretty near an equality of P and U. I get P quite strong at first and then there was a shoot of U, but not extreme. Then attention fluctuated back and forth and P and U fluctuated. Now there is no difference between them. It is hop, skip, and jump—and it's all over." [95] The common-sense type of report "is characterized by common sense statements about the object of experience, usually the stimulus-object. There are two subtypes which we shall call the objective and the subjective. In the objective type, P and U are referred or attributed to the object, e.g. 'the object is P,' 'the U is from the object,' 'this is a P object,' etc. The subjective type is characterized by statement of an attitude toward the object, e.g. 'I like the object,' or by the effect of the object upon me, e.g. 'the object displeases me.' " [96]

Although reports of the psychological type were by far the more frequent, they contained no mixed feelings. These reports, according to Young " . . . contain the statement that P and U alternated or fluctuated—sometimes slowly, sometimes rapidly, sometimes so completely 'jumbled' that a full report is impossible—but there is not a single case of coexisting P-U to be found in the reports of the psychological type." [97] As to reports of the "common sense statement about the object of experience" type, those of the subjective sub-type did not contain any mixed feelings either. Those of the objective sub-type, however, did in some cases mention the occurrence of mixed feelings. Instances of such reports are as follows: "(U memory, perfume) 'Here were two things in consciousness. There was the U situation in which I was all keyed up. I felt very tense about it and was almost on the verge of tears. Then on the borderline of consciousness was an odor which I recognized as slightly P. The U of the memory was still there' (F 72) . . . (Buttered toast, odor stale cheese) 'P from the toast. An increase in P due to amusement. Then a slight flash of U coexisting with P' (K 254)." [98]

These data indicated in Young's opinion that pleasant and unpleasant objects may coexist, but that there can be no coexistence of pleasant and unpleasant *affections* in the sense of elements or groups of elements having hedonic tone as an attribute. Reports of the objective sub-type are ambiguous, since they tell nothing about experience. "If a subject reports 'the object was P' we, of course, cannot doubt that the meaning of pleasantness attaches to the object. But what guarantee have we that pleasantness was felt?" [99] The fact then, that mixed feelings occur in common sense reports of the objective type is no proof of the coexistence of P and U, but only of the coexistence of meanings of P and meanings of U. Indeed, this distinction between "meaning affection" and "process affection" is frequently made by the observers themselves. One observer reports: "The ugly one gave me an incipient shrinking in the stomach like nausea. That meant U, but didn't seem to be U." [100] It follows that " 'Mixed feelings' involve a confusion between the meaning of pleasantness (or unpleasantness), which is referred to an object, and affective experience." . . . They "involve the awareness of an object to which the meaning of pleasantness or unpleasantness is attached. . . . Pleasantness and unpleasantness are not felt at the same time." [101]

In 1919, A. Wohlgemuth published a monograph entitled "Pleasure-Unpleasure" in which he described an extensive experiment carried out by him from 1915 to 1917 in the psychological laboratory of University College, London.[102] The purpose of this experiment was "to obtain as much information as possible about feeling by the impression method."[103] The stimuli were very numerous and varied: 6 tactile, 6 visual, 6 olfactory, 4 gustatory, 6 auditory and 3 painful. These stimuli were presented singly and in pairs, the observers being instructed to concentrate their attention on the hedonic side of their experiences and to describe them as well as they could in words. Before the beginning of the experiment, and occasionally during it, the observers were made to read a questionnaire which included the following question: "What view do you hold respecting the coexistence or fusion of two feelings in consciousness? Do you hold the view on experimental, i.e. introspective, evidence or on theoretical grounds? Is that view necessary to fit in with any theory or system you hold?" [104] This procedure was carried out in order to ascertain the various biases of the observers and to keep them interested in certain points of importance without asking questions.

Of the four observers, one experienced mixed feeling from the very beginning; two experienced none at the beginning of the experiment but definitely did report some towards the end; and one was sure of having experienced mixed feelings but once, usually reporting them with some qualification expressing doubt. Wohlgemuth concludes as follows:

"Two or more feeling-elements may coexist in consciousness; they may be like or they may be unlike.

"There is some indication that it may be easier for two

pleasant feeling-elements to coexist than for two unpleasant ones.

"Great individual differences obtain in the apprehension of the coexistence of feeling-elements.

"The ability to apprehend the coexistence of feeling-elements is improved with practise." [105]

J. P. Nafe, in his "Experimental Study of the Affective Qualities" (1924), examined the reports of his observers with respect to the occurrence of mixed feelings. Not a single case was reported.[106] The conditions of the experiment were not such, however, as to favor the occurrence of mixed feelings, and consequently Nafe's result cannot be given much weight.

In an article published in 1925 in the British Journal of Psychology, Young analyzes the results, secured by Wohlgemuth in 1919, which led the latter to conclusions directly opposed to those of Young.[107] He found that "in every case of so-called co-existing and localized feeling, one or more of the feelings is referred to an object or cause or to some other phase of experience." [108] Such reports, he points out, are ambiguous as to what was felt and as to the temporal relations of affective experience. He concludes that Wohlgemuth's own results do not bear out his conclusions that two or more feeling-elements may coexist in consciousness. This criticism called forth a prompt reply. In an article published in 1926, Wohlgemuth[109] contended that, even if an observer at the time of his report is dealing with "meaning of P or U," "in order to have obtained that knowledge he must have had the affective experience, must have *felt* the feeling during the introspective period. If he is a trained and careful observer he *knows* whether two feelings were felt simultaneously or whether a feeling whilst it was being felt was localized, however he may describe his experience afterwards, whether in forms resembling judgments or as objective references." [110] Wohlgemuth concludes that Young's distinction between "meaning of P and U" and "processes of P and U," although it may sometimes refer to experiences, usually refers to form of

report alone, and consequently that the objective reports
of mixed feelings secured by both Young and himself indicate that pleasure and displeasure may coexist in consciousness.

Is it possible to arrive at a solution of the problem of
mixed feelings which will be in accord with all of these
data? Inspection of the table below, in which I have listed
the experiments, together with their conclusions, would appear to dictate a negative answer. Such is indeed the
opinion to which was ultimately led one of the men whose
work figures prominently in the table, namely P. T. Young.
In an article published in 1927, he contends that the data

TABLE X

Do mixed feelings occur?

1903	Orth	No
1905	Hayes*	No
1906	Johnstone	Yes
1907	Alechsieff	No
1909	Nakashima	Yes
1911	Koch	Yes
1915	Kellogg	Yes
1916	Henning	Yes
1918	Young	No
1919	Wohlgemuth	Yes
1924	Nafe	No

*Published in 1918 by Young.

on mixed feelings, together with those on a number of other
problems concerning hedonic tone, are so dependent upon
the observer's training and the experimenter's bias that
they are entirely devoid of value.[111] I do not think, however, that this pessimism is warranted. Indeed, I think
that Young himself, in his article of 1918, provided the
correct solution of the problem. His results, it will be remembered, showed that pleasant and unpleasant objects
were reported to coexist in experience, albeit infrequently,
but that coexistence was never reported of pleasant and

unpleasant affections, in the sense of elements or groups of elements having hedonic tone as an attribute. These findings suggest a ready explanation for the divergence of conclusions in the list above. They suggest, namely, that the experimenters who have concluded against the occurrence of mixed feelings have been led to do so by critical rejection of reports of Young's objective sub-type, whereas the experimenters who have concluded in favor of the occurrence of mixed feelings have been misled into doing so by uncritically interpreting such reports as indicating coexistence of opposed affections. This suggestion is well borne out by examination of the work of the various experimenters. Both Orth and Alechsieff introduce their data by long and critical discussions of the nature of affections.[112] Hayes, Young and Nafe all did their experiments at Cornell under Titchener, well known for his insistence upon critical evaluation of reports.[113] These five men are the ones who concluded against the occurrence of mixed feelings. Johnstone, on the other hand, bases his view on cases which, according to Titchener, were "not above suspicion." [114]   Nakashima cites as possible cases of mixed feeling two reports which are obviously of the objective sub-type.[115]   Kellogg supports his conclusions with many such reports.[116]   Koch does likewise,[117] and Wohlgemuth, as has been pointed out by Young, supports his conclusions wholly upon such reports.[118]

If we accept this explanation there is no longer any reason for the pessimism voiced by Young in 1927. All of the data on mixed feelings may be considered to support the conclusion which he reached in 1918—the conclusion that there are no mixed feelings in the sense of coexistence of pleasant or unpleasant elements or groups of elements with hedonic tone as an attribute. They must also be considered, however, to support a further conclusion, unrelated to the problem of mixed feelings. This further conclusion is that it is possible under particularly favorable conditions, for a pleasant object and an unpleasant one to be experienced simultaneously.

CLEARNESS, LOCALIZATION AND EXTENSITY
OF AFFECTIONS

Besides the experiments on mixed feelings, there are three other groups of experiments dealing primarily with some one characteristic of affections, in the sense of the elements or groups of elements having hedonic tone as an attribute. These groups of experiments are concerned with the clearness of affections, their localization, and their extensity. We shall deal with them in the present section in the order named.

Clearness as a Characteristic of Affections.— W h a t appears to have been the first experiment bearing upon this problem was published in 1893 by Külpe.[119] As far as can be judged from a very scanty account, sphygmographic records were taken in the case of a single observer under two different sets of conditions: under "normal" conditions, and when the observer had been instructed to attend to the affections occasioned by various supposedly pleasant and' unpleasant stimuli. "The subject," Külpe wrote, "often insisted that the feeling had altogether disappeared under attention, and that it was very difficult, in any case, to attend to pleasantness or unpleasantness. Feeling has too little objectivity and substantiality for the attention to be directed and held upon it. It is focussed for a moment, and then other processes, especially organic sensations, interpose and take possession of the conscious fixation point." [120]

In 1894, Titchener published some experiments which led him flatly to deny the possibility of attending to affections.[121] I use the term "experiments," however, only because Titchener has done so in a subsequent reference to this publication.[122] Otherwise I should use the expression "series of casual self-observations." At all events, the conclusion reached was that "We cannot attend to pleasure-pain as such." [123]

The first experiment upon the problem of which there is an adequate record is that of Zoneff and Meumann, published in 1901.[124] The main feature of this experiment was an attempt to establish a correlation between hedonic tone and characteristics of the pulse and of respiration. Having succeeded in this attempt to their own satisfaction (though not to that of others, as we shall see later), Zoneff and Meumann sought to utilize their knowledge in order to establish the relation of attention to feeling. Their general procedure was to present a pleasant or unpleasant stimulus, to have the observer attend now to the stimulus-object, now to the affections which were aroused, now to some other object, and to infer from changes in the observer's pulse and respiration the effect upon the affections of these various directions of attention. The results were interpreted by the authors as follows: "Simple direction of attention to feeling strengthens the latter; if, however, the feeling becomes the object of a psychological analysis, and in this sense the object of attention, it is markedly weakened, or even wholly obliterated . . ." [125]

This conclusion, like that of Külpe above, is by no means univocal with respect to the clearness or lack of clearness of affections. It is obvious that both conclusions may be interpreted as consistent with the occasional clearness of affections, at least when attention is not "analytical." Titchener, however, has argued that they support the conclusion of his own experiment.[126] His argument rests essentially upon two points. In the first place, he contends that in the conclusions of Zoneff and Meumann the expression "simple direction of attention" means really not attention to affections, but attention to pleasant or unpleasant objects. In the second place, he tacitly assumes that when Külpe writes of attention to affections "weakening" them, and when Zoneff and Meumann ascribe the same effect to analytical attention, these writers are really referring to complete obliteration of affections. He is thus able to cite both experiments in support of the thesis "that affections lack, what all sensations possess, the attribute of clearness." [127]

Whatever the logical validity of Titchener's argument, it is difficult to conciliate his conclusion with the data secured subsequently by Wohlgemuth and Nafe. Among the experiments published by Wohlgemuth in 1919 is one directly concerned with the relationship of affections to attention.[128] His observers were first made to read the four following quotations, selected from standard psychological works:

"1. 'Attention to a sensation means always that the sensation becomes clear; attention to an affection (i.e. feeling element) is impossible. If it is attempted, the pleasantness and unpleasantness at once eludes us and disappears, and we find ourselves attending to some obtrusive sensation or idea that we had not the slightest desire to observe.'

"2. 'A weakly pleasurable feeling is intensified by the direction of the attention upon its concomitant sensations, and an impression which stands on the borderline between pleasantness and unpleasantness may be made unpleasant by intense concentration of the attention upon it. In a certain sense, then, attention is a favorable condition for the feeling as it is for the sensation.'

"3. 'A mere direction of the attention to the feeling intensifies the feeling. If, however, the feeling is subjected to a psychological analysis and in this way becomes the object of attention, it is considerably weakened or even destroyed.'

"4. 'We can intensify a pain (i.e. unpleasure) or pleasure by attending to it as such.' "[129]

The observers were asked to make a preliminary statement on these views, and then were subjected to a variety of stimuli with instructions to vary attitudes at will and to give introspective reports. Finally they were again asked to state what they had meant, in their reports, by attention and attending.

The reports of two observers indicated that affections had greater *intensity* and *clearness* when attended to directly than when attention was on cognitive content or lacking completely. A third observer, however, could not fix his attention on affections. These individual differences, corresponding to differences between the views of different authors, were explained in Wohlgemuth's opinion by reference to the statements of the observers concerning their use of the expression "attending to." The first two meant attention to the pleasant or unpleasant object, the last meant attention to affections per se. Wohlgemuth checked this interpretation by carrying out another experiment in which the two observers who had reported ability to attend to affections were instructed "to analyze out the feeling-element, to focus the attention upon it to the exclusion of everything else as he would do with a cognitive content of consciousness." [130]   Of these observers, one was entirely unable to assume the attitude, and the other found that it destroyed hedonic tone.

Wohlgemuth concludes as follows: "If a feeling element is attended to as belonging to a cognitive content or as a part of a situation or complex, it is *intensified* and becomes *clearer;* but if an attempt be made to focus the attention upon it to the exclusion of its cognitive concomitant, the feeling-element is destroyed." [131]

These results are entirely confirmed by those of Nafe in his experiment on the nature of affection published in 1924—to which we have already had occasion to refer. Nafe found evidence that: "The affective qualities are palpable, that is, they stand up under observation. All of our Os were able to observe both P and U, but none could attend to either to the total exclusion of the sensory experience. The affective quality may be the dominant part of the total experience, however, and the O may know more about it for report than he does about the sensory process." [132] Some of the introspections upon which Nafe bases these statements are as follows:

Obs. H. (Pyridine 1 U) " . . . Attention to the object of stimulation in its U-character seems to be most favorable for affective experience. I don't know if that means I'm attending to the affection, but it surely is the object as a U object,—not just U and not just object, but attention covers the affective nature of the object."

(Salt 1 U) "I couldn't attend exclusively to the affection and I don't know if I did primarily; but U forced itself to the fore in attention, a sort of oscillation. Towards the end the affective part was fairly attended to."

Obs. M. (Ammonium Valerianate 19 U) "I don't know whether to say they are beaten up or just lying there side by side; for I can get the affection so clear and dominant that I tend to forget the sensation, though I don't ever really."

(Asafoetida 20 U) "I can isolate th∘ U, but it's always there with the sensory." [133]

When it comes to drawing a geneial conclusion from these five experiments, we are in a quandary. The conclusions of one experiment—that by Titchener—are against the clearness of affections. The conclusions of two experiments—those of Külpe and Zoneff and Meumann—are ambiguous with respect to the problem. The conclusion of the two last experiments—those of Wohlgemuth and Nafe —are in favor of the clearness of affections. The latter solution has a slight statistical advantage—but frequency of opinion is surely no measure of its correctness. It seems wiser to consider the problem to be as yet unsolved.

Localization as a Characteristic of Affections. — Another problem which has led investigators to widely divergent conclusions is that of the localization of affections. Orth[134] in 1903 and Alechsieff[135] in 1907 concluded from experimental data that affections *are not* localized. Nafe in 1924 concluded that they are *never definitely* localized, and rarely localized at all.[136] Nakashima[137] in 1909, Koch[138] in 1913, Kellogg[139] in 1916 and Wohlgemuth[140] in 1919 concluded that affections *are* localized. Nafe in 1927 accepted the latter view, attributing the failure of his earlier observers to localize affections well to lack of specific instructions upon this point.[141]

I shall not describe these experiments because they have already been dealt with in connection with the problem of mixed feelings. This circumstance itself, however, deserves particular attention. In 1908, E. B. Titchener, in his "Psychology of Feeling and Attention" referred to the problem of mixed feeling as that of "inner localization,"[142] and discussed it as a special case of the problem of the localization of affections. Whether or not the occurrence of mixed feelings implies localization of affections, as Titchener seems to believe, need not detain us. There can be no doubt that the two problems are closely related. Consider the following table in which are listed the various experiments bearing upon the localization of affections mentioned above. The column marked "localization" shows the conclusions with respect to localization, a + sign indicating that affections were localized, a — sign indicating that affections were never localized. Similarly, + and — signs in the column marked "mixed feelings" indicate that the conclusions with respect to the occurrence of mixed feelings are positive or negative. It will be observed that the correspondence of results with respect to mixed feelings and localization is very great.

TABLE XI

Experimenter	Localization	Mixed Feelings
Orth (1903)	—	—
Alcchsicff (1907)	—	—
Nafe (1924)	+	—
Nakashima (1909)	+	+
Koch (1913)	+	+
Kellogg (1915)	+	+
Wohlgemuth (1919)	+	+

Indeed the only exception to a one to one correlation is the work of Nafe, whose conclusions with respect to localization have been somewhat variable. This correspondence suggests that disagreement between the conclusions of different investigators might be due to the same causes in both cases.

That such is the case is the view advanced in an article upon the localization of affections published in 1918 by P. T. Young.[143] Examining the data which he had secured in his study of mixed feelings, he found that "The relationship of localized feeling to mixed feeling is shown quantitatively by several facts. In the first place, the same subjects report both: unequivocal mixed feeling is reported by F(4), H(21), O(2); unequivocal localized feeling is reported by F(17), H(51), K(4). In the second place, the distribution of localized feelings and mixed feelings is of the same type; both occur in sporadic groups throughout the course of the experiment and throughout the single experimental hour. In the third place, the group of localized feelings and mixed feelings overlap; both occur on the same days. In the fourth place, the percentages of mixed feelings and localized feelings are almost identical, although the overlapping is only partial. There are 3.2% mixed feelings and 3.4% localized feelings in the experiment as a whole." [144]

Young further found that his observers reported four main types of localization:

1. Localization in the place of the stimulus-object. Example: (Taste of salt solution) "U, a drawn up feeling . . . localized in the mouth." [145]

2. Organic localization, remote from the stimulus-object. Example: (Perfume, H_2S) "P, localized along the spinal cord." [146]

3. Localization involving radiation from a given center. Example: "A slightly nauseating U particularly in the stomach. It spread itself out to most of the body." [147]

4. Localization involving the whole body. Example: "U, the whole body revolted; I felt it all over." [148]

The suggestion which to Young seemed implicit in these four types of reports was that the observers were localizing not affections, but sensory correlates of affections. This suggestion was definitely verified in the case of two observers. In the course of the experiment, one of these observers was asked whether, when speaking of feeling, he meant muscular and organic sensation. He replied: ". . . The P actually seems to come from the chest region; it seems to be there." Two days later he said: "It seems that the organic sensation *is* the P localized." [149] This observer was then instructed to "abstract from organic sensation and report the feeling." Throughout the rest of the experiment he never again repor.ed localized feelings, except on one single day. As to the other observer who had localized feelings at the place of the stimulus when the stimuli were odors, tastes, pain, tones, etc., he stopped reporting localized feelings as soon as pictures were used as stimuli. Furthermore, during the latter part of the experiment, his reports instead of being of the "common sense statement" type, became "psychological," i. e., feeling was reported for its own sake, with no reference to the object.

Young drew the conclusion that localization, like coexistence with an entity of opposed hedonic tone, is a characteristic of the "unanalyzed object-feeling of common sense"; that when affections are regarded independently, localization is no more reported than coexistence of opposed affections, and consequently that "affections are not localizable." [150]

In 1927, Young reported another experiment upon the localization of feelings.[151] The results were extremely similar to those just described. Five observers were presented single stimuli including perfumes, candy, auditory stimuli such as crumpling of paper near the ear, and clangs from tuning-forks, tactual stimuli such as sandpapering of the chin and placing cotton on the cheek. They were instructed "to describe the quality and the spatial characteristics of the feeling, noting especially the place where it is located." [152] At the close of the experiment, the following questions were asked:

"1. Judging from your observation in this experiment, are P and U experienced at some place?

"2. How do you understand the instruction to describe 'the spatial characteristics of the feeling, noting especially the place where it is located?' " [153]

The general results were as follows: One observer never reported localized feelings. Another reported localized feelings, but at the close of the experiment gave the opinion that they were non-localizable when experienced alone. Two observers reported localized feelings and also agreed to the reality of such localizations at the end of the experiment. One observer reported localized feelings, but was not questioned at the end of the experiment.

Examination of the protocols showed that the term "feeling" was used by the observers in three different senses, namely to indicate "(a) Clear sensory processes, especially organic and kinaesthetic processes; (b) sense-feelings as, for example, an odor which has the character of P or which means U, or which possibly is a fusion of sensory processes; and (c) non-sensory, non-clear affective processes, P and U, differing in quality, intensity and in temporal course. . . . When the observers used the term 'feeling' in the sense of (a) or (b), localization in perceptual space was sometimes reported. In the sense of (c), localization was not reported." [154]

These results are similar to those of Young's earlier experiment, but the conclusion he drew is quite different. This conclusion is that the disagreement of his observers depends upon the ambiguity of the terms "feeling" and "localize"; that "these terms may be understood in a manner justifying the conclusion that 'P and U are not localizable'; in another manner the conclusion follows that 'P and U are localizable' "; and that "The experiment brings to clear light the question of the existence and nature of the traditional affective processes, and a serious difficulty with the introspective technique." [155] As to his earlier conclusion, that of 1918, Young felt that it presupposed "a certain systematic position regarding the nature of the affective processes—the position which was in the air at Cornell University in 1917-18. Starting from the view that there exist non-clear, non-sensory affective processes, which vary in quality (P and U), in intensity, and in temporal course, the papers I wrote have a certain validity. The validity is relative to the postulates which underlie these studies. Given another set of postulates, the results might be reversed. The answer to the question of localization may be 'yes' or 'no' according to what one understands by 'feeling' and 'localization.' " [156]

The language in which Young couches his conclusion of

1927 suggests that he does not consider it to be a satisfactory solution of the problem.[157] I believe, on the contrary, that it is a very satisfactory solution. In the first place, it is perfectly definite: pleasant and unpleasant objects of experience can be localized; pleasant and unpleasant "sensory processes" can also be localized; pleasant and unpleasant special affective elements cannot be localized. In the second place, it offers an excellent explanation of the divergent conclusions reached by other investigators. Orth and Alechsieff, for instance, were dealing critically with affections as special elements different from sensations. It is natural, therefore, that they should have concluded against localization. In the preceding section we saw reason to believe that Nakashima, Koch, Kellogg and Wohlgemuth uncritically interpreted reports concerning objects of experience to be reports concerning affections. As for Nafe, the conclusions of his experiment make it obvious that he was dealing with affections in the sense of patterns of sensations. It is natural, therefore, that these latter men should all have concluded that affections are localizable. We may conclude, therefore, reformulating slightly the conclusion of Young, that—besides the occurrence of localization in the case of pleasant and unpleasant objects—affections in the sense of sensory elements or groups of elements having hedonic tone for an attribute are subject to localization, but that affection in the sense of special affective elements are not subject to localization.

Extension as a Characteristic of Affections.—The question whether or not affections are extended is one which has been taken up but recently by experimentalists. In his research published in 1924, J. P. Nafe found that "P and U are both extended, voluminous; and all Os describe P as larger, more extended, more voluminous than U. One affection may be larger or smaller than another, and may itself expand or contract." [158]

In an experiment published in 1927, P. T. Young likewise found that some of his observers ascribed extensity to affections. One, for instance, reported: "The U seems to begin in the mouth and to spread out around. It spreads out in rays. It goes out in one plane. It is a flat thing. Some of it goes outside me and some of it is in me. These rays seem bits of more intense U." And another observer said: "There was a momentary U, diffuse and not localized anywhere; a general feeling of U." [159] This was true, however, of only four out of five observers. The fifth never could observe extension or voluminousness of affections. Examinations of the reports led Young to the conclusion that when volume and extension are reported, they are sensory in nature.[160]

These data are obviously insufficient to warrant any but a very tentative conclusion. They indicate, however, that volume and extension, like localization, are attributes of affections in the sense of sensory elements, or groups of elements, but not of affections in the sense of special affective elements.

GENERAL CONCLUSION

Let us for a moment review the data presented above on the relation of hedonic tone to mental elements. In the first place, we dealt with the work upon the tridimensional theory proposed by Wundt. There we found that in spite of numerous experiments by Wundtians and Titchenerians stretching over a period of nearly twenty years Wundt remained unshaken in his convictions that special affective elements were qualitatively three-dimensional, while Titchener remained equally convinced that they were qualitatively uni-dimensional. In view of the fact that there were experimental data supporting both of these views, it seemed as though the problem of the qualitative dimensions of the affective element were experimentally equivocal—as though special affective elements could be tridimensional in Leipzig and uni-dimensional at Cornell.

We then turned to the general experiments upon the existence of special affective elements. There we found four experimenters reaching four different conclusions. Alechsieff believed his data showed the existence of special affective elements; Koch concluded that affections were sensory in nature; Yokoyama concluded that at least in the case of judgments by paired comparison affections were meanings, i. e., special patterns of sensations, and Nafe maintained that in his experiment affections turned out to be patterns of bright and dull pressure. Nafe's establishment of a relationship between hedonic tone and bright and dull pressure received confirmation by Hunt, but not his conclusion as to the nature of affection. There were, indeed, two experimenters whose results led to the same conclusion, namely Nakashima and Young. This conclusion, however, was that introspective reports upon the nature of affections vary from one observer to another in accordance with previous psychological training. It seemed obvious here again that we were faced with a problem which was experimentally equivocal.

Finally we took up the work which had been done upon four characteristics of experience in an attempt to learn whether or not they were attributes of affections. In the case of the first of these characteristics, coexistence of opposed affections, we found the evidence to agree that it was not a characteristic of affection in the technical sense of the word, namely in the sense of elements or groups of elements with hedonic tone as an attribute. We did find evidence, however, that pleasant and unpleasant objects of experience may occasionally coexist. In the case of the second proposed characteristic of affections, clearness, we found reason to consider the problem as unsolved. As to the last two characteristics dealt with, namely localization and extension, we found evidence that they were indeed characteristics of affections in the sense of sensations or combinations of sensations, but not of affections in the sense of special affective elements. It was also incidentally shown that pleasant and unpleasant objects could be localized.

P. T. Young has summarized this equivocal situation remarkably well, and drawn from it a very definite conclusion. In an article published in 1927, after giving data of his own upon a number of the individual issues, he wrote:

"Some of the conditions which determine the report in affective psychology are (a) the O's education in psychology which includes the kind and amount of his information, (b) the O's bias determined in part by his theoretical reflections, (c) the O's understanding of words and his habits of speech, and (d) the suggestions which happen to reach him from various sources.

"These factors, except possibly suggestion, may be grouped together under the term 'training.' Introspective investigators of feeling usually recognize the importance of training. . . . But perhaps it is too important. . . . It is so important that through training one can apparently demonstrate in affective psychology almost anything one likes. I will guarantee to train a group of unsophisticated Os to report uniformly that P and U are non-sensory affective processes, or meanings, or pressures, or bodily reactions, or something else. I will guarantee to train a group of naïve Os to localize P and U or to declare that these processes are non-localizable, to report mixed feelings, or to declare that mixed feelings do not exist, to describe qualitative diversity within the qualities of P and U or to report lack of qualitative diversity within the qualities of P. and U. The only requirement I make is that my Os be young and plastic. . . .

"The present situation can be cleared up only by the frank recognition of the complete relativity of so-called fact to the logical system which is the product of training. It is important to find common ground which is independent of training. In the search for data which are independent of training I see hope; not in further training of trick Os." [161]

Everything that we have found in studying the relation of hedonic tone to mental elements—what is generally called the "nature of the affective processes"—favors our acceptance of Young's conclusion. The conclusion is not, however, a solution. Such acceptance raises a further issue: Is the dependence of available data upon training due to the nature of the problem, or is it due to faulty technique? Should we entirely give up attempts to establish the relation of hedonic tone to mental elements, or should we merely give up attempts to do so by means of current methods? It seems to me that this question can be answered by examining the history of a similar problem in a more thoroughly developed field, namely the history of the nature of sensation. Until 1910, the prevailing opinion among psychologists was that sensations were *actual* elements of experience *constituted* of certain attributes. Külpe in his "Grundriss" wrote: "The sensations are those simple conscious processes which stand in relation of dependence to specific nervous organs, both peripheral and central. Despite the qualitative simplicity of a sensation one can discover in it various attributes as a result of comparison with other sensations." [162]   And Titchener in his "Textbook" expressed the same view: "Sensations are, of course, the characteristic elements of perception, of the sights and sounds and similar experiences due to our present surroundings. . . (The mental elements) are simple, it is true, in the sense that they are mental experience reduced to its lowest terms; but they are still real processes, still actual items of mental experience. Hence, like the chemical elements, they show various aspects or attributes—present different sides, so to speak—each of which may be examined separately by the psychologist. It is by reference to these attributes that introspection is able to classify them under different headings." [163]

In spite of this agreement concerning the general nature of these actual elements of consciousness, psychologists, peculiarly enough, could not agree at all concerning the attributes of sensations. Titchener in his "Textbook" wrote: "A sensation, as the term is used in this book, may be defined as an elementary process which is constituted of at least four attributes—*quality, intensity, clearness* and *duration.*" [164]   Külpe, on the other hand, maintained that only *two* attributes belonged to all sensations, namely *quality* and *duration.* Two further attributes, *intensity* and *extensity,* belonged according to him to certain sensations, but not to others. As for Wundt, the teacher of both Titchener and Külpe, he considered sensations to have only two attributes, namely *quality* and *intensity.* Extensity and duration were for him attributes of *ideas.* Thus a spatial idea was a "three dimensional compound whose parts are fixed in their location with reference to one another, but capable of indefinite variation in their location with reference to the ideating subject." [165]

Why so striking a disagreement concerning the attributes of sensation? The answer was provided by Rahn in 1913. In a monograph published in that year, Rahn attacked Titchener's conception of sensation on experimental grounds.[166] Külpe, in his now famous abstraction experiments, had shown that an observer has much difficulty in reporting upon any attribute other than that for which he has been instructed.[167] Rahn pointed out that this was fatal to the notion of sensation as a datum.

The evidence from Külpe, together with certain other points raised by Rahn, was so compelling that Titchener, in replying to Rahn, conceded that for psychology sensations were not *data,* but logical constructions. He wrote: "It would be a great simplification of psychology if a sensation, *tota, teres, atque rotunda,* would stand before us under a single comprehensive determination and allow us adequately to observe it as a whole. But that, if it ever happens, happens only after we have made many separate observations of its distinguishable aspects. The sensation of classification is the *logical resultant* of many observations. . . . We group certain attributes together in our classification because, having observed one attribute under a certain determination, we thereafter invariably light upon certain other attributes when, with a shift of determination, but with excitation unchanged, we undertake to observe them." [168]

Titchener's change of view with respect to the nature of sensation was the forerunner of a widespread change of view among psychologists. Not only were Rahn's arguments telling, but the notion of an "actual" sensation was subjected to a withering fire of criticism by the Gestalt school. To-day, it is generally accepted that the term sensation refers not to a constituent of experience, to a datum, but to a conceptual entity constructed from experience. If this be so, it is clear that the equivocality of experiments upon the relation of hedonic tone to mental elements is due not merely to faulty technique, but to the very nature of the problem. The conceptual entities constructed by psychologists depend upon general systematic backgrounds. As this background varies from one psychologist to another, the conceptual entities will vary likewise. The conceptual entities being different, the relation of hedonic tone to these conceptual entities will likewise be different. Thus observers with different backgrounds must, by the very nature of the problem, give reports which are to some extent conflicting. Likewise, experimenters with different backgrounds must interpret their data in ways which yield conflicting conclusions. The views that hedonic tone is an attribute of sensations, of complexes of sensations, of qualitatively unidimensional affective elements, of qualitatively pluridimensional affective elements, are not inconsistent descriptions of experience, but alternative hypotheses constructed from experience. Again the views that affections may and may not give rise to mixed feelings, are and are not clear, localized, or extended, do not constitute pairs of contradictory characterization of a single entity, but independent characterizations of different entities. The problem of the relation of hedonic tone to mental elements does not involve merely the data secured upon it, but the general theory of psychology.[169]

This fact naturally does not imply the final insolubility of the problem. It does, however, make the validity of any solution contingent on the validity of the underlying doctrine concerning psychological elements. This necessary basis would seem for the present to be a quicksand. Complete lack of agreement concerning the question of psychological elements is amply demonstrated by the variety of existing views upon the relation of hedonic tone to mental elements. It is even more obvious, because explicit, in the controversies between Neo-Titchenerians and Gestalt psychologists. Rather than embark in haste upon the construction of elements whose adequacy must long remain problematical, it would seem wiser to refrain—at least for a time—from constructing any elements whatever. It would therefore seem best to close our discussion of the relation of hedonic tone to mental elements by concluding that the problem does not at present exist.

This conclusion, however, requires a postscript. The experiments which we have considered in the present chapter brought to light certain incidental data—data not bearing upon the main problem at issue—whose interpretation is not at all dependent upon controversial systematic issues. In denying the existence of the general problem, we must not overlook the conclusions indicated by these incidental data. These conclusions, the first of which has considerable systematic significance, are as follows:

1. There is a high correlation between the hedonic tone of an object and the brightness-dullness of the pressure experiences which may accompany it. (Nafe and Hunt.)

2. The coexistence in experience of two objects, the one pleasant, the other unpleasant, is rare, but does occasionally occur. (Young.)

3. Objects characterized by hedonic tone may be localized. (Young.)

FOOTNOTES AND REFERENCES

[1] W. Wundt. Beiträge zur Theorie der Sinneswahrnehmung, Leipzig, 1862, XIV.

[2] W. Wundt. Grundriss der Psychologie, 14th edit., Stuttgart, 1920, 31.

[3] E. B. Titchener. A Textbook of Psychology, New York, 1919, (1909), 255-6.

[4] W. Wundt. Grundriss der Psychologie, 14th edit., 1920, 99.

[5] Th. Ziehen. Introduction to Physiological Psychology, London, 1895, 134-135.

[6] C. Stumpf. Ueber Gefühlsempfindungen, Z. f. Psychol., 44, 1907, 1-49.

[7] Th. Lipps. Leitfaden der Psychologie, Leipzig, 1903, 268 ff.

108 RELATION TO MENTAL ELEMENTS

[8] J. Royce. Outlines of Psychology, New York, 1903, 177.

[9] W. Wundt. Grundriss der Psychologie, Stuttgart, 1896.

[10] For the historical development of Wundt's view cf. E. B. Titchener, Lectures on the Elementary Psychology of Feeling and Attention, New York, 1908, 125 seq.

[11] O. Vogt. Zur Kenntnis des Wesens und der psychologischen Bedeutung des Hypotismus, 2nd continuation, *Z. f. Hypnotismus,* 4, 1896, 123

[12] *Ibid.,* 128.

[13] *Ibid.,* 128.

[14] E. B. Titchener. Zur Kritik der Wundt'schen Gefühlslehre, *Z. f. Psychol. und Physiol. d. Sinnesorgane,* XIX, 1899, 321.

[15] *Ibid.,* 326.

[16] W. Wundt. Bemerkungen zur Theorie der Gefühle, *Philos. Stud.* 15, 1899, 149.

[17] P. Mentz. Die Wirkung akustischer Sinnesreize auf Puls und Atmung, *Philos. Stud.,* 11, 1895, 61.

[18] A Lehmann. Die körperlichen Auesserungen psychischer Zustände I, Plethysmographische Untersuchungen, Leipzig, 1919; II, Atlas, Kopenhagen, 1898.

[19] W. Wundt. *Op. cit.,* 163.

[20] W. Wundt. Physiologische Psychologie, 5th edit., II, Leipzig, 1902 272.

[21] E. B. Titchener. Ein Versuch die Methode der paarweisen Vergleichung auf die verschiedene Gefühlsrichtungen anzuwenden, *Philos Stud.,* 20, 1902, 382.

[22] *Ibid.,* 405.

[23] J Orth. Gcfühl und Bewusstseinslage, Berlin, 1903.

[24] *Ibid.,* 78.

[25] S. P. Hayes. A Study of the Affective Qualities, *Am. J. Psychol.* 17, 1906, 358.

[26] *Ibid.,* 389.

[27] N. Alechsieff. Die Grundformen der Gefühle, *Psychol. Stud.,* 3 1907, 156.

[28] *Ibid.,* 264.

[29] *Ibid.,* 270.

[30] W. S. Foster and K. Roese. The Tridimensional Theory of Feeling from the Standpoint of Typical Experience, *Am. J. Psychol.,* 27, 1916, 157

[31] Wundt died in August, 1920.

[32] Titchener died in 1927. I omit posthumous editions.

[33] N. Alechsieff. Die Grundformen der Gefühle, *Psychol. Stud.,* 3 1907, 156.

[34] T. Nakashima. Contributions to the Study of the Affective Processes, *Am. J. Psychol.,* 20, 1909, 157.

[35] *Ibid.,* 161.

[36] *Ibid.,* 166.

[37] *Ibid.,* 179.

[38] *Ibid.,* 180.

[39] B. Koch. Experimentelle Untersuchungen über die elementare Gefühlsqualitäten, Leipzig, 1913.

[40] M. YOKOYAMA. The Nature of the Affective Judgment in the Method of Paired Comparison, *Am. J. Psychol.*, 32, 1921, 357-370.

[41] B, D, F and P are the initials of the observers.

[42] *Ibid.*, 369.

[43] *Ibid.*, 369.

[44] J. P. NAFE. An Experimental Study of the Affective Qualities, *Am. J. Psychol.*, 35, 1924, 507.

[45] *Ibid.*, 510.

[46] *Ibid.*, 517.

[47] *Ibid.*, 543-544.

[48] *Ibid.*, 542.

[49] J. P. NAFE. The Psychology of Felt Experience, *Am. J. Psychol.*, 39, 1927, 387.

[50] J. P. NAFE. The Sense of Feeling, in The Foundations of Experimental Psychology, Worcester, 1929, 411.

[51] P. T. YOUNG. Studies in Affective Psychology, III, The "Trained" Observer in Affective Psychology, *Am. J. Psychol.*, 38, 1927, 175.

[52] *Ibid.*, 185.

[53] J. P. NAFE. *Am. J. Psychol.*, 35, 1924, 544.

[54] P. T. YOUNG. Studies in Affective Psychology, IV, The Logic of Affective Psychology, *Am. J. Psychol.*, 38, 1927, 176.

[55] *Ibid.*

[56] W. A. HUNT. The Relation of Bright and Dull Pressure to Affectivity, *Am. J. Psychol.*, 43, 1931, 87-92.

[57] *Ibid.*, 90.

[58] *Ibid.*, 92.

[59] *Ibid.*, 92.

[60] *Ibid.*, 92.

[61] Hunt's experiment confirms Nafe's results insofar as these are interpreted as indicating a connection between hedonic tone and brightness of pressure. It does not, however, confirm Nafe's conclusion that hedonic tone is an attribute of patterns or pressures.

[62] E. B. TITCHENER. A Textbook of Psychology, New York, 1919, 235-236.

[63] A. BAIN. Emotions and the Will, 3rd Edit., 1876, 12-13.

[64] O. KÜLPE. Outlines of Psychology, transl. by E. B. Titchener, New York, 1895, 264-265.

[65] W. McDOUGALL. Outline of Psychology, New York, 1923, 349.

[66] J. ORTH. Gefühl und Bewusstseinslage, Berlin, 1903.

[67] *Ibid.*, 118.

[68] *Ibid.*, 127.

[69] P. T. YOUNG. An Experimental Study of Mixed Feelings, *Am. J. Psychol.*, 29, 1918, 239.

[70] C. H. JOHNSTONE. The Combination of Feelings, *Harvard Psychol. Studies*, II, 1906, 159.

[71] *Ibid.*, 177.

[72] *Ibid.*, 178.

[73] N. ALECHSIEFF. Die Grundformen der Gefühle, *Psychol. Stud.*, 3, 1907, 259 seq.

[74] T. NAKASHIMA. Time Relations of the Affective Processes, *Psychol. Rev.*, 16, 1909, 303.

110   RELATION TO MENTAL ELEMENTS

[75] *Ibid.*, 319.
[76] T. NAKASHIMA. Contributions to the Study of the Affective Processes, *Am. J. Psychol.*, 20, 1909, 184.
[77] *Ibid.*, 179.
[78] *Ibid.*, 184.
[79] B. KOCH. Experimentelle Untersuchung über die Elementaren Gefühlsqualitäten, Halle, 1913, 89.
[80] C. E. KELLOGG. Alternation and Interference of Feelings, *Psychol. Monog.*, XVIII, 1915, 1-94.
[81] *Ibid.*, 21.
[82] *Ibid.*, 21.
[83] *Ibid.*, 32-33.
[84] *Ibid.*, 89.
[85] H. HENNING. Der Geruch, II, *Z. f. Psychol.*, 74, 1916, 379; also Der Geruch, Leipzig, 1916.
[86] H. HENNING. Der Geruch, 172.
[87] P. T. YOUNG. An Experimental Study of Mixed Feelings, *Am. J. Psychol.*, 29, 1918, 237-271.
[88] *Ibid.*, 241.
[89] *Ibid.*, 242.
[90] *Ibid.*, 242.
[91] *Ibid.*, 241.
[92] *Ibid.*, 244.
[93] *Ibid.*, 248.
[94] *Ibid.*, 252.
[95] *Ibid.*, 252.
[96] *Ibid.*, 253.
[07] *Ibid.*, 253.
[98] *Ibid.*, 250-251.
[99] *Ibid.*, 258.
[100] *Ibid.*, 261.
[101] *Ibid.*, 271. Young's distinction between "meaning affection" and "process affection" is very similar—as has been pointed out by Young himself—to a distinction between two types of affections drawn as far back as 1905 by G. Störring. In that year, Störring reported an experiment in which he sought to determine the characteristics of two different types of pleasure which he called "Empfindungslust" and "Stimmungslust." (G. STÖRRING. Experimentelle Beiträge zur Lehre vom Gefühl, *Arch. f. ges. Psychol.*, VI, 1905, 316-356.) His method of arousing "Empfindungslust" was to give the observer a taste solution and have him keep it in his mouth while describing the experience. To arouse "Stimmungslust" on the other hand, he instructed the observer to "swallow the solution and then to disregard the sensation, to consider the taste stimulus as brought to an end by the swallowing." (*Ibid.*, 317.)
[102] A. WOHLGEMUTH. Pleasure-Unpleasure, an Experimental Investigation of the Feeling Elements, *Brit. J. Psychol., Monogr., Suppl.*, VI, 1919, 1-252.
[103] *Ibid.*, 13.
[104] *Ibid.*, 15.
[105] *Ibid.*, 190.

[106] J. P. NAFE. *Am. J. Psychol.*, 35, 1924, 252.

[107] P. T. YOUNG. The Coexistence and Localization of Feeling, *Brit. J. Psychol.*, XV, 1925, 356.

[108] *Ibid.*, 356-357.

[109] A. WOHLGEMUTH. The Coexistence and Localization of Feeling, *Brit. J. Psychol.*, 16, 1925, 116.

[110] *Ibid.*, 117.

[111] P. T. YOUNG. *Am. J. Psychol.*, 38, 1927, 186.

[112] *Cf* J. ORTH. Gefühl und Bewusstseinslage, 33-34 and N. ALECHSIEFF, *Psychol. Stud.*, 3, 1907, 158-161.

[113] *Cf.* E. B. TITCHENER. Description vs. Statement of Meaning, *Am. J. Psychol.*, 23, 1912, 165.

[114] E. B. TITCHENER. Lectures on the Elementary Psychology of Feeling and Attention, New York, 1908, 55.

[115] T. NAKASHIMA. *Am. J. Psychol.*, 20, 1909, 184.

[116] C. E. KELLOGG. *Psychol. Monogr.*, 18, 1915, 43-55.

[117] B. KOCH. Experimentelle Untersuchungen ueber die Elementaren Gefühlsqualitäten, 20, 35-38, 51, 55.

[118] P. T. YOUNG. *Brit. J. Psychol.*, 15, 1925, 356.

[119] O. KÜLPE. Grundriss der Psychologie, Leipzig, 1893, 267.

[120] O. KÜLPE. Outlines of Psychology, trans. by E. B. Titchener, New York, 1895, 260.

[121] E. B. TITCHENER. Affective Attention, *Philos. Rev.*, 3, 1894, 429.

[122] E. B. TITCHENER. Lectures on the Elementary Psychology of Feeling and Attention, New York, 1908, 71.

[123] E. B. TITCHENER. *Philos. Rev.*, 3, 1894, 433.

[124] P. ZONEFF and E. MEUMANN. Ueber Begleiterscheinungen Psychischer Vorgänge in Athem und Puls, *Philos. Stud.*, 18, 1901, 1.

[125] *Ibid.*, 173.

[126] E. B. TITCHENER. Lectures on the Elementary Psychology of Feeling and Attention, New York, 1908, 69-77.

[127] *Ibid.*, 69.

[128] A. WOHLGEMUTH. *Brit. J. Psychol., Monogr. Suppl.*, VI, 1919, 17-18 and 222-225.

[129] *Ibid.*, 18. The excerpts are from the following authors: 1, TITCHENER. Lectures on the Elementary Psychology of Feeling and Attention, 1908, 69. 2, KÜLPE. Outlines of Psychology, 1895, 258. 3, ZONEFF and MEUMANN. Uber Begleiterscheinungen Psychischer Vorgänge in Athem und Puls, *Philos. Stud.*, 18, 1903, 73. 4, J. SULLY. *Human Mind*, 1892, I, 77.

[130] *Ibid.*, 224.

[131] *Ibid.*, 224.

[132] J. P. NAFE. *Am. J. Psychol.*, 35, 1924, 533.

[133] *Ibid.*, 533-535.

[134] J. ORTH. Gefühl und Bewusstseinslage, Berlin, 1903, 75-127.

[135] N. ALECHSIEFF. *Psychol. Stud.*, 3, 1907, 264.

[136] J. P. NAFE. *Am. J. Psychol.*, 35, 1924, 544. Nafe's Os failed to localize affections definitely, but did occasionally localize them within the body, or as projected from the body, or as referred to some more or less well-defined part of the body.

[137] T. NAKASHIMA. *Am. J. Psychol.*, 20, 1909, 264.

112 RELATION TO MENTAL ELEMENTS

138 B. Koch. Experimentelle Untersuchung über die Elementaren Gefühlsqualitäten, 90.

139 C. E. Kellogg. *Psychol. Monogr.*, XVIII, 1915, 77.

140 A. Wohlgemuth. *Brit. J. Psychol., Monogr, Suppl.*, VI, 1919, 207.

141 J. P. Nafe. The Psychology of Felt Experience, *Am. J. Psychol.*, 39, 1927, 371.

142 E. B. Titchener. Lectures on the Elementary Psychology of Feeling and Attention, New York, 1908, 45.

143 P. T. Young. The Localization of Feeling, *Am. J. Psychol.*, 29, 1918, 420-430.

144 *Ibid.*, 422.

145 *Ibid.*, 426.

146 *Ibid.*, 426.

147 *Ibid.*, 427.

148 *Ibid.*, 427.

149 *Ibid.*, 429.

150 *Ibid.*, 430.

151 P. T. Young. Studies in Affective Psychology, I. The Localization and Spatial Character of Pleasantness and Unpleasantness, *Am. J. Psychol.*, 38, 1927, 157-167.

152 *Ibid.*, 158.

153 *Ibid.*, 158.

154 *Ibid.*, 164.

155 *Ibid.*, 165.

156 *Ibid.*, 166.

157 That this is indeed so is proved by another paper by Young, published in the same journal. Young there asserts that certain data concerning hedonic tone are so ambiguous as to be valueless, and includes among these data those on localization of affections (Cf. P. T. Young, *Am. J. Psychol.*, 38, 1927, 188).

158 J. P. Nafe. *Am. J. Psychol.*, 35, 1924, 523.

159 P. T. Young. *Am J. Psychol.*, 38, 1927, 159-161.

160 *Ibid.*, 165.

161 P. T. Young. *Am. J. Psychol.*, 38, 1927, 187-189.

162 O. Külpe. Grundriss der Psychologie, Leipzig, 1893, 30.

163 E. B. Titchener. A Textbook of Psychology, New York, 1928 (1909), 48-50.

164 *Ibid.*, 52.

165 W. Wundt. Outlines of Psychology, transl. by C. H. Judd, Leipzig, 1902, 114.

166 C. Rahn. The Relation of Sensation to Other Categories in Contemporary Psychology, *Psychol. Monogr.*, 16 (No. 67), 1913.

167 O. Külpe. Versuche ueber Abstraktion, *Ber. ü. d. I. Kongr. f. exper. Psychol.*, Leipzig, 1904, 56-68.

168 E. B. Titchener. *Am. J. Psychol.*, 26, 1915, 262.

169 Since writing this chapter I have read E. G. Boring's remarkable article on "The Psychologist's Circle" (*Psychol. Rev.*, 38, 1931, 177-182). This article states in a fully generalized form the point that I here try to make with reference to sensation and affection alone. It also states the point in its full historical setting.

Chapter IV

Hedonic Tone in Relation to Primary External Stimuli

INTRODUCTION

Long before experimental psychologists became interested in the relation of hedonic tone to mental elements—an unfortunate occurrence, as we have seen—experimental aestheticians were dealing extensively with another relation of hedonic tone, namely with its relation to stimuli external to the organism—to physical objects. Work in this field started with Fechner—it was he who first supplied the necessary methods. The initial experiments certainly antedate 1871, for it was in that year that Fechner published his first results.

As is true of all investigations of the relation between phenomena and stimuli, these experiments involve three fundamental variables or groups of variables. One variable, obviously, is hedonic tone. Another, obviously again, is some characteristic of stimuli. In addition—and this is not so obvious—these experiments involve all other variables related in any way to hedonic tone, for unless all such variables be kept constant the observed co-variation of hedonic tone and of a characteristic of stimuli may be no index at all of their co-relation.

In the early days of hedonic psychophysics, the variables of this third group were practically unknown. Clearly the only way to make sure that results would be significant was to attempt to hold these variables constant by holding the general condition of the experiment absolutely constant. Today, many of the variables of the third group are known, but this knowledge does not dispense the experimenter from holding general experimental conditions constant. Indeed, so marked has turned out to be the dependence of hedonic tone upon characteristics such as direction of attention and needs that constancy of general conditions seems today to be more necessary than ever before.

With respect to the second variable mentioned above, the stimulus-variable, it is desirable to distinguish between primary and secondary stimuli. The work of the Gestalt school during the past fifteen years has shown beyond a doubt that any part of experience, any phenomenon, is usually dependent not merely upon the the particular stimulus corresponding to it—the primary stimulus—but also upon secondary stimuli, upon the rest of the present stimulus-field and past stimuli. Thus Wertheimer found that the introspective position of a line in space was dependent not only upon the position of the corresponding physical line, but upon other present and past stimuli corresponding to introspective "anchorage points." [1] If the observer's entire visual field were objectively slanted by means of a mirror, a similarly slanted objective line tended to appear vertical. Even after this objectively slanted field had been replaced by a homogeneous surface, a line slanted as before still tended to be seen as vertical. We shall deal with the relations of hedonic tone to these two classes of stimuli successively, beginning with the relations to primary stimuli.

Before turning to the actual experiments, however, I should like to say a word concerning terminology. Most of the work on the relation of hedonic tone to stimuli has been done without proper definition of the stimuli involved—without describing them in terms of their physical variables. Experimenters have as a rule thought it enough to define stimuli in terms of corresponding phenomena. This practice has led to the use of terms such as "red," "salt," etc., to denote not only characteristics of phenomena, but correlated characterisitcs of stimuli. Thus one reads of red stimuli, salt stimuli, etc. Definition of a stimulus in terms of corresponding phenomena is bound to be inaccurate. If, however, one is obliged to resort to such definitions, simplicity and clarity of exposition require that one adopt likewise the terminology mentioned above. Structure of sentences is obviously much simplified if the expression "stimulus corresponding to red phenomena" is replaced by "red stimulus."

As the present chapter deals very largely with stimuli defined only in terms of corresponding phenomena, I propose to use such terms as red, green, etc., in two senses: First, in their strict sense, as denoting psychological characteristics of phenomena; secondly, in an elliptical sense, as denoting the characteristics of stimuli which correlate with these psychological characteristics. Which of these senses is involved in any particular case should be perfectly clear from the context.

Hedonic Summation

Before we inquire into the relations of hedonic tone to the various characteristics of primary stimuli, it is necessary that we ascertain whether there is *hedonic summation,* i. e., whether given two stimuli α and β corresponding singly to phenomena whose hedonic tone is a and b, the hedonic tone of the phenomenon corresponding to the combination of the two stimuli is equal to a + b. The reason why we need to investigate this problem at the very outset is that if such summation should hold, we should be justified in confining our attention to the relation of hedonic tone to the characteristics of simple stimuli, confident that the resulting data, together with the principle of additiveness, would enable us always to infer the hedonic tone correlated with the characteristics of complex stimuli.

This problem, like so many others, is one which arose out of the doctrine of mental elements. "Wundt, in his analysis of affective fusion, declares that the characteristic of feeling lies in the fact that all feelings present in consciousness at a given moment tend to fuse into a unitary manifold, a 'Totalgefühl' which, nevertheless, is not a mere sum of its components, but has a unique property of its own. Külpe, McDougall and Titchener, on the other hand, hold

that the affection of any given moment is the algebraical
sum of the affections attaching to all the various sensory
processes that constitute the mind at that moment." [2]
The early experimental literature upon this problem is
very meagre.[3] The first experimental investigation dealing
directly with the issue is that of L. R. Geissler in 1917.[4]
The subject-matter of Geissler's inquiry was the relation
between the hedonic tone of color combinations and the
hedonic tone of the same colors experienced singly. Using
7 Milton-Bradley pigment colors, he first had 122 observers
rank them hedonically by the method of paired comparisons, and then had the same observers rank all pairs of
these colors (i. e., $\dfrac{7 \times 6}{2} = 21$ pairs) by the same method.
To avoid time errors, the order of the two parts of the experiment was reversed in the case of 32 observers, i. e., they
judged the single colors last. The two sets of data were
then compared in the following fashion:
In the case of the single colors, the frequencies of preference for the various colors was first computed for each
observer. In the case of one observer, for instance, one
might find for colors a, b, c, d, e, f, g, the frequencies 6, 5
4, 3, 2, 1, 0; in the case of another, however, two or more
colors might have the same number of frequencies: 5, 5
4, 4, 2, 1, 0. Frequencies 5 and 6 were then arbitrarily taken
to represent "most pleasant," frequencies 2, 3 and 4 "medium pleasant," and frequencies 0 and 1 "least pleasant.'
(Cf. schema below.)

TABLE XII

Frequencies	Colors for Observer			Ratings
	A	B	etc.	
6	a	a,b		Most pleasant
5	b			
4	c	c		Medium pleasant
3	d	e		
2	e	d		
1	f			Least pleasant
0	g	g,f		

Thus each color was classed in the case of each observer in one of three classes—most pleasant, medium pleasant, or least pleasant.[5] The problem at issue was then restated in the following terms: "What degree of pleasantness will result for color-pairs if they are composed of (a) two most pleasant colors, (b) a most and a medium pleasant color, (c) two medium pleasant colors, (d) a most and a least pleasant color, (e) a medium and a least pleasant color, and (f) two least pleasant colors?" The de-

TABLE XIII

(*From Geissler*)

Class	Frequencies of Pref. of colors entering into combinations	Average of Frequencies of Pref. of combination	Average of Frequencies of Pref. of combinations for entire class
Most + Most	6 + 5 5 + 5	15.1 ± 3.7 14.7 ± 3.3	14.9
Most + Med.	6 + 4 6 + 3 5 + 4 6 + 2 5 + 3 5 + 2	14.1 ± 3.5 13.4 ± 3.2 12.8 ± 3.4 12.1 ± 3.5 11.9 ± 3.5 10.5 ± 3.7	11.1
Med. + Med.	4 + 4 4 + 3 4 + 2 3 + 3 3 + 2 2 + 2	11.4 ± 3.4 11.2 ± 3.7 10.8 ± 3.9 10.6 ± 3.5 8.8 ± 3.9 7.8 ± 3.9	10.2
Most + Least	6 + 1 6 + 0 5 + 1 5 + 0	11.5 ± 4.1 10.9 ± 2.6 9.3 ± 3.7 8.7 ± 3.8	9.7
Med. + Least	4 + 1 4 + 0 3 + 1 3 + 0 2 + 1 2 + 0	8.7 ± 3.6 8.2 ± 3.5 7.2 ± 3.1 7.7 ± 3.2 7.2 ± 3.4 6.6 ± 3.6	7.6
Least + Least	1 + 1 1 + 0	6.4 ± 3.5 6.1 ± 3.5	6.2

grée of pleasantness of each of these 6 classes of color-pairs was then determined by averaging for each the frequency of preference of all the color-pairs falling into this class. The results are shown in the table on the preceding page, which partially reproduces a table given by Geissler. Geissler believes that these results "force upon us the general conclusion that the pleasantness of the color-pairs increases directly with the pleasantness of the colors taken individually.[6]

Geissler consequently formulates the following law with respect to the hedonic tone of color-pairs: "The greater the pleasantness of the individual constituents, the greater will be the pleasantness of the combination." [7]

In 1921, Washburn, Haight and Regensburg published a quasi-repetition of Geissler's experiment in which, however, the method of single stimuli (scale of 1-7) was used instead of the method of paired comparison, and in which furthermore instead of using only 7 single colors differing only in hue, there were used 64 colors differing in hue, saturation, and brilliance.[8] Each of two experimenters used 32 ot these colors singly and 16 combinations of them. The relation between the pleasantness of the colors and that of the combination was established as follows: "The total affective value of every color, when shown alone, was determined by adding the numbers by which the observers expressed their judgments of its pleasantness; . . . then the sums thus obtained for each of two colors that were shown in combination were added. . . . This being done for each of the pairs of colors, it was possible to arrange them in an order representing their pleasantness as determined solely by their appearance singly. Then the numbers which represented the affective judgments of the observers on the combinations as such were added, and the combinations arranged in the order of the size of these sums. Evidently the rank difference correlation between these two arrays will give the degree of relationship between the pleasantness of a color combination and the individual pleasantness of its component colors." [9]

The correlation in question was found to be plus .747 ± .0119. The authors conclude that "It is clear that to a very considerable extent the pleasantness of a color combination depends upon the pleasantness of the individual colors." [10] The authors do not feel, however, that this indicates simple summation of affections. Were the latter true, a combination of two pleasant colors would be more pleasant than either judged singly; and a combination of two unpleasant colors should be more unpleasant than either judged singly. In their experiment, however, out of 861 cases where component colors, when judged singly, were both found agreeable, there were 263 cases, i. e., 30.5%, where the combination was found positively disagreeable. Likewise, out of 465 cases where the component colors, judged singly, were both judged disagreeable, there were 72 cases, i. e., 15.4%, in which the combinations were judged agreeable. The authors conclude that besides summation, some other factor is operative, which they suggest may be particularly prominent when attention is directed to total effect rather than to the separate colors in a combination.

In the same year, M. Yokoyama published a research in which he studied the "simultaneous effect of two aspects of a simple sensory material in conditioning affective tendency, and the nature of the affective resultant." [12] His stimuli were 49 colored forms representing combinations of each of 7 colors with each of 7 forms. In a first part of the experiment the stimuli were arranged into seven series in each of which form was constant but color varied. The relative hedonic tones corresponding to the members of each of these series were determined for 5 observers by the method of paired comparison with instructions to attend to the colors alone. In a second part of the experiment, the stimuli were arranged in seven series in each of which color was constant but form varied, and the relative hedonic tones corresponding to the members of each of these series were determined for the same five observers by the method of paired comparison with instructions to attend to the

form alone. In a third part of the experiment, the relative hedonic tones corresponding to all 49 stimuli were
determined by the method of paired comparison for the
same 5 observers with instructions to attend to the "color-
forms."

A comparison of the hedonic rank orders of the 7 colors in the case of each of the 7 forms, as determined in
part one with instructions to attend solely to color and as
determined in part three with instructions to attend to
"color-forms" showed a striking agreement. Likewise, high
agreement was found between the rank orders of the 7
forms in the case of each of the 7 colors, as determined in
part two with instructions to attend solely to form, and as
determined in part three with instructions to attend to
"color-form." These facts according to Yokoyama indicate "that both color and form were effective in conditioning the pleasantness of a colored form when the attention
was directed by instruction upon both the color and the
form aspects, and that color and form operate simultaneously in conditioning affective judgment in the same manner that each operates when attended to separately." [13]

The relative effectiveness of each color in conditioning
the hedonic tone corresponding to the color-forms in part
three was measured in terms of the inverse of the M. V.
of the hedonic tones corresponding to the seven forms with
which it was combined. The relative effectiveness of each
form was similarly determined. This relative effectiveness
of each of the 7 forms and 7 colors was then compared to
their hedonic tone as determined in Parts I and II. It was
found that the extremes, i. e., the most pleasant and the
least pleasant colors and forms were the most effective.
This shows, according to Yokoyama, "that the relative effectiveness of color and form in simultaneous operation is
dependent upon the effectiveness of each when operating
under attentive isolation." [13]

But according to Yokoyama, "To say that color and
form thus work independently and simultaneously to establish affective tendency in the way in which each works sepa-

rately is to state that the two summate." [13] He consequently concludes that "Within the dimension of pleasantness and unpleasantness, the affective tendency of color-form varies approximately with the algebraic sum of the affective tendencies of its constituent color and form." [14]

These three experiments, whose results agree and are uncontroverted by any other data, indicate that in the case of complex phenomena whose parts correspond to spatially distinct stimuli, the hedonic tone of the composite phenomenon varies directly with the sum of the hedonic tones of the phenomena corresponding to the single stimuli. This is not, however, to assert that hedonic summation holds, as Yokoyama's conclusions indicate. Such summation, to be proved, would require the use of a method involving quantitative determination of hedonic tone, not merely the establishment of hedonic rank orders. But the only one of the three experimenters above who used a method adequate to give such quantitative determination is Miss Washburn, and we have seen that she considers her results to be definitely opposed to summation. Furthermore, J. Cohn has shown that in the case of color combinations whose components are equally pleasant, certain combinations are definitely preferred, namely those in which the components are markedly different.[15] Summation cannot possibly be made consistent with this fact unless it be argued that these results show the operation of a third factor besides the hedonic tone of the components, a factor of "similarity." But the operation of this third factor is itself deduced on the assumption that the law of summation holds, and consequently it cannot be invoked to save the law of summation.

In the case of combinations of stimuli which correspond to relatively unitary phenomena—in the case of clangs, for instance—the correlation stated above does not hold. Ziehen, in his "Leitfaden der Psychologie," has pointed out that "Certain combinations both of simple tones and of clangs—of piano tones, for instance—possess an incomparably greater pleasingness (Wohlklang) than simple tones or tones accompanied only by overtones. These are the so-called consonant intervals." [16] More definite still in their implications are results recently published by K. Danzfuss.[17] Danzfuss carried out a large number of experiments, both by the method of paired comparison and by the method of single stimuli, on clangs, successive intervals, chords, and series of chords presented to adults and children. He tried to deduce the feeling effect of richly organized musical structures from the combined effect of the elements, in particular of the clangs, but was obliged to conclude that "both in the case of judgments of pleasantness and in the case of characterization of mood-content, it is apparent that the complex structures cannot be considered as nothing but the sum of their components." [18]

The data above lead to three definite conclusions:

(a) Hedonic summation does not obtain.

(b) In the case of combinations of stimuli which correspond to heterogeneous composite phenomena, the hedonic tone of the composite phenomenon varies more or less directly with the hedonic tone corresponding to the single stimuli.

(c) In the case of combinations of stimuli which correspond to relatively homogeneous phenomena, the co-variation mentioned above does not hold.

These conclusions in turn imply that in the study of the relation of hedonic tone to primary stimuli it is not sufficient to deal with the cases involving simple stimuli, but that it is further necessary to investigate the cases involving combinations of these simple stimuli.

HEDONIC TONE IN RELATION TO CHARACTERISTICS OF STIMULI CORRELATED WITH SENSORY QUALITIES

Simple Color-Stimuli.—The first thoroughgoing experiment on the relation of hedonic tone to color-stimuli is that of J. Cohn, published in 1894.[19] Cohn worked by the method of paired comparison. His stimuli were primarily gelatine-plates illuminated from behind with white light. He studied the relation of hedonic tone to all three qualitative attributes of color. His results led him to the following conclusion:

"In the case of two shades (Nuancen) of the same color the more saturated is the more pleasing. Likewise in the case of a series of different colors the more saturated ones are in general preferred. In the case of colors of approximately the same saturation preference appears to rest on wholly individual inclinations. Yellow alone seems to rank below the other colors for a majority of observers, even when fully saturated. . . . In the comparison of different achromatic colors the only relatively clear result was the preference of white over gray and black." [20]

This experiment was followed by that of Major in Titchener's laboratory, published in 1895.[21] Major used the method of single stimuli. His stimuli were Bradley papers. Except for matters of methodology, the only positive conclusion of Major is "that the whole question of the affective tone of colors is a very difficult one." [22] He was unable to confirm Cohn's rule that the more saturated colors are the more pleasant, nor that yellow was displeasing to the majority of persons. With his observers also hue preferences seemed to be a matter of individual inclination.

Major's experiment was repeated by Cohn and the results were published in 1899.[23] Cohn found that the greater number of observers preferred saturated colors, but that a few (3 out of 16 in his experiment) did indeed prefer unsaturated colors. It would seem that these latter results of Cohn are typical of the general relation of hedonic tone to the complexity of the visual stimulus. E. J. G. Bradford[24] and M. Luckiesh[25] have both confirmed them. In Luckiesh's experiment, for instance, the stimuli were 15 of Wundt's colored papers, presented on a white surface. The method was that of order of merit. The instructions to the observers (15 in number) were "Choose them in the order of preference for color's sake alone." His results are indicated in the graph below, taken from his article. The colors are in spectral order as far as possible, and consequently the middle region of the graph corresponds to colors of low saturation. Blue-gray at the extreme right was also low in saturation.

He concludes: "It appears to the writer from these and other observations that, when colors are chosen 'for colors' sake alone,' the saturated colors are almost invariably chosen." [26]

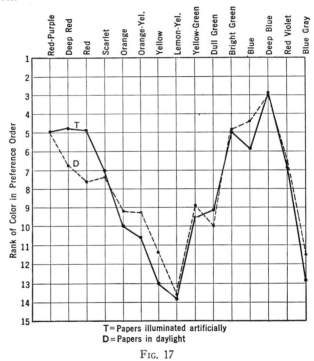

T = Papers illuminated artificially
D = Papers in daylight

FIG. 17
(From Luckiesh)

Cohn's second conclusion was that except for the unpleasantness of yellow—which, incidentally, is very unsaturated even in the spectrum—the relation of hedonic tone to hue is a matter of personal inclination. This second conclusion does not seem borne out by subsequent experimentation, although the data on this point are by no means conclusive.

Quite a few experiments apparently deal with the relation of hedonic tone to hue. Some, however, like those of Jastrow[27] and Bradford,[28] involve the use of stimuli varying markedly not only in hue, but in saturation. Although these experiments yield definite average rank orders of colors according to hedonic tone, they yield no light on the relation of hedonic tone to hue, for they do not make it possible to isolate the part played by hue from that played by saturation.

One of the most thoroughgoing attempts to determine the role of hue alone in determining color preference is that of Miss Washburn, published in 1911.[29] Using the method of single stimuli, Miss Washburn had 35 observers judge each of three sets of Milton-Bradley papers. One set consisted of saturated colors, one of tints and one of shades. The average rank orders of these three sets were as follows:

TABLE XIV

Saturated Colors	Tints	Shades
Red (most P)	Blue (most P)	Yellow-green (most P)
Green-blue	{ Red-violet	Blue
Orange-red	{ Violet	{ Red
Violet	Blue-violet	{ Violet-blue
{ Orange-yellow	Violet-blue	{ Blue-violet
{ Blue-violet	Yellow-green	{ Green-blue
{ Blue	Green	{ Green
{ Violet-blue	{ Orange-red	Violet
Violet-red	{ Green-blue	{ Red-orange
Red-orange	{ Blue-green	{ Orange-red
Blue-green	{ Red-orange	Violet-red
Yellow-orange	{ Red	{ Red-violet
Yellow	Yellow-orange	{ Green-yellow
{ Green	{ Yellow	{ Yellow-orange
{ Red-violet	{ Orange-yellow	{ Orange
{ Yellow-green	Orange	Blue-green
{ Orange	Green-yellow	Orange-yellow
Green-yellow (least P)	Violet-red (least P)	Yellow (least P)

Luckiesh in an experiment published in 1915 presented 15 highly saturated Zimmerman papers to 26 students.[30]

Each student was instructed to select the most pleasing color, then the next most pleasing, etc. The averaging of results yielded the following rank order according to decreasing pleasantness:

TABLE XV

1. Dark blue (most P)
2. Blue
3. Red-purple
4. Green
5. Violet-purple
6. Deep red
7. Orange-red
8. Crimson
9. Dull yellow-green
10. Orange
11. Orange-yellow
12. Dull green
13. Slate blue-grey
14. Yellow
15. Lemon-yellow (least P)

Geissler, in his work on hedonic summation, had 122 observers judge 7 Milton-Bradley colors by the method of paired comparison. His colors appear to have been fully saturated. He found the following average orders for 61 men, 61 women, and 122 men and women combined (the lines indicate marked differences in position) :[31]

TABLE XVI

Rank	61 Men	122 Men & Women	61 Women
Highest	Blue	Green	Green
	Purple	Purple	Red
	Green	Red	Blue-green
Intermediate	Red	Blue	Purple
	Yellow	Yellow	Yellow
	Blue-green	Blue-green	Orange
Lowest	Orange	Orange	Blue

It is clear that the results of these investigators do not accord well with one another. The fact that Luckiesh's rank order does not agree with that of Geissler nor that established by Washburn for saturated colors is in itself unimportant, for Luckiesh was not using the same stimuli as the other two investigators. It can be taken for granted that the saturation of his stimuli was not quite the same as that of the stimuli of Washburn and Geissler, and this, according to Washburn's results, should markedly alter the affective rank order of the colors. Washburn found, for instance, that red ranked first when fully saturated and compared with other saturated colors, third when less saturated and darker (when a "shade"), and eighth when less saturated and lighter (when a "tint"). The fact, however, that Geissler's rank order for women does not agree with the rank order of saturated colors according to Washburn is a serious criticism of the validity of one of the two rank orders. Both experimenters used saturated Milton-Bradley colors, and Washburn's observers were women. Washburn, however, used the method of single stimuli, whereas Geissler used the method of paired comparison; Washburn used 18 stimuli, Geissler, only 7; and we have no grounds to believe the illumination to have been identical in the two experiments. It is quite possible, therefore, that the difference in results is due not to equivocacy of the relationship being investigated, but to a difference in technique. It certainly seems unlikely that Geissler's rank order for 122 observers should have been due entirely to chance. Before any definite conclusion can be drawn, however, it will be necessary to verify the results of one at least of the two experiments.

Whether or no there is, besides the relation of hedonic tone to saturation, also one to hue, it is a fact that the variability between hedonic judgments by different observers upon identical stimuli is extremely great. A good example of this variability is given by the following table from an investigation of the color preference of 1006 negroes by F. M. Mercer. The table indicates for each of 7 colors the number of observers who assigned to it a given rank. Thus

134 under red and opposite 1 means that red was given first place 134 times out of a possible 1006.[32]

TABLE XVII

(*After Mercer*)

	Red	Blue	Violet	Green	Orange	Yellow	White
1	134	348	143	114	124	71	57
2	149	197	152	129	142	115	118
3	132	148	127	185	168	156	92
4	138	104	154	177	183	178	77
5	125	93	148	181	168	177	125
6	147	67	171	137	143	207	133
7	181	49	111	83	84	102	404

It is clear that the hedonic tone of colors depends on vastly more than the mere primary stimulus. Indeed, although there is undoubtedly a general relation between hedonic tone and saturation, and likewise probably one between hedonic tone and hue, one cannot but agree with G. J. v. Allesch, who closes the publication of a long series of experiments on the aesthetic appearance of colors with the paragraph: "The final result, however, is that the old-fashioned talk of beautiful and ugly colors has only a relative sense. No color is beautiful, none is ugly, but rather each can be anything, if it occurs at the right moment and in the right place in the dynamic structure of the aesthetic process."[33]

Peculiarly enough, there does not seem to be anything like as much variability in the hedonic judgments of a single observer at different times. E. J. G. Bradford[34] determined the hedonic rank orders of 15 colored stimuli in three series of observations separated by intervals of 2 weeks and 11½ months.[35] Bradford stated his results in a table which is reproduced below. In this table, "1st," "2nd" and "3rd" symbolize respectively the series determined in the first set of observations, the series determined in the second set of observations two weeks later, and the series determined in the third set of observations 11½ months after the second, and consequently 12 months after the first. The table gives for each pair of the three series of observations the coefficients of correlation for each observer between the rank orders determined in the two series.

TABLE XVIII

Coefficients of Correlation

Subjects	1st & 2nd	1st & 3rd	2nd & 3rd
H. S.	.81 ± .06		
E. B.	.94 ± .02	.87 ± .04	.88 ± .04
H. S.	.94 ± .02	.81 ± .06	.83 ± .05

It should be noticed that in this table the coefficients of correlation between series 1 and 2 are higher than those between series 1 and 3. This fact suggests that the uncontrolled determinants involved in this experiment operate to some extent cumulatively.

More recently, M. Yokoyama[36] determined the affective rank order of 7 colored squares in two sets of observations separated by an interval of 5 months.[37] Yokoyama states his results in the form of a table, which is reproduced below.[38] The table gives, for each observer, the degree of agreement between the rank orders, determined in the two sets of observations, in terms of a scale extending from — 100 to 100, in which — 100 indicates complete dissimilarity and 100 complete agreement.

TABLE XIX

Observers	Agreement
B	64.3
D	90.5
F	100
P	92.9

Yokoyama's conclusions were as follows: "The preferential orders of colors . . . are relatively permanent during a period extending over 5 months." [39]

Further data upon this question are yielded by a group experiment upon color-preferences published in 1926 by R. M. Dorcus.[40] Using the method of paired comparison, he presented each of two sets of Munsell colored papers in all possible binary combinations (15) and in both spatial orders. A few minutes later he repeated the same procedure. Dorcus gives a table which shows, for each of the fifteen pairs of colors, the percentage of observers who reversed their choice on the second presentation. There were six groups of observers: aged people, psychopathic patients, college students, children ten years old, children nine years old, children eight years old. Each group was again subdivided into males and females. The table below, which summarizes a part of the table given by Dorcus, deals only with the results from college students, as these alone are significant with respect to the problem of general variability discussed by us. The table shows, for each of the two sets of Munsell colors, and for 430 men and 401 women students, the average of the percentages of observers who reversed their judgments on each of the fifteen pairs of colors.

TABLE XX

Average % of college students reversing judgments of preference on pairs of colors

	Saturated Colors	Unsaturated Colors
Women	23%	20%
Men	30%	28%

It is impossible to compare these results accurately with those of Bradford and Yokoyama because the measures of variability are not the same. It seems likely, however, that the variability for Dorcus's observers is far greater than for those of the other two investigators. As the latter observers were presumably more used to making judgments of preference upon colors [41] it seems likely that the high constancy which they displayed was in part at least due to training. This view is further supported by the lesser variability shown by women students, who are accustomed to deal with the hedonic tone of colors with respect to dress. The conclusions which we have drawn concerning the relation of hedonic tone to simple color-stimuli may be summarized as follows:

1. Pleasantness varies directly with saturation, in the case of most observers. For a few, however, the reverse appears to be the case.

2. There seems to be a relation between hedonic tone and hue, although available data are too scanty to allow a definite conclusion. It appears that the extremes of the spectrum (R & B) are preferred to the middle (Y & G).

3. Individual differences are extremely marked in hedonic judgments upon colors.

4. In the case of a single observer, on the other hand, who is made to judge the same colors at different times, there is a marked constancy in hedonic judgments. This relative constancy appears to be in part dependent upon training in judging the hedonic tone of colors.

Combinations of Two Color-Stimuli.—Cohn, in the investigation referred to above, studied not only the hedonic tone of simple colors, but that of binary combinations of colors. His results led him to believe that "Presupposing equal pleasantness of components, the greater the difference between the components . . . of a combination of two colors, the greater the pleasingness of the combination"; and that "The greater the difference between two achromatic colors, the better they accord with each other."[42] He concluded by formulating the following general law: "In the realm of visual sensations, the greater the difference between neighboring sensations, the greater the efficacy in arousing pleasure."[43]

Cohn's conclusion concerning the greater pleasantness of contrasting *chromatic* colors has been controverted by the results of four subsequent investigations by three different experimenters. Baker, working with binary combinations of 24 colored papers and using the method of order of merit, concluded as follows: "The traditional view regarding the preference of complementaries in color combinations is unfounded. . . . With minor exceptions our results tend to confirm the view that the most pleasant combinations are not between complementary colors, but between colors of less difference in quality." [44] In a later experiment concerned with the same problem, Miss Baker used spectrally pure colors in binary combinations. The results substantiated those secured with pigment colors— there was found to be little justification for the old dictum of the maximum pleasantness of pairs of complementaries. A subsequent study from the same laboratory in which there were used not merely colors of the same saturation, but also tints and shades, confirmed the conclusion of Miss Baker.[46] Finally, Geissler, in his experiment upon the affective tone of color combinations mentioned above,[47] found no evidence of the hedonic influence of complementariness.

Cohn's conclusion with respect to the greatest pleasantness of contrasting *achromatic* colors (i. e., greys) has been controverted by recent findings of J. T. Metcalf.[48] Metcalf used 20 stimuli consisting of all possible combinations of one black, three greys and one white as centre and background. Thus one stimulus might be a black square as centre on a larger light grey square as background, another a light grey centre on a white background, etc. All of these stimuli, consisting of centre and background, were presented to the observer on a white field under artificial illumination. The hedonic tone of these stimuli was determined by the method of paired comparison for 24 observers. The results showed that the majority of observers *preferred relatively small degrees of contrast,* thus directly contradicting the conclusions of Cohn. On the other hand, two of the 24 observers did find brightness differences pleasant in proportion to the degree of brightness difference between the components, and three observers also showed a preference for the black-white combinations.

It would seem that there are indeed marked relationships between hedonic tone and types of color-combinations, but that these relationships are much more complicated than was thought by Cohn. Grouping together the results of the experiments by E. S. Baker, S. A. Chown, and F. L. Barber, all of them carried out in the psychological laboratory of the University of Toronto, we can say the following:

1. Grouping equally saturated colors, combinations approaching the complementary relation, though not actually complementary, are the most often preferred.[49] There is "a slight but decided preference for the 'warm' side of the manifoldness of color. The 'centre of gravity' of the combinations seems always to be not in the middle point of the color circle, but somewhere towards the side of the purple, orange, and yellow."[50]

2. For combinations of chromatic colors with greys, "the so-called warm and cold colors have aesthetically a decided advantage. The best aesthetic effect is obtained with red and with blue. . . . Tints seem to harmonize more easily with colorless light than colors in full saturation, and these more easily than shades. Nevertheless the effect of greatest pleasantness is mostly obtained with full colors and shades. . . . The emotionally indifferent colors, yellow, yellow-green, and green, and to a lesser degree violet and purple also, furnish with uncolored light indifferent or even unpleasant combinations; and the more so, the less light intensity the components show. . . . The much discussed, but experimentally never verified, assumption of the aversion to yellow probably has its foundation in the fact that yellow does not harmonize easily with colorless light."[51]

3. For combinations of colors with tints and shades, "there seems to be a consensus of judgment that colors of great contrast (though not complementaries) and colors of small intervals form pleasant combinations. (a) When there is a considerable intensity and saturation contrast, the tendency is towards the small interval of quality (e. g., shades with tints, etc). (b) When the saturation contrast is practically eliminated and the intensity contrast largely reduced, for instance in colors, tints or shades each combined with themselves, the wide interval aesthetically predominates (e. g., between yellow-green and red)."[52]

Are these principles laws which allow prediction of individual cases, or are they laws representing the central tendencies of results of great variability, as are those relating to the hedonic tone of single colors? Let us examine Miss Baker's experiment upon the hedonic value of binary combinations of 24 Prang standard pigment colors. In each trial there were presented to the observer simultaneously the 23 binary combinations into which one of the Prang colors could enter, with the instruction to pick out first those combinations which were pleasant, and then from among these that combination which was most pleasant. The number of observers was 30. Miss Baker, besides giving her results in tabular form, displayed them in the form of graphs. Each graph indicated for one of the 24 colors the number of times that each of the 23 combinations into which it could enter was judged pleasant, and the number of times that it was judged most pleasant. The figure below represents these graphs for three colors—purplish-red, red, and orange-red. These particular graphs are representative of the 21 others and were chosen arbitrarily because they were the first three given by Miss Baker. In each graph, the upper curve represents the number of times that the various combinations were judged pleasant, and the lower the number of times that they were judged most pleasant. It is difficult to determine variability from inspection of the upper curves, for the number of combinations judged pleasant varied from trial to trial. On the other hand, the lower curves do indicate variability very well, for there was but one combination judged most pleasant in each trial. If there had been no variability at all, a single one of the 23 color combinations would have received all of the judgments most pleasant, and the values of each curve would have been zero for all but one abscissa-value, namely that corresponding to the color which was involved with the fundamental color of the graph in the most pleasing combination. A mere glance at the graphs shows that this is far from being the case. For combinations involving purplish-red, the number of judgments most pleasant distributed over these combinations was 172. Of these only 20 were made upon the statistically most pleasant com-

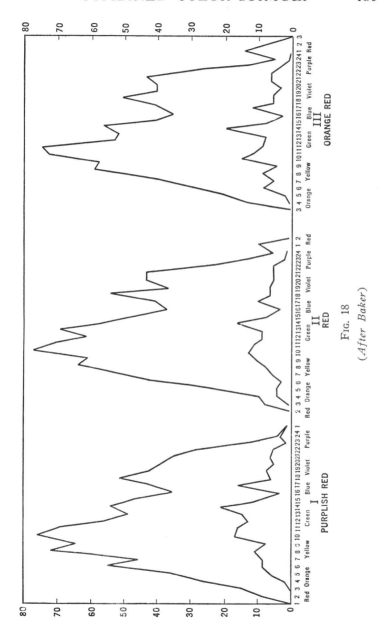

Fig. 18
(*After Baker*)

bination. Only 3 of the 23 combinations failed to be judged most pleasant on some occasion, and 7 of these combinations were judged most pleasant at least half as often as the statistically most pleasant combination. In the case of combinations involving red, 118 judgments most pleasant were distributed over these combinations. Of these, only 16 were made upon the statistically most pleasant combination. Only 3 of the 23 combinations failed to get at least one judgment of most pleasant, and 4 were judged most pleasant at least half as often as the statistically most pleasant combination. In the case of combinations involving orange-red, 130 judgments most pleasant were made upon these combinations. Of these, only 19—i. e., about 1/6—were made upon the statistically most pleasant combination. Only 3 combinations failed to get any judgment most pleasant and 3 combinations were judged most pleasant at least half as often as the statistically most pleasant combination. The principles formulated by Miss Baker, then, are statements of central tendencies of results of very great variability.

Is this variability—which appears not only in the results of Miss Baker, but in those of Chown and Barber—due primarily to individual differences? This question cannot be answered with certainty, as none of the experimenters give the data for their individual observers. Certain indirect evidence, however, makes it extremely likely that the answer should be affirmative. K. Gordon, in 1923, published a study of the variability of preference judgments upon colored plates of oriental rugs.[53] The stimuli were 50 in number, divided into two series of 25 each, and there were 207 observers. The method used was that of order of merit. The results show two very striking facts. In the first place, there was a great variation of opinion as to the relative merits of the rugs. Miss Gordon writes: "Every rug without exception was rated very high by some persons and very low by others, that is, it was put within 3 places of the top and the bottom of the series respectively. Nearly every rug was put quite at the top and at the bottom by different judges. The following distributions of choices will illustrate the variations:

TABLE XXI

Distribution of Choices on Rugs

Place Given	Rug 1 No. of Persons	Rug 5 No. of Persons	Rug 8	Rug 17	Rug 22	Rug 25
1	24	6	29	2	0	1
2	25	6	12	4	2	3
3	24	8	12	4	2	1
4	21	16	11	3	3	1
5	11	18	6	6	4	3
6	20	15	4	5	2	2
7	14	12	6	6	7	2
8	9	10	3	3	11	5
9	4	12	8	12	1	1
10	6	8	9	10	5	3
11	7	8	4	14	7	6
12	2	7	7	9	7	8
13	6	11	1	10	8	2
14	3	6	5	9	12	5
15	5	7	7	15	7	5
16	4	10	7	13	13	3
17	4	3	6	15	17	12
18	3	7	3	10	18	6
19	1	9	4	13	12	11
20	3	5	5	14	12	7
21	1	6	8	9	14	12
22	2	5	8	4	10	16
23	1	3	14	8	9	14
24	0	2	13	2	10	29
25	0	1	9	1	7	43

"In this table the first column at the left gives the places assigned in an order of merit to the rugs. The remaining six columns show the number of persons who assigned a given rug to such places. For example, Rug No. 1, which had the highest average position in this series, was given first place by 24 persons, second place by 25 persons, third place by 24 persons, etc., whereas Rug 25, which had the lowest average position, was assigned first place by 1 person and last place by 43 persons. Rug 8 is illustrative of a small group which showed bi-modal distribution. There were a few cases in which the distributions were similar to those of pure chance." [54]

The second striking fact was the considerable consistency of the judgments of single observers on two different occasions. Miss Gordon secured a second trial of the two series for 38 observers, the time interval between the trials being not less than three weeks. She measured the agreement between the observer's preferences on the two occasions by correlating the rank order of the rugs in the two trials by means of the Spearman formula. She writes: "For Series One the coefficients ranged from —.23 to +.94, with a mean of +.71 and standard deviation .185. For Series Two the range was —.17 to +.96, mean +.72, S. D. .157. It is clear from these figures that in some cases a person's second arrangement of the pictures had no significant correlation with the first. But these cases are exceptional, and the greater number showed a fair degree of self-consistency." [55] In view of these results it seems reasonable to infer that in the case of simple binary combinations of colors, as in the case of single colors, variability of hedonic judgments is primarily due to individual differences, and not to lack of consistency in succeeding judgments by single individuals.

Auditory Stimuli. —The article published by D. R. Major in 1895, which contained the first formulation of the method of single stimuli, also described the first experiment upon the hedonic tone of simple tonal stimuli. The method used was naturally that of single stimuli, with a scale of 1 (very pleasant) to 7 (very unpleasant). Each of three observers was made to give 8 judgments upon each of 14 single tones aroused with tuning forks of the following frequencies (simple vibrations): 512, 576, 640, 682, 768, 853, 960, 1024, 1250, 1536, 2048, 2304, 2560, 2792. Major presents his results in the form of three charts, one for each observer. Each chart indicates the averages of the 8 judgments made in connection with each stimulus, these averages being recorded in the same order as the stimuli listed above. The three charts are reproduced below:

Major draws the obvious conclusion that "individual differences exist here, as for sight." [59]

The general tendency of later psychologists has been to

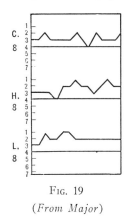

Fig. 19

(*From Major*)

interpret these results as indicating *nothing* but individual differences. Thus Ziehen, in his "Leitfaden," writes: "Within wide limits tonal quality is without influence on feeling-tone. Only very high and very low tones, other things being equal, are more readily accompanied by negative feeling-tones." [58] It is very possible, however—indeed to my mind likely—that data from observers sufficient in number to allow statistical elimination of individual differences would yield a definite relationship between hedonic tone and frequency of simple tonal stimuli.

The hedonic tone of combinations of notes has received far more attention than that of single notes. In an experiment published in 1913, C. W. Valentine established an order of preference for the 12 intervals which can be played on the piano within one octave. [59] His method was that of single stimuli, the observers being instructed to judge whether a given interval were "very displeasing," "displeasing," "slightly displeasing," "indifferent," "slightly pleasing," "pleasing," "very pleasing," and the judgments then being translated into a series of numbers for purposes of calculation. The series of numbers chosen to correspond to the judgments was: — 2, — 1, — $\frac{1}{2}$, 0, $\frac{1}{2}$, 1, 2. The total scores for the various intervals are indicated in the table below, copied from Valentine.[60]

TABLE XXII

Major third	324	Tritone	153
Minor third	261	Fifth	139½
Octave	246½	Major second	— 99
Major sixth	243	Minor seventh	— 162
Minor sixth	214	Major seventh	— 316
Fourth	157½	Minor second	— 368

The existence of individual differences is apparent in the next table of Valentine's article in which he gives side by side the results for men and women alone. This table is reproduced below.[61] The numbers in brackets represent the votes of the men increased proportionately to make them comparable with those of the women.

TABLE XXIII

Men (62 subjects)			Women (84 subjects)	
Major third ...	141½	(187)	Major third	183½
Octave	118½	(148)	Minor third	156½
Major sixth ...	105	(140)	Major sixth	138
Minor third ...	104½	(139½)	Octave	128
Minor sixth ...	103½	(138)	Minor sixth	110½
Tritone	67½	(91)	Fourth	93½
Fourth	64	(85)	Tritone	86
Fifth	61½	(83)	Fifth	78
Major second ..	— 41	(— 55)	Major second ...	— 58
Minor seventh..	— 67½	(— 90)	Minor seventh ..	— 95
Major seventh..	— 120½	(— 160)	Major seventh ..	— 196
Minor second ..	— 152	(— 202)	Minor second ...	— 216½

Evidence that these individual differences involve two main types of observers is yielded by an experiment upon fusion published in 1921 by C. C. Pratt.[62] This investigator gives separately for each of 5 observers the hedonic tones of 12 intervals as determined by the method of paired com-

parison. These hedonic tones are indicated in the graph
below, in which the ordinates represent frequencies of preference, the abscissae the 12 intervals in order of decreasing
average hedonic tone, and the five lines the various frequencies of preference corresponding to the various intervals for the five observers. It will be noticed that the
curves fall into two well-defined groups, which may be taken
to represent two distinct types of observers. Pratt was able

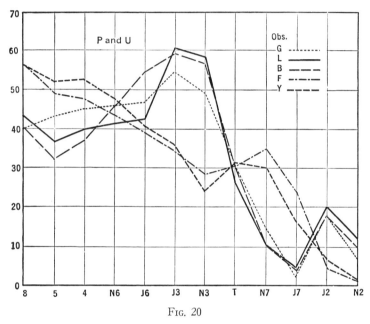

Fig. 20

Rank-order of tonal intervals under instructions for *P* and *U*. Curves
for five *O*'s.

(*From Pratt*)

to correlate these types with definite attitudes on the part
of the observers, the type which includes observers G, L,
and B corresponding to an attitude in which hedonic judgments are on *meanings,* that which includes F and Y to an
attitude in which hedonic judgments are on *smoothness* and
roughness. We shall return to these correlations when we

discuss the relation of hedonic tone to cognitive attitudes. It is obvious from the foregoing that there is some relationship between the fusion of an interval and its hedonic tone. An experiment of A. M. Brues, however, proves that this relationship is far from being one of co-variation.[63] As stimuli Brues used not only the usual musical intervals, but also "12 intervals so chosen that each one, as a ratio, was the geometrical mean between two of the musical intervals, i. e., at intervals of 50, 150, 250 cents., etc." [64] Hedonic tone and degree of fusion were determined by the method of paired comparison and also in the case of the latter, by the method of single stimuli. Furthermore, certain additional data were secured by qualitative introspection. Brues found in the first place that his observers agreed better as to the hedonic tone of the intervals than as to their degree of fusion. He found in the second place that in many cases pleasantness was wholly unrelated to fusion.[65]

Major and minor modes have also been compared with respect to hedonic tone. It has been maintained in the past that the former is more pleasant than the latter. "Rameau and d'Alembert . . . founded the cause of consonance on the existence of upper partial tones. The fact that every resonant body audibly produces at the same time as the 'generateur' its twelfth and next higher third as 'harmoniques' led them to designate the major chord as the *most natural* of all chords. The minor chord, although prescribed by nature, was not as natural and not as perfect as the major. The fact that the major triad was the more natural and the more perfect chordal structure made it, by a certain cosmic fundamentality and necessity, the more beautiful, the more pleasing, and hence the more desirable." [66] Recent evidence makes it very doubtful that the two modes involve any such intrinsic difference in pleasantness. Heinlein, from whom I have quoted the passage above, had observers characterize major and minor chords and compositions in the two modes with respect to certain emotional characteristics. He found that "Reaction to major and

minor chords in conformity with the joyful-melancholy dimension of feeling is dependent upon training to react in
this specific manner. . . . The mode in which a composition is written has little relation to the type of feeling which
the composition may arouse. Minor compositions may be
reacted to by both trained and untrained subjects as bright,
happy, cheerful, joyful and exuberant, whereas major compositions may be reacted to as gloomy, plaintive, melan-
choly, and mournful. Any fixity of feeling-tone in relation
to a given mode is dependent upon training to react in a
specific manner to a purely intellectual discrimination." [67]

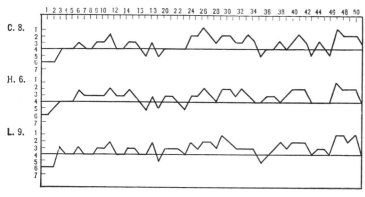

Fig. 21
(*From Major*)

Cutaneous Stimuli.—Very little is known concerning
the relations between hedonic tone and cutaneous quality.
Major in the experiment which he published in 1895 determined the hedonic tone of a number of complex tactual
stimuli by the method of single stimuli for three observers.[68]
His results are given in the form of three charts, one for
each observer. Each chart indicates for each stimulus the
average of between 6 and 9 judgments made upon it. These
averages are recorded in relatively arbitrary order, but the
order is the same for all observers. The charts are reproduced above:

An examination of the hedonic values attributed to the

various stimuli led Major to conclude that softness and smoothness are more pleasant as a rule than stiffness, roughness and coarseness. The most important result, however, is the relatively high agreement of the observers. Major points out that individual differences here are much less striking than in the case of simple tones.

This does not mean, however, that individual differences are wholly lacking. Wohlgemuth has shown that pain stimuli, although usually unpleasant, are by no means invariably so. He subjected 4 observers to various stimuli including the prick of a bristle 0.4 mm. in diameter and exerting a maximal pressure of about 32 gr., the pressure, on deep tissues, of a glass rod 7 mm. in diameter with rounded ends, and the pinch exerted by a forceps. Three of the four observers reported cases in which pain was accompanied by a pleasant feeling tone.[69]

Gustatory Stimuli.—The only reliable data on the relation of hedonic tone to the qualitative characteristics of gustatory stimuli are to be found in a research of R. Engel published in 1928.[70] Using various concentrations of four sapid substances, he determined for each concentration of each substance the number of "pleasant," "indifferent," and "unpleasant" judgments made upon it by from four to seven observers. The optimum concentration of sugar yielded 100% "pleasant" judgments, that of acetic acid 66%, that of salt 54%, that of quinine sulphate only 24%. Engel drew the tentative conclusion that the hedonic order of tastes is sweet, sour, salt, bitter.

He then set out to check this conclusion. Selecting the optimum concentration (in water) of the four sapid substances, namely 9% of cane sugar, .28% of acetic acid, 2% of cooking salt, and .0007% of quinine sulphate, he presented these stimuli in all possible orders to seven observers, with instructions to judge whether the tastes were pleasant, indifferent or unpleasant. The total number of judgments with each stimulus was 66. Engel gives his results in the form of a histogram, which is reproduced below. For the sake of comparison the figure likewise shows, by means of a continuous line, the percentages of pleasant judgments secured in the original experiment, when the four optimum concentrations were presented with other concentrations. It will be seen that the results of the two experiments are wholly in accord. As a further check Engel determined the hedonic tone of the four optimum concentrations by the method of paired comparison. The results, expressed in percentages of times preferred, are shown on

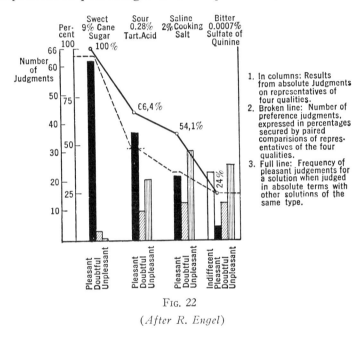

Fig. 22

(*After R. Engel*)

the figure by the broken line. The results of this third experiment completely accord with those of the first two. Engel consequently felt entitled to accept as final the tentative conclusion of his first experiment, namely that the hedonic order of tastes is, beginning with the most pleasant: sweet, sour, salt, bitter.

Is this rank order valid for all observers? The data supplied by Engel on the variability of the position and degree of optima for given types of solutions in the case of different observers—data which we shall mention in discussing the relation of hedonic tone to the intensity of the stimulus—make any such universal validity extremely unlikely. Only in one case, however, does Engel give the individual data of a single observer for two types of solutions, and this one case happens to be one agreeing with the statistical rank order stated above.

Olfactory Stimuli.—In his monograph upon olfaction, Henning has a very interesting chapter on the relation of hedonic tone to odors.[71] Among other topics he discusses the various types of incense and perfumery used by different races and in different ages. The hedonic tone of odors depends to some extent, he believes, upon racial peculiarities. The Phoenicians, for instance, mixed pepper in their perfumes. Orientals like valerian, which is disliked by most Europeans. "For the Japanese, camphor and borneol is *the* perfume so much so that in the world market no natural borneol is available except for Japanese, and this in spite of the fact that Japan itself has enormous areas of camphor forests and imports considerable quantities of artificial Borneo camphor from Germany."[72] Among primitive peoples women use butter and rancid fat as hair oil. The hedonic tone of odors depends also, he believes, upon custom—the "mode." In illustration of this point he submits the following schema of preferred perfumes:

Style of Louis XIII: Eau des Anges and similar mixtures involving musk, civet, myrtle and iris.
Style of Louis XIV: Forbidding, harsh, spice, resins, incense-like aromatics.
Style of Louis XV: Primarily rose.
First Empire: Eau de Cologne, rosemary, later exotic odors.
After 1830: Mixtures of patschouli and flowers (lavender, wall-flower).
After 1870: Harsh musk and patschouli odors; later, novelty mixtures and flower odors.
Recent times: Simple flower odors for young women, heavy novelty mixtures for older ones.

In spite of these and other factors making for individual differences, he believes it possible to establish certain gen-

eral relationships between hedonic tone and olfactory qualities. "A secant plane divides the olfactory prism in a pleasant half and an unpleasant half. On the pleasant side lie
the first four classes of odors (spicy, flowery, fruity and
resinous), on the unpleasant the two last (putrid and
burnt). Indifferent odors would lie along the section." [73]
In 1924, A. E. Findley published a study of Henning's
system of olfactory qualities in which, among other things,
she sought to test Henning's contention that the odors on
the putrid-burnt edge of the prism are unpleasant, while
those on the ethereal-fragrant-resinous-spicy face are
pleasant. [74] Findley used the method of single stimuli
(ascription of numerical values of — 2, — 1, 0, 1, 2, to

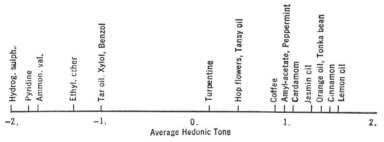

FIG. 23

(*Data from Findley*)

odors which were respectively "very unpleasant," "more unpleasant than pleasant," "indifferent," "more pleasant than
unpleasant," and "very pleasant"). Her results are indicated above in graphical form. Findley concludes that
Henning is in general correct, i. e., that fragrant, ethereal,
spicy and resinous odors are usually pleasant; putrid and
burnt odors usually unpleasant.

Findley did not in her article deal with the variability
of hedonic judgments upon odors. This topic has, however, been investigated by three other experimenters. P. T.
Young in 1923 published an experiment in which he presented 8 olfactory substances to 4 observers three times a

week for five weeks, with instructions to report hedonic tone
in terms such as very pleasant or unpleasant, moderately
pleasant or unpleasant, weakly pleasant or unpleasant, and
indifferent.[75] The data in verbal terms were then translated into numerical terms (scale of — 3 to + 3) in order
to make possible mathematical treatment. Comparison of
the average hedonic tone of the odors for the 4 different
observers showed that the subjects agreed about the quality of five out of eight odors, three being unpleasant for

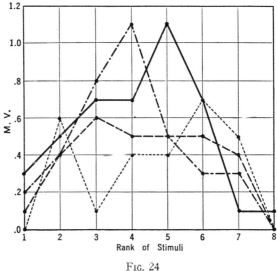

Fig. 24

(*Data from Young*)

all, and two being pleasant for all; that two of the remaining three odors were judged pleasant by all but one subject; and that one odor was weakly pleasant for two subjects and weakly unpleasant for the other two. As to the
successive hedonic judgments of individual observers, they
showed relatively low variability. This is indicated in the
graph above, in which there are given for each observer
the m.v. (ordinates) of the judgments which he made upon
the stimuli which for him had an average effective rank of

1, 2, 3, etc. (abscissae). Each of the four lines represents the results for one of the four observers. It will be noticed in the first place that the greatest average m.vs. are only 1.1, which is only a little more than a sixth of the entire scale (— 3 to 3). Young draws from these results the general conclusion that "the most variable odors are in the region of indifference, while the most constant are either 'very P' or 'very U.'" [76] In a more recent article, however, Young has pointed out that this conclusion does not follow from the data, as it is already implicit in the method of measurement employed: high average hedonic tone is possible only with a low m.v., and conversely, a high m.v. implies a low hedonic tone.

A re-examination of the data, taking this statistical artifact into consideration, leads him to revise his conclusion and to state that "daily variations in affective judgment are about the same in all regions of the scale." [77]

The relation between hedonic tone and variability seems to be worthy of further investigation. The proper procedure, in order to avoid the pitfalls met by Young, would be as follows: first, determine the hedonic tone of a set of stimuli in such a way that the measurements are not based upon variability of single judgments—by the method of paired comparison, for instance, using stimuli sufficiently spaced with respect to hedonic tone to avoid variability of judgments upon different pairs; second, determine the hedonic tone of the stimuli by a method involving variability of judgment—the method of single stimuli —and compute the m.vs for the different stimuli; third, examine the relationship between these m.vs and the hedonic tone of the stimuli as determined by the first method.

By far the most striking illustration of individual differences in hedonic judgments upon odors is to be found in an article by Kate Gordon on the recollection of odors.[78] Miss Gordon caused 200 observers to rank 10 odors in order of preference. She then made out for each odor a frequency diagram showing how many observers had given

it each of the 10 possible ranks. The figure below reproduces the diagrams for the (statistically) first, fifth and
tenth odors.

H. J. Kenneth published in 1928 an experiment involving the comparison of hedonic judgments upon 12 olfactory
substances made by a single observer (himself) at four
years' interval.[79] Two methods were used, that of single
stimuli and that of order of merit. The results of the lat-

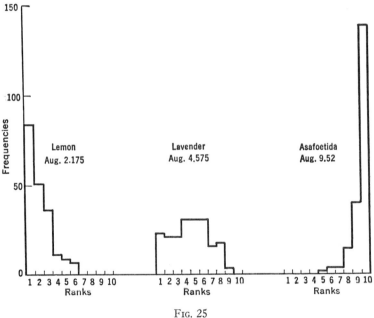

Fig. 25

(*From Gordon*)

ter method are indicated in the table below. The figures
indicate for the stimuli arranged along the top of the table
their median preferential positions in a number of different
trials. The table also shows the median preferential positions of the same stimuli for a large number of men and
women.

TABLE XXIV

Median Preferential Position

	Amyl alcohol	Camphor	Cassia oil	Cedarwood oil	Citronella oil	Menthol	Musk	Origanum oil	Pine oil	Rose oil	Sandalwood oil	Xylol
Mr. Kenneth 1922.	12	7	9	2	4	6	8	5	3	1	11	10
1927.	12	7	9	2	5	6	8	3	4	1	10	11
Men	12	8	2	5	7	3	9	6	4	1	10	11
Women	12	6	2	10	5	3	9	4	7	1	11	8
M. & W.	12	7	2	8	5	3	9	4	6	1	11	10

This table shows on the one hand certain differences between the average preferential order for large groups of men and women, and also even greater differences between the preferential orders for Mr. Kenneth and for the group of men. On the other hand, it shows marked similarity between the two preferential orders for Mr. Kenneth established at an interval of four years.

Further light is shed on the relation between these two forms of variability by the data which I secured in an investigation of hedonic habituation. In the course of the experiment I determined the hedonic rank orders of 14 olfactory substances for each of 8 observers in each of three experimental series.[80] The first experimental series (Series I) was separated from the second series (Series II) by two weeks, and the second from the third (Series III) by four and one-half to seven months. During intervals between the three series the observers participated in experiments upon hedonic habituation involving presentation of a large number of olfactory substances including the 14 referred to above.

In Table XXV will be found, for each of Series I, II and III, the average, range and standard deviation of the twenty-eight coefficients of correlation secured by intercorrelating the rank orders of the 14 stimuli for the 8 observers. The table also shows the average of the averages of the coefficients of correlation for all three series, and the total range of these coefficients.

TABLE XXV

Correspondence of Rank Orders for Different Observers

	Average	Range	S.D.
Series I	.54	.21 to .88	.21
Series II	.33	.43 to .86	.33
Series III	.39	.16 to .81	.26
Avg. of Avgs.	.42	Tot. Rge. .43 to .88	

In Table XXVI will be found, for each pair of series, the average, range and standard deviation of the coefficients of correlation between the rank orders of the 14 stimuli as determined for each observer in the two series. The table also shows the average of the averages of the coefficients of correlation for the three pairs of series and the total range of these coefficients.

TABLE XXVI

Correspondence of Rank Orders for Same Observers on Different Occasions

	Average	Range	S.D.
Series I and II	.83	.69 to .96	.09
Series II and III	.83	.58 to .99	.13
Series I and III	.75	.50 to .94	.14
Avg. of Avgs.	.80	Tot. Rge. .50 to .99	

Comparison of these two tables shows clearly[81] that for intervals up to seven and one-half months the correspondence between hedonic rank orders of a single set of olfactory stimuli established at different times for a single observer is much greater than is the correspondence between hedonic rank orders of such a set of stimuli established for different observers.

The tables also yield information concerning the parts played by "nature" and "nurture" in relative affective judgments upon odors. Table XXVI shows that the correspondence between rank orders established at different times for the same observer is greater between Series I and II and between Series II and III than it is between

Series I and III. The differences involved have a certain statistical significance, being respectively 2 times and 1.7 times their P.E.[82] As the temporal order of the series was I, II and III, this result indicates a gradual shift in the relative hedonic judgments of an observer as a function of repeated stimulation. Table XXV shows that the correspondence between rank orders for different observers is greatest for Series I. The differences involved have considerable statistical significance, that between Series I and II being 4 times its P.E., and that between Series I and III 3 times its P.E. This result indicates that the gradual shift mentioned above is in the direction not of greater agreement among different observers, but of greater disagreement. Although these results need confirmation—especially those in Table XXVI—it seems reasonable to conclude tentatively that in the case of relative hedonic judgments by different individuals upon a single set of olfactory stimuli agreement is primarily dependent upon like organic constitution, whereas disagreement rests in the main upon unlike past experiences.[83]

Stimuli Corresponding to Different Modalities. — An interesting question, and one of considerable systematic importance, is that concerning the relative hedonic effectiveness of stimuli belonging to *different* modalities—of colors and sounds, for instance. From a theoretical point of view the first step in dealing with this question would obviously be to compare, for a constant physical intensity or for a constant psychological intensity, the distribution of hedonic judgments secured by complete variation, with respect to characteristics correlated with qualities, of the various stimuli corresponding to the chief psychological modalities. This step, however, is for the present impossible. Constant physical intensity could not be maintained, for the simple reason that we are too ignorant of the process of stimulation in the case of taste and smell to measure its intensity even approximately. As for constant psychological intensity, it is also out of the question due to our ignorance concerning cross-modality judgments. For many years to come we shall have to be satisfied with comparisons of distributions of hedonic judgments secured with arbitrary selections of stimuli having an apparently normal intensity. Indeed for the moment we must be satisfied with the results of a single experiment, by Babbit, Woods and Washburn, on the distribution of hedonic judgments upon a very limited number of visual and auditory stimuli.[84]

In this experiment a large group of observers was made to give absolute hedonic judgments on a variety of colors, tones and articulate sounds. From these judgments there were computed, for each observer and for each type of stimulus, an "index of affectivity" consisting of the ratio of the number of judgments "indifferent" to the number of judgments "very pleasant" and "very unpleasant." For the three types of stimuli the numbers of indices below unity (indicating more judgments "very pleasant" or "very unpleasant" than judgments "indifferent," and consequently greater "affectivity") were as follows:

For tones 64
For colors 60
For syllables 29

Again, for the three types of stimuli the numbers of observers who made no judgments "indifferent" upon stimuli of a given type were as follows:

For tones 10
For colors 1
For syllables 1

Finally, the number of observers who, in judgments upon one type of stimulus, never made any judgments "very pleasant" or "very unpleasant" were:

For tones 0
For colors 0
For syllables 6

The authors concluded that their results "show that affective sensitiveness to tones is greater than that to colors, but only slightly, and that affective sensitiveness to articulate sounds is markedly less than to either tones and colors." [85]

It is a pity that this experiment deals only with visual and auditory stimuli, for these two types of stimuli seem to be far more alike than is either to olfactory, gustatory or cutaneous stimuli. The theoretical importance of the issue would seem to warrant further work in this field, in spite of the impossibility of securing entirely reliable results. If it could be demonstrated, for instance, that the so-called "lower" senses are actually more conducive to extremes of hedonic tone than are the higher ones, this would constitute evidence in favor of a theory of hedonic tone emphasizing motor response—a theory like that of Lange, for instance. This is because the higher senses are known to involve fewer reflexes than do the lower.

General Conclusion. —It is apparent from the preceding discussion that in its general features the relationship between hedonic tone and the "quality"-characteristics of the stimulus is the same in the case of all classes of stimuli. These general features may be described as follows:

1. The hedonic tone of a phenomenon is a definite function of those characteristics of the corresponding stimulus which correlate with sensory quality.

2. This relationship allows only of statistical prediction, not of prediction in individual cases, because of marked individual differences. These individual differences, in turn, indicate that the hedonic tone of a phenomenon is but very partially determined by the nature of the corresponding stimulus.

3. The hedonic judgments of a single individual vary little over periods of time as long as a year. They appear to vary least in the case of observers familiar with the stimuli. What variation occurs appears to be cumulative and in the direction of lesser agreement among different

observers. These facts clearly suggest that hedonic tone is partially determined by learning.

HEDONIC TONE IN RELATION TO SPATIAL CHARACTERISTICS OF STIMULI

Area of Stimulus.—The only experiment that I know which deals with the relation of hedonic tone to the area of the stimulus is that of Clark, Goodell and Washburn, published in 1911.[86] These investigators used two sets of colored paper squares. The squares in one set were 5 cm. a side, in the other, 25 cm. a side. Each set involved 6 saturated colors and the lighter tint and darker tint of each of these colors—18 colored papers in all. The observers, 23 in number, observed each square of both sets for ten seconds and recorded their affective judgment in numerical terms, using the numbers 1 to 7 to indicate 7 degrees of hedonic tone ranging from very unpleasant to very pleasant. The data were treated in two different ways. First there were computed in the case of each color the number of observers who assigned higher hedonic tone to the larger square than to the smaller one, and the number of observers who assigned a lower hedonic tone to the larger square. Comparison of these numbers showed the following results:

1. For saturated colors, more observers preferred the *smaller* area in the case of all colors except red. In the case of red, more preferred the larger area.

2. For tints, a slight majority preferred the *larger* area.

3. For shades, a majority likewise preferred the *larger* area, though this majority was small for green and violet.

Secondly, there was computed in the case of each color the ratio of the sum of the hedonic tones assigned by all the observers to the larger square to the sum of the hedonic tones assigned by all observers to the smaller square. Examination of these ratios showed the following:

1. For saturated colors, the *smaller* area is more pleasant except in the case of red.

2. For tints, all the *larger* areas were slightly preferred except in the case of green.

3. For shades, the *larger* areas were preferred except in the case of green.

The investigators drew the following conclusions: "(1) Saturated colors are preferred in smaller area, with the exception of saturated red, which is preferred in larger area; (2) the larger area of tints is slightly preferred; and (3) the larger area of shades is preferred, the preference being least in the case of green and violet." [87]

Washburn and her collaborators unfortunately do not give any figure from which one might determine whether the preference for smaller areas of saturated colors is statistically very significant or not. It might be that there was a general trend to prefer larger areas, but that this trend happened to be offset in Washburn's experiment by chance factors. One would also like to know how much of a decrease from a dimension of 5×5 cm. would still be accompanied by a change in hedonic tone, and likewise how far above 25×25 cm. the factor of area would be operative in altering hedonic tone. It would be very helpful to have this experiment repeated and extended.

It might be that increase in the area of a stimulus correlates not so much with *arithmetical* increase of the corresponding hedonic tone as with its *algebraic* increase. In other words, it might be that the main effect of increasing area is to increase both pleasantness *and* unpleasantness. Such was apparently the case in the experiment above, for the investigators wrote: "There was no correspondence between the absolute affective value of a color and the preference for it in larger or smaller area." [88] It is not clear from the article, however, to what extent the data were examined from the point of view of this problem. The problem is of sufficient importance to warrant further investigation.

Form of Stimulus.—The relation of hedonic tone to

the form of a visual stimulus was the subject of the first
work of Fechner in experimental aesthetics. It was also
studied extensively by some of his disciples, by Witmer, for
instance. The most important result of these investigations
was to establish the hedonic superiority of the *golden section*, of *the proportion in which the smaller section bears
the same relation to the larger section that the larger does
to the whole*. In such a proportion the ratio of the smaller
section to the larger is roughly 3/5 and more approximately 21/34. (3/5 is roughly equal to 5/(3 + 5) and
21/34 is more approximately equal to 34/(21 + 34)).
Fechner, in his "Vorschule der Aesthetik," gives data showing that in the case of rectangles of equal area but of varying ratios of height to length the rectangle preferred by
the greatest number of observers is the one in which the
ratio of height to length is 21/34.[89] Witmer extended the
field of investigation to many other figures. He studied
the preference of observers for various proportions in the
case of lines divided into two parts, of right angles, of vertical lines perpendicular to the centre of a horizontal line,
of two lines intersecting each other at right angles, and of
certain closed figures, namely rectangles, ellipses and triangles. Witmer summarizes his results as follows: "In the
case of all observers and of all figures there were found
but two ranges corresponding to maxima of feeling. The
one lay around equality, the other around a proportion,
which with few exceptions lay between the proportions $\frac{1}{2}$
and $\frac{2}{3}$ and usually approached the golden section with a
slight deviation towards the proportion $\frac{1}{2}$."[90]
    The results of both Fechner and Witmer were in gen-
eral confirmed in the later work of Angier and Thorndike.
Angier published in 1903 a thoroughgoing investigation of
the optimal bisection of a straight line. The average of the
bisections preferred by his nine observers was "surprisingly
close" to the golden section.[91] Thorndike published in 1917
an investigation of preferred proportions for rectangles,
triangles, crosses and designs.[92] He found that the most
liked rectangles had as the ratio of height to base, 1.83

to 1 and the most liked triangles the similar ratios of 1.6
to 1 and 1.7 to 1 (in the case of the triangles two propor-

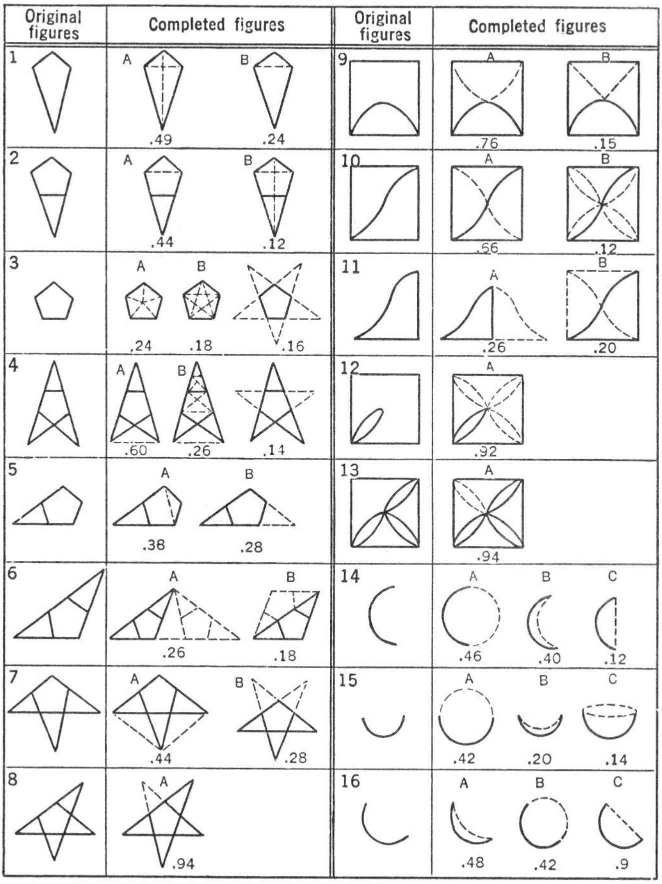

FIG. 26. COMPLETION OF SOME OF THE FIGURES USED IN SET A

The numerals below the figures indicate the number of times (expressed
in percentages) these particular completions occurred.

(*From Lund and Anastasi*)

tions tied for first place). These ratios were quite close
to the golden section which, expressed in corresponding
form, is 1.6 to 1. In the case of the crosses, however, there

was no preference for a proportion akin to the golden section. "The most liked of the crosses had a bar half of the length of the upright so as to leave one-fourth above and three-fourths below. A bar two-fifths of the length of the upright is nearly as well liked." [93]

Another important condition of the hedonic tone of phenomenal forms is *completeness*. In an experiment published in 1923, Lund and Anastasi studied the principles according to which observers complete figures when instructed to do so in such a manner as to secure maximal aesthetic effect.[94] In a first part of the experiment, they

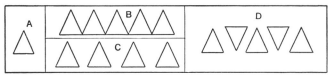

Fig. 27

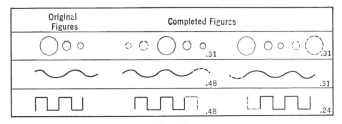

Fig. 28

(*After Lund and Anastasi*)

presented to their observers a variety of simple figures together with the following instructions: "Add to each figure such lines or elements as will give to the presentation the most satisfactory, pleasing or aesthetic effect, without making the completion too great a departure or elaboration of the given elements." The results showed a strong tendency to complete figures *in accordance with some familiar object* and in accordance with *balance and symmetry*. Figure 26 above shows some of the stimuli used, together with the most frequent types of completion. The frequency with which a certain completion occurred is indicated by a number below the completed figure.

In a second part of the experiment, the figures presented involved repetition of similar elements, and the instructions called for completion through the addition or duplication of elements given in the figure. A few of the stimuli, together with the more frequent results, are given in Fig. 28. The results showed *a preference for symmetry and balance.*

In a third set of experiments, the observers were made to indicate their order of preference for series of stimuli involving one element alone and various combinations of such elements. Thus one such series involved the four stimuli in Fig. 27. The results showed a decided preference for several combinations compared with single figures. Lund and Anastasi draw the general conclusion that, in the case of visual patterns, the importance of "preparedness-facilitation" in determining pleasantness is extremely great.

This experiment in itself is extremely interesting. It suggests, however, another of equal or even greater interest. Lund and Anastasi required their observers to *complete* certain figures, and then determined what *form of completion* was most pleasing. Is it not possible that completion per se correlates with pleasantness? In order to answer this question it would only be necessary to repeat the experiment of Lund and Anastasi, using instructions which require not *completion,* but merely the addition of further elements. Such an experiment was carried out in the Harvard Laboratory by Mr. F. W. Swift.[95] The results were surprisingly conclusive. The completions secured by Lund and Anastasi were found to occur in about the same frequency, even though no mention of completion was made in the instructions. It seems clear, then, that hedonic tone, besides varying with symmetry in the case of complete figures, likewise varies with the completeness of the figures— the more *complete* the figure, the more pleasing.

Completeness, however, is a phenomenal characteristic, not a characteristic of stimuli. To what physical characteristics does it correspond? So far are we from being able to answer this question that we are not even sure of its correspondence to *any* characteristic of the stimulus. If the Gestalt school is right in its insistence that configurations are dependent not wholly upon learning, but upon the configuration of stimuli,[96] we may hope some day to answer this question. This hope is my reason for dealing with completeness in connection with the relation of hedonic tone to stimuli.

Any discussion of the hedonic correlates of spatial form would be incomplete without reference to the recent work of the mathematician, G. D. Birkhoff. In a paper presented in 1928 at the Sixth International Congress of Mathematics, Birkhoff seeks to establish a relationship between the "feeling of pleasure or aesthetic measure" correlated with an object and the nature of that object.[97] Commonsense, together with the aesthetic principle of "unity in variety," suggest, he believes, that such a relationship is given by the equation

$$M = \frac{O}{C}$$

in which M represents the aesthetic measure of the object, O its orderliness, symmetry or harmony, and C its complexity. Birkhoff then shows that in the case of polygons, of designs, and of the form of vases it is possible to define univocally O and C in such a way that the forms which to his mind rank high aesthetically within their class (e. g., the class of polygons) also rank high in terms of the aesthetic measure M. In the case of vases, for instance, Birkhoff considers the plane figure representing the contour of the vase (its axis being vertical) as an adequate representation of the vase itself. He then defines C as the sum of the following *characteristic points:* "(1) the four points terminating the contour, (2) the points on the contour where the tangent to the contour has a vertical or horizontal direction, (3) the points where this direction changes suddenly, (4) the points of inflection where the curvature passes through zero, (5) the centres of the vase

situated on the axis at the points where the horizontal
straight lines of maximal or minimum length cross the
axis." O is defined as the sum of four magnitudes, H, V,
HV and T, themselves defined as follows: H is the number
of mathematically independent relations of the type x = y
or x = 2y in which x and y are vertical distances between
horizontal lines drawn through symmetrical characteristic
points; V is the number of like relations in which x and y
are total lengths of such horizontal lines; HV is the number of mathematically independent relations of the type
x = y in which x is the vertical distance between two of
the horizontal lines referred to above, and y the length of
these lines; T is the number of cases in which tangents to
characteristic points on one side of the vase are perpendicular to one another, parallel to one another, horizontal
or perpendicular to a line passing through one of the centres (points where horizontal lines of maximal or minimal
length cross the axis). With C and O thus defined Birkhoff goes on to compute the aesthetic value M of a number of Chinese vases illustrated in a work by Hobson on
Chinese Art.[98] He also gives an example—in the form
of an illustration—of a vase designed by himself in such a
fashion that its aesthetic value M is greater than that of
any of the Chinese vases selected from Hobson's work.
The Chinese vases having a high aesthetic value M do indeed appear more attractive to me than the others, and
the vase designed by Birkhoff himself according to formula
strikes me as extremely graceful.

Is this most interesting and ingenuous procedure valid?
The answer must wait upon experimental verification. According to Birkhoff, M is not merely a quantity defined in
terms of certain characteristics of objects, but it represents
also the "feeling of pleasure or aesthetic measure" which
rewards the "preliminary effort necessary properly to per-
ceive the object." This latter assertion is subject to experimental verification—indeed, it requires such verification. It is to be hoped that someone will soon establish
the correlation, for various classes of objects, between their

aesthetic value in terms of M and their aesthetic value in terms of the preference judgments of an adequate group of observers.

The relation of hedonic tone to spatial characteristics of stimuli is subject to very marked individual differences. In the experiments of Fechner, mentioned above, preferences were by no means confined to the golden section. Indeed, but 34% of the preferences fell to the lot of the rectangle representing the golden section, while 2.74% fell to the lot of the square, statistically the least liked figure. Again in the experiment of Witmer, individual differences were sufficiently striking to be discussed in a special section of the article. With the experiment of Angier, these individual differences become the main topic of discussion. Each observer was made to give not one judgment (as with Fechner), but a large number of judgments. As stated above, the *average* of the bisections of a line preferred most frequently by the different observers was surprisingly close to the golden section. Only in two cases, however, out of a possible eighteen, did the mode of the preferences of an observer coincide with the golden section, whereas in five cases the golden section was entirely outside the distribution of preferences. Angier concludes that "the records offer no one division that can be validly taken to represent 'the most pleasing proportion' and from which interpretation may ensue." [99] With Thorndike individual differences are likewise the main issue. Again, they turn out to be very marked: "In the case of the rectangles it will be observed that 27, 28, and 29, those most liked, still have some ratings in the lowest position of all; and that 33, the one least liked, still has ratings in the highest position. In only 3 cases out of 144 do over 25% of the ratings give a rectangle the same position. In the case of the triangles, there is a pronounced drift of opinion against the tall triangles, but even so almost every position has votes in the case of each. This is still more the case with the crosses. In the case of the designs, where the sequence by proportions is more hidden, the variability becomes enor-

mous. Although any one person may feel very decided preferences, these are never shared by enough of his fellows
to make anything like universal agreement. In the series
of 12 designs, not one has 25% of ratings in any one position. In the series of 24 designs, in only about one case
out of thirty are there 10% or more of ratings in any one
position." [100]

Judgments made by single individuals, however, again
show remarkable constancy. In the experiment mentioned
in connection with hedonic summation, Yokoyama determined the hedonic order of 7 geometrical forms in two
sets of observations separated by an interval of five months.
The results are stated in the form of a table, which I reproduce below. The figures represent the agreement between the rank orders determined in the two sets of
observations in terms of a scale extending from — 100
(complete disagreement) to 100 (complete agreement).[101]

TABLE XXVII

Observers	Agreement
B	90.5
D	95.2
F	100
P	88.1

HEDONIC TONE IN RELATION TO THE INTENSITY
OF STIMULI

The Curve.—The relationship between hedonic tone
and the intensity of stimuli is stated in a good many text-
books in the form of a curve. The curves vary slightly
from textbook to textbook, but are sufficiently similar so
that but a single illustration need be given. The curve below is taken from Ziehen's "Leitfaden der Physiologischen
Psychologie." It is explained by the author as follows:
"The continuous lines of the appended drawing. . . represent the relationship between the intensity of sensation
and that of the stimulus. Intensities of stimulus are represented as abscissae. R_s represents the absolute threshold,

R_h the intensity of the stimulus. The continuous curve represents the variation of intensity of sensation as the intensity of the stimulus increases. The broken curve represents the intensity of hedonic tone. That part of the broken line which lies above the axis of abscissae indicates positive hedonic tone, i. e., pleasant feeling; that part which

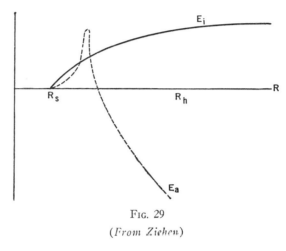

FIG. 29

(*From Ziehen*)

is beneath the axis represents negative hedonic tone, i. e., unpleasant feeling." [102]

Hedonic tone is notoriously difficult of measurement. What remarkable quantitative data are at the basis of this curve? Ziehen refers back to Wundt.[103] In the "Physiological Psychology" of 1902, we find the same curve, but we further find that this curve is not a graphic representation of data, but only a schematic representation of casual observation. Very intense sensations, Wundt points out, are unpleasant, and this unpleasantness increases with increase in the intensity of the sensation. Moderately intense sensations, on the other hand, are usually pleasant, and this pleasantness decreases with decrease of intensity of the sensation until it becomes liminal near the lower absolute limen. "Hence," writes Wundt, "the general dependence of hedonic tone upon intensity of sensation should probably be represented as follows": And he gives the figure reproduced by Ziehen. The reader is warned not to take this figure too seriously: "As feelings, unlike sensations, are not subject to exact measurement, nothing can be said concerning the detailed form of this curve of feeling." [104]

Rough Experiments.—For many years Wundt's view that hedonic tone is not subject to exact measurement remained uncontroverted as far as experiments are concerned, and knowledge of the relationship between hedonic tone and intensity of stimulus seemed doomed to remain schematic. Not that experiments upon this relationship were lacking, but their data never involved hedonic tone in units of amount. Kiesow, for instance, published in 1899 an experiment in which he sought to determine variations in hedonic tone correlated with variations of the intensity of sweet sensations. [105] His procedure was first to determine for local stimulation of two equally sensitive areas of the tongue the relationship between intensity of taste, expressed in j.n.d's, and the intensity of a sweet stimulus, expressed in terms of concentration. He then established in his observers criteria of pleasantness and unpleasantness by presenting to them highly affective stimuli of various sorts. After these preliminaries, he secured from his observers judgments of pleasantness or unpleasantness with the stimulus-values corresponding to the successive D.L.'s of taste sensitivity. Kiesow states that the curve representing his results "Begins at the threshold with a stage of indifference. It then increases very slowly until there is reached another stage of indifference. The curve then inclines towards unpleasantness and decreases rather fast." He adds, however, that "for reasons beyond my control I have not yet been able to complete this research, and must consequently postpone until later the publication of results, which are not yet sufficiently well established." [106] I have never discovered this promised amplification of results. As far as the results published in the 1899 article are concerned, they support Wundt's schematic curve except with respect to the second stage of indifference. They do not, however, involve data in units of amount which would allow this curve to be considered anything more than a schema.

Another interesting experiment on the relation between hedonic tone and stimulus-intensity is that described by Lehmann in his "Hauptgesetze." [107] The particular relationship with which he dealt was that between hedonic tone and the temperature of a cutaneous stimulus. He caused two observers to dip the outer phalanges of two fingers into water whose temperature was increased in 2 minutes and

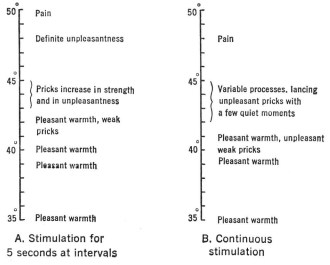

A. Stimulation for
5 seconds at intervals

B. Continuous
stimulation

Fig. 30

(*After Lehmann*)

20 seconds from 35° to 50° (Centigrade). In one case, the observers were made to dip their fingers into the water for 5 seconds at various temperatures whose hedonic correlate Lehmann desired to determine. In a second set of trials the observers were made to keep their fingers in the water for the whole of 2 minutes and 20 seconds. The observers were required to describe their feelings. The results of this little experiment are indicated in the preceding figure. These results, however sketchy, are interesting in that they

show that from 35° to 40° the hedonic tone was pleasant, while between 40° to 42° it became unpleasant and increased in degree of unpleasantness up to 50°. This supports the Wundtian schema in a general way, but again it does not support it with respect to the transition from pleasantness to unpleasantness. According to the Wundtian schema this transition should involve indifference. None was reported by Lehmann's observers. Furthermore, as with Kiesow's work, the data are quantitative only in the most general sense of the term.

Experiments Involving Measurement. —In the last few years two experiments have been published on the relation of hedonic tone to the intensity of the stimulus which have changed our knowledge of the relationship *from · being merely schematic to being definitely quantitative.* These experiments are those of Saidullah and Engel. Saidullah's research sought to establish the relationship between hedonic tone and the intensity of salt-solutions, measured in terms of their concentration.[108] His stimuli were 18 salt-solutions, varying in concentration from 0.5% to 30%. These solutions were presented to the observer singly, the observer being instructed to judge the hedonic tone of the resulting taste by stating whether it was: 1, indifferent; 2, pleasant; 3, very pleasant; 4, unpleasant; or 5, very unpleasant. There were 8 observers. The results in the case of solutions at 9° Centigrade are indicated in figure 31 below. The curves represent for each stimulus (abscissae) the number of judgments of each of the 5 categories made by all observers upon that stimulus.

Saidullah further sought to determine what effect variation of temperature would have upon the hedonic judgments of his observers. He consequently repeated the experiment with solutions at 18° and 36° Centigrade. The results of all three experiments are indicated in figure 32 below. In this figure, each curve indicates for each stimulus the difference between the total number of pleasant judgments made upon that stimulus by all observers and the total number

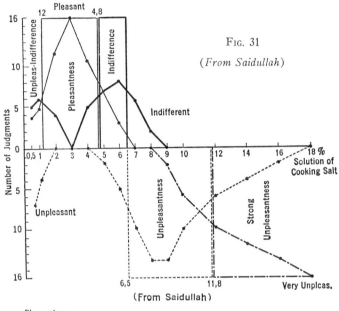

FIG. 31

(*From Saidullah*)

(From Saidullah)

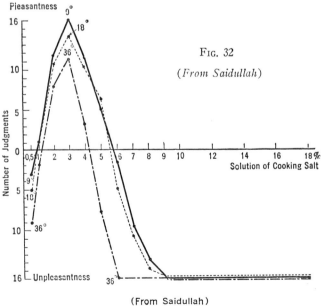

FIG. 32

(*From Saidullah*)

(From Saidullah)

of unpleasant judgments. The three curves represent the
three temperatures used. Saidullah concludes that in the case of salt-solutions
the *Wundtian schema must be changed to show in certain
cases an unpleasant phase preceding the pleasant phase,* and
further that the pleasant phase and succeeding unpleasant
phase are separated by a large region of indifference. In
this latter respect, however, his data do not entirely support his conclusion. For no concentration in this region
of transition is the number of indifferent judgments greater
than the sum of the pleasant and unpleasant judgments.
He further concludes that the *optimal concentration—the
most pleasant one—is independent of temperature, but that
increase of temperature tends to shift the hedonic tone of
all solutions towards unpleasantness.*

Engel's experiment was similar to that of Saidullah, but
more complete.[109] Instead of investigating the co-variation
of hedonic tone and of intensity of the stimulus in the case
of salt solutions alone, he did so for salt solutions, bitter
solutions, sweet solutions and sour solutions. The method
employed by Engel, a special case of the method of single
stimuli, was similar to that used by Saidullah. He presented
to his observers a given type of solution in different concentrations—a salt solution, for instance, in concentrations
varying from 0.5 to 10%—and had his observers make an
absolute judgment upon the taste determined by each individual concentration. This method differed from that of
Saidullah, however, in that the observers were not instructed
to distinguish degrees of pleasantness and unpleasantness,
but merely to state whether a given experience were pleasant, indifferent or unpleasant. In the case of salt solutions,
Engel also made use of the method of paired comparison.
The solutions were in all cases at room temperature, i. e.,
between 16° and 18° Centigrade. The total results for the
various solutions are indicated graphically in the following
figures. "Total results" is here used in a strict sense.
The curves represent not averages of the judgments of the
different observers, but sums of the judgments of all
observers.

The results for salt solutions are indicated in figures 33 and 34.   Figure 33 represents not only the total number of pleasant, indifferent and unpleasant judgments made in connection with each stimulus, but also what the writer calls "ideal regions"—ranges of concentration in which judg-

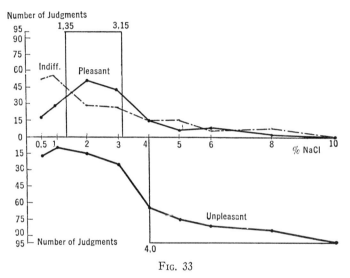

FIG. 33

Curve representing the hedonic tone of cooking salt solutions for 7 observers in 7 sittings. Also ideal regions of pleasantness and unpleasantness.

(*From Engel*)

ments of a particular type predominate.   The figure shows that for concentrations around 0.5% the judgments of indifference preponderate.   Then occurs a predominantly pleasant range of concentrations with an optimum at 2%. This in turn is followed by a predominantly unpleasant range for concentrations of 4% and more.   Figure 34, representing results secured by the method of paired comparison, again shows an optimum for concentration of 2%.   In the trials involving the method of paired comparison, Engel had his observer make an additional absolute judgment upon that member of each pair which was preferred.   The re-

sults in terms of these absolute judgments are indicated
in figure 34 by "ideal regions." The close correspondence
of these "ideal regions" with those indicated in figure 33
constitutes a strong confirmation of the results represented
in the latter figure, particularly since the observers involved
were not the same.

In his experiment with salt solutions, Engel further

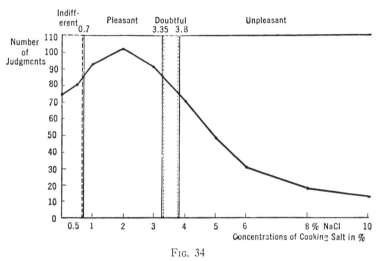

Fig. 34

1. Curve representing the preference judgments of 7 observers in paired
comparisons of solutions of cooking salt. 2. Ideal regions calculated from
absolute judgments of the same stimuli.

(*From Engel*)

sought to test Saidullah's conclusion that, when the temperature of salt solutions is varied, the position of the
optimum remains unchanged, but the degree of unpleasantness increases for all concentrations with increase of temperature. Engel's experimentation had so far been done
with solutions at room temperature. He now repeated his
work with salt solutions, using two new temperatures,
namely 0° C. and 54° C. For the low temperature the results were practically identical with those described above
for room temperature. For the high temperature, Engel

found a decrease of pleasant judgments distributed over the majority of stimuli, although the beginning of the unpleasant range remained at 4%. This confirms the results of Saidullah.

Figure 35 shows the total results secured by the method of single stimuli for bitter solutions. The results for a concentration of 0% are partly hypothetical, as this concentration was not included in the range of stimuli for all observers. This fact is indicated in the figure by a vertical line. The curve shows an optimum for concentrations around 0.0007, but this optimum is much less marked than

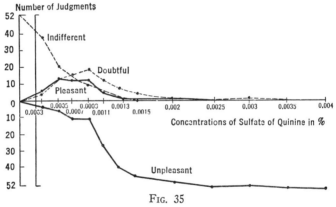

Fig. 35

Curve representing the hedonic tone of solutions of Sulfate of Quinine for 10 observers in 6 sittings.

(*From Engel*)

for salt solutions. The unpleasant region begins at 0.0011, and the degree of unpleasantness increases indefinitely with the increase in concentration of the solution. It will be noticed that the transition from pleasantness to unpleasantness (around .09) involves a preponderance not of *indifferent* judgments, but of *doubtful* judgments. These judgments refer, according to Engel, to feelings characterized by "ego-warmth" (Ich-Wärme), and consequently not strictly indifferent, but nevertheless not such that they can be called pleasant or unpleasant. Unfortunately Engel does not go further into the definition of this fourth category of judgments.

The total results for sour solutions are represented in figure 36. They show the optimum is at a concentration of 0.28%, and that this optimum involves a higher degree of pleasantness than do the optima of salt and bitter (opt. for Sour, 66.4% P judgments; opt. for Salt, 54% P judgments; opt. for Bitter, 24% P judgments). It is noteworthy that there is no sharp transition from pleasantness to unpleasantness, both types of judgments occurring in the case of all but two stimuli. It is also noteworthy that at

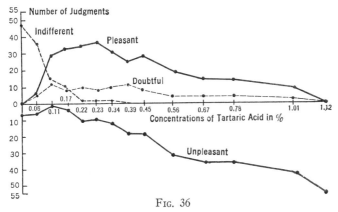

Fɪɢ. 36

Curve representing the hedonic tone of solutions of tartaric acid for 7 observers in 6 sittings.

(*From Engel*)

the statistical transition between pleasantness and unpleasantness at the concentration where these two classes of judgments balance there is not a single judgment of indifference recorded, and only a few doubtful ones.

The total results for sweet solutions are indicated in figure 37. The most striking feature of this curve is the great preponderance of pleasant judgments over all others for all but the lowest concentrations. Engel ascribes the occurrence of unpleasant judgments for concentrations of 0% and 1% to contrast. Concentrations around 9%, at which the pleasant curve becomes asymptotic, correspond, according to Engel, to the concentrations usual in foods and beverages.

What is the consequence of these results with respect to the validity of Wundt's schema? In a very general way they support the schema. They show that, *as a rule,* when the intensity of the stimulus increases from a liminal value

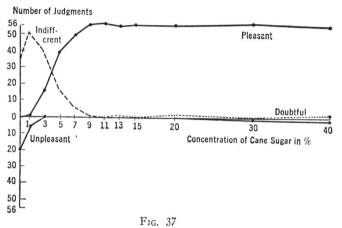

FIG. 37

Curve representing the hedonic tone of solutions of Cane Sugar for 10 observers in 6 sittings.

(From Engel)

to a very high value, the hedonic tone of the corresponding phenomenon starts with indifference, goes through a maximum of pleasantness and then becomes unpleasant. In matters of detail, however, Engel's results fail to support Wundt. In the first place, in the case of sugar, even extremely high concentrations fail to yield unpleasantness or even lesser pleasantness. It would seem here that the curve does not go through a maximum, but becomes asymptotic to an ordinate representing maximal pleasantness. Again, the Wundtian transition from pleasantness to unpleasantness through indifference is opened to question. According to the Wundtian schema the results should show for substances which involve a transition from pleasantness to unpleasantness, a preponderance of indifferent judgments for concentrations corresponding to the transition. What the results actually show, however, is that for both salt and sour the sum of the indifferent and "doubtful" judgments never exceeds the sum of the pleasant and unpleasant judgments in regions of transition. Indeed, in the case of sour the sum of the indifferent and doubtful judgments is not as great, in the region of transition, as either the number of pleasant judgments or the number of unpleasant ones.

The fact that Engel's results cast doubt upon the oc-

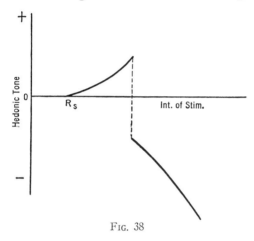

Fig. 38

currence of indifference in the transition between pleasantness and unpleasantness is important. We have seen that an earlier rough experiment by Lehmann had done the same. Both of these experiments suggest the possibility that the function relating hedonic tone to intensity of stimulus is discontinuous, and should be represented not as in the Wundtian schema, but as in the graph above.[110] Neither the data of Lehmann, which were extremely rough, nor those of Engel, which did not involve *degrees* of pleasantness and unpleasantness, can be considered as more than merely suggestive. On the other hand, the only data supporting the Wundtian continuous curve are also far from conclusive. Kiesow's work was never reported in full, and Saidullah's results, as we pointed out, do not involve an actual preponderance of indifferent judgments for any of the concentrations in the region of transition. In view of the systematic importance of the issue, it would be well to repeat Engel's experiment upon salt, sour and bitter substances, but to require from the observers judgments of *degree* of pleasantness and unpleasantness. If in the region of transition the ratio of extreme judgments (very pleasant, very unpleasant) to intermediate judgments (pleasant, indifferent, unpleasant) *decreased* for all three substances, the function relating hedonic tone to intensity of stimulus could be considered definitely to be continuous, as in Wundt's schema. If, on the other hand, the ratio remained constant for all substances, the function could be considered to be discontinuous.

All of the curves above indicate total results for all observers. Are they representative of the judgments of individual observers? Of the majority of individual observers, yes. Of all, decidedly no. Engel writes as follows: "The experiments above suggest that there is considerable agreement between individuals in contrast with the general exaggeration of individual differences. The curves for individual observers agree completely with the curves presented above, and it would seem that under constant conditions all normal individuals react in much the same way. . . . Nevertheless there are always extreme types for which a given quality produces either an excess of pleasantness or excess of rejection." [111] Engel illustrates this latter point by giving curves showing for each of three sapid substances the distribution of pleasant, indifferent and unpleasant judgments of an observer liking the substance and of an observer disliking it. The curves are reproduced on the following page.

As regards sweet solutions, he gives no graphic comparison of results for different observers. He does state, however, that two observers who professed a dislike for sweets showed an optimum for concentrations of 1%, followed by a doubtful region extending to concentrations of

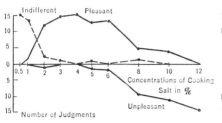

Type A. Liking salt.
Judgments of solutions of
cooking salt by Obs. Ch.K.
(From R. Engel)

Type B. Disliking salt.
Judgments of solutions of
cooking salt by Obs. K.B.
(From R. Engel)

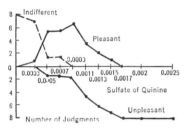

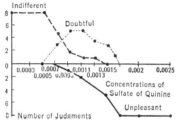

Type A. Liking bitter.
Judgments of solutions of
sulfate of quinine by Obs. A.K.
(From R. Engel)

Type B. Disliking bitter.
Judgments of solutions of
sulfate of quinine by Obs. Ch.K.
(From R. Engel)

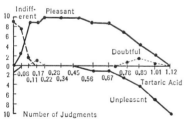

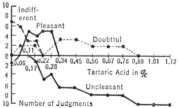

Type A. Liking sour.
Judgments of solutions of
tartaric acid by Obs. W.T.
(From R. Engel)

Type B. Disliking sour.
Judgments of solutions of
tartaric acid by Obs. I.R.
(From R. Engel)

Fig. 39
(*From Engel*)

9%, which in turn was followed by a predominantly unpleasant region covering all concentrations above 9%. Both observers reported excessive consumption of sweets in their youth.

Weber's Law and Fechner's Law.—It was with reference to a characteristic closely related to hedonic tone that was formulated the first psychophysical equation—an equation destined, in slightly different form, to play an important role in psychology under the name Fechner's law. In the early eighteenth century, mathematicians were much interested in problems relating to gambling—owing no doubt to their frequent dependence upon rich patrons for whom gambling was an important pastime. These problems were discussed in terms of *value* to the players involved, but the value of a given chance of gain in a game was always assumed to be the same for any player, provided the objective conditions were the same. In other words, value of gain and chance of gain were assumed to be identical. This assumption was flatly rejected by Daniel Bernouilli [112] in a paper, entitled "Specimen theoriae novae de mensura sortis," published in 1738, in the proceedings of the Imperial Academy of Sciences of St. Petersburg.[113] A rich man, argued Bernouilli, secures less *advantage* from winning a given sum than does a poor man. The true state of affairs is best represented, according to Bernouilli, by the proposition "that any gain, however small, determines an advantage (emolumentum) which is inversely proportional to the fortune already at hand." [114] This proposition he later formulated in the equation

$$dy = \frac{b \, dx}{x}$$

in which dy represents an increment in advantage, dx an increment in fortune, x the original fortune, and b a constant. This differential equation implies that there must be between x (total fortune of a man) and y (advantage of this fortune to a man) a relationship of the form

$$y = b \log x + C$$

in which log x represents the natural logarithm· of x, and C a constant, for differentiation of the latter equation leads to the former differential equation.[115] The latter equation is the mathematical expression of Fechner's law, and thus Bernouilli may be considered to have maintained that the relationship between "advantage from fortune" and "fortune" followed a law whose mathematical expression was the same as that of Fechner's law.

Laplace[116] in his "Théorie analytique des probabilités," published in 1812, follows the same line of thought as Bernouilli, except that instead of speaking of "advantage from fortune" in relation to "fortune" he speaks of "moral fortune" in relation to "physical fortune." [117] By "physical fortune" Laplace means the totality of goods in the possession of a man. By "moral fortune" he means the value of these goods to their owner. After distinguishing the absolute value of a good from its relative value, i.e., its value to a particular individual, Laplace states that it is natural to suppose the relative value of an infinitely small sum to be directly proportional to its absolute value but inversely proportional to the total wealth of the individual involved. "For," he writes, "it is clear that a franc means little to him who possesses many, and that the most natural manner of estimating its relative worth is to suppose this worth to be inversely proportional to the number of francs possessed." [118] Laplace then proceeds to give this proposition a mathematical form: "According to this principle, x being the physical fortune of an individual, the increment dx which it receives, produces for the individual a moral good which is the reciprocal of this fortune. The increase of his moral fortune can consequently be expressed by $\frac{k \, dx}{x}$, k being a constant. Thus if one designate by y the moral fortune corresponding to the physical fortune x, one has

$$y = k \log x + \log h,$$

h being an arbitrary constant to be determined by means of a value of y corresponding to a given value of x." [119] Here again we have for the relationship between "moral fortune" and "physical fortune" the equation which is the mathematical expression of Fechner's law (h being a constant, log h is obviously also a constant and can be represented equally well by C).

The fact that the relationships established by Bernouilli and Laplace may be expressed in a mathematical form identical with the psychophysical function which he had derived from Weber's law led Fechner to consider these relationships as special cases of Weber's law. He wrote: "The physical goods which we own (physical fortune) have no value and no meaning for us as dead objects, but only insofar as they are means of arousing in us a sum of valuable sensations (moral fortune), with respect to which a thaler has much less value for the rich man than for the poor one, and while it makes a beggar happy a whole day long, the increment which it represents in the fortune of a millionaire is hardly appreciable to him. This may be subsumed under Weber's law." [120] But if the relationship between "moral fortune" and "physical fortune" is a special case of Weber's law, may one not infer that hedonic tone follows Weber's law? This has indeed been done by many psychologists. Titchener, for instance, in supporting his view that "there is some little evidence that affection, on its intensive side, obeys Weber's law," [121] first discussed the relation of hedonic tone to insistence, and then wrote: "At any rate, it is true as a general rule that what gives us pleasure or displeasure is roughly proportional to our income, our age and status, our ambition, our standard of comfort. If I am starting a library with a hundred volumes, and a single book is given to me, I am as pleased—other things being equal—as I should be by the addition of ten volumes to a library of a thousand." [122]

Is Fechner right in considering the relationships established by Bernouilli and Laplace to be special cases of Weber's law? It could well be objected that these relationships are based not on experimentation, but on casual observation. Such an objection, however, would not be conclusive. Experimentation might substantiate the relationship. There is another objection, however, which is indeed conclusive. Weber's law involves relationships between psychological magnitudes and *physical* magnitudes— magnitudes of *stimuli*. The relationships established by Bernouilli and Laplace are between psychological magni-

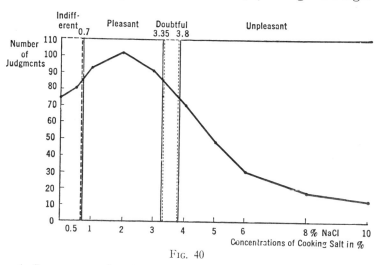

Fig. 40

1. Curve representing the preference judgments of 7 observers in paired comparisons of solutions of cooking salt. 2. Ideal regions calculated from absolute judgments of the same stimuli.

(From Engel)

tudes and *economic* magnitudes, magnitudes of money. Whether money is to be defined as purchasing power or in some other way, it is certainly not to be defined as a stimulus. The same stimulus—a silver coin, for instance— may at different times correspond to many different amounts of money, and the same amount of money may correspond to many different stimuli—e.g., to a cheque, to a bond, etc. It must be recognized, I think, that the relationships established by Bernouilli and Laplace, however similar their mathematical formulation may be to that adopted by Fechner for his extension of Weber's law, are in no wise special cases of Weber's law, and consequently are in no wise evidence that Weber's law holds in the case of hedonic tone.

Is there any other evidence that Weber's law holds for hedonic tone? No. There are, however, certain considerations which suggest that evidence of a limited applicability of Weber's law might be secured with proper experimental technique. Engel, it will be remembered, in studying the relation between hedonic tone and concentration of salt sub-

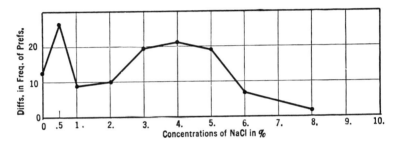

FIG. 41

(*Data from Engel*)

stances, established the frequencies of preference of ten different concentrations by the method of paired comparisons. The frequencies which he found are given in the curve on the preceding page.

At first sight it would seem that such a curve, with a distinct maximum, certainly precludes the applicability of Weber's law. Weber's law, however, says nothing about unidirectional variation in the psychological dimension correlated with physical intensity—it merely states that for all differential limens $\dfrac{\triangle R}{R} = K$. If now we plot differences in frequency of preference of adjacent concentrations regardless of sign beginning with the lowest concentration, we find that these differences decrease—though very irregularly—

as the concentration increases (cf. Fig. opposite). This makes it very likely that the hedonic differential limens, if they were established for different concentrations, would be found to increase with increase in concentration except in the case of concentrations near the optimum. Whether such an increase would conform to that required by the equation $\dfrac{\triangle R}{R} = K$, cannot be predicted in the absence of data, but it is a distinct possibility.

Although it is possible that Weber's law holds for hedonic tone in the case of concentrations other than optimal, it is quite certain that Fechner's law does not hold at all. Whereas it is conceivable that the equation $\dfrac{\triangle R}{R} = K$ might hold in the case of hedonic tone for all but optimal intensities in spite of the existence of a hedonic maximum, such a maximum absolutely precludes the applicability of the function $H = k \log R + K$ (in which H stands for hedonic tone). We have seen, however, that Engel's work makes it possible that the function relating hedonic tone to intensity of stimulus is *discontinuous*. Should this indeed be the case, and should Weber's law turn out to hold for hedonic tone, the function between hedonic tone and intensity of the stimulus would be of a form similar to that of Fechner's function, namely $|H| = k \log R + K$, in which $|H|$ stands for amount of hedonic tone without regard to sign.

Hedonic Tone in Relation to the Temporal Characteristics of Stimuli

Duration of Stimuli.—The relationship between hedonic tone and duration of stimulus was investigated by T. Nakashima in a series of experiments published in 1909.[123] In a first experiment, Nakashima sought to ascertain the *latent time* of hedonic tone, i.e., the minimal time necessary for the arousal of an experience characterized by hedonic tone. The assumption underlying this work was that if observers could give hedonic judgments upon each of a number of stimuli presented in immediate succession, the duration of each stimulus must be sufficient to allow the arousal of an experience characterized by hedonic tone. Otherwise, displacement of the experience by a new one would preclude hedonic judgment. As stimuli, Nakashima used 32 pairs of Milton-Bradley colored papers exposed in immediate succession with six different durations of exposition, varying from 6.3″ to .84″. His observers, 8 in number, were instructed to judge the hedonic tone of each experience in terms of the numbers 1 to 7, representing 7 values from very pleasant (1) to very unpleasant (7). The data showed that with a decrease of the time of exposure there occurred a marked increase in the number of indifferent judgments and a tendency for the hedonic value of colors to converge towards indifference. They also showed that all observers reported pleasant or unpleasant experiences even for the shortest time of exposure, namely 0.84″. Some of the observers, however, were of the opinion that their hedonic judgments for exposures of 0.84″ and 0.98″ might have been made from memory, although all agreed that for exposures of 1.26″ the experiences were definitely pleasant or unpleasant. Nakashima concludes that "affective intensity decreases with decrease of time of exposure" and that "the shortest time necessary for an affection to arise varies from 0.84 to 0.98 sec." [124] In both these experiments all observers "were certain that there was no single case in which affection appeared simultaneously with, or earlier than, the sensation. It always appeared distinctly later than the cognition of the impression." [125]

In a further experiment, Nakashima sought to determine not the latent time of hedonic tone, but its *action-time*, i.e., the shortest duration of exposure adequate to arouse an experience characterized by pleasantness or unpleasantness. The stimuli were 55 pictures. Each picture was presented singly by means of a tachistoscope. By the method of limits Nakashima determined for 10 observers the minimal time of exposure adequate to arouse pleasant, indifferent and unpleasant experiences. It was found that the average minimal exposure-time varied for the different observers from .390″ to .515″, while that for indifference varied from .390″ to .500″. (Indifference referred in this experiment to characteristics of feelings other than pleasantness or unpleasantness, e.g., strain.) Thus it is seen that these times are much the same for pleasantness, unpleasantness and indifference. Nakashima further points out that they are of the same order of magnitude as those for sensory reactions, but a little longer.[126] He also found in general that "All the observers agreed that although feeling appeared only after a more or less clear perception of the stimulus, the temporal disjunction was in most cases very slight." [127]

In a third set of experiments, Nakashima sought to determine hedonic reaction-times to various stimuli and to compare these to sensory reaction-times for the same stimuli. The averages of the reaction-times for color stimuli and for tonal stimuli were as follows:

TABLE XXVIII

Color Stimuli

Obs.	Sensory R.-T. in sec.	Hedonic R.-T. in sec.
R	.343	.471
P	.470	.697
G	.441	1.043

Tonal Stimuli

Obs.	Sensory R.-T. in sec.	Hedonic R.-T. in sec.
G	.344	.783
P	.304	.579
W	.392	.632
K	.375	.679

Nakashima points out that the times for hedonic reactions are in all cases decidedly longer than for simple cognitive reactions, a result which agrees with those of the former experiment, which showed the minimal time of exposure for the arousal of pleasant, indifferent or unpleasant experiences to be longer than that for the arousal of purely cognitive experiences. Again in this experiment there was found no case in which hedonic tone appeared before cognitive content.

Nakashima's general conclusions from the three sets of experiments described above were essentially as follows:

1. The arousal of an hedonic experience requires longer than that of a purely sensory experience.

2. Hedonic times and their variability are either abso-

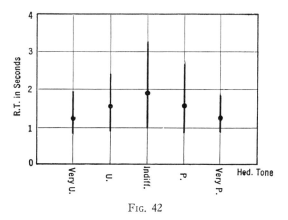

Fig. 42

(*After Potter, Tuttle and Washburn*)

lutely or relatively of the same order as sensory times and their variability.

Another investigation of hedonic reaction-times was published in 1914 by Potter, Tuttle and Washburn.[128] The results confirmed in general those of Nakashima, but also yielded interesting information on the relation of hedonic reaction-times to the degree of hedonic tone. The stimuli were colored papers. The observers, 25 in number, were instructed to judge whether the colors—which were presented singly—were pleasant, indifferent or unpleasant. They were also told that they might add. "very pleasant" or "very unpleasant" when such was the case. The time elapsing between exposure of the color and the making of the judgment was recorded in the case of each presentation. The results are shown in the graph opposite. Ordinates indicate reaction-times in seconds. The five types of hedonic judgments are represented along the axis of abscissae. In the case of each type of judgment, the range of reaction-times for all observers is represented by a line, and the average by a dot. From these results the investigators draw the following conclusions:

1. "There is no difference whatever between the average time required for judgments of pleasantness and that required for judgments of unpleasantness.

2. "It takes on the average .3 sec. longer to make judgments of moderate pleasantness or unpleasantness than to make an extreme judgment under either category.

3. "It takes about .3 sec. longer to make a judgment of indifference than to make one of moderate pleasantness or unpleasantness." [129]

Two further experiments upon hedonic reaction-times have been reported by F. L. Wells. In the first, Wells studied hedonic reaction-times to visual stimuli,—to 40 pictures of women's faces, 20 beautiful and 20 ugly.[130] The observers were shown the pictures singly, with instructions to raise the right hand if a picture were attractive, the left if it were unattractive. The time between exposure of the picture and the raising of the hand was recorded. Wells summarized his results as follows: "The average times (σ) observed ranged between 500 and 850, a central score being about 700. These findings are thus in substantial agreement with Nakashima's despite the difference in procedure." He concludes: "The general evidence of these findings is that affective reactions, even in the minor intensities here dealt with, are not uncommonly established within periods of the order of four-fifths of a second." [131]

In a second experiment, Wells investigated hedonic reaction-times to olfactory stimuli.[132] Ten odors, 5 presumably pleasant, 5 presumably unpleasant, were presented singly to 11 observers, with instructions to judge the hedonic tone of the corresponding experiences. The observers wore pneumographs, and the reaction-times were calculated from breathing curves recorded upon a kymograph. The reaction-time was defined as the interval between the beginning of the inspiration immediately following the beginning of stimulation, and the beginning of the irregular breathing movements accompanying vocalization of the judgment. Wells gives the results in the following statement: "The general average time of reporting a stimulus as pleasant or unpleasant approximates 0.88 sec. after the beginning of inspiration. The average time of every S's reactions ranges between 0.7 and 1.38 sec., the mean variation of these quantities is 0.22 sec. There was no determinable difference between the reaction-times for the pleasant and unpleasant odors, indeed the averages for the ten odors differ little, ranging from 0.83-0.96 sec., with mean variation of 0.05 sec." [133]

In a subsequent repetition of the experiment, 9 of the preceding 11 observers reacted again to the same stimuli, but their reaction-times were measured in a different way. The observers were instructed to *sniff* of the stimuli, and to indicate the resulting hedonic tone by a reaction with the right hand if the experience were pleasant and with the left hand if the experience were unpleasant. The beginning of the sniff was registered by a pneumograph which "made" a circuit through a galvanometric chronograph, and the beginning of the hand-movement was registered by release of a telegraph key, resulting in a "break" of the chronograph circuit. This second procedure yielded hedonic reaction-times markedly shorter than had the first. Wells writes: "The general average of the choice times in these observations is 555 sigma. The individual averages range between 369 and 905 sigma. The average of their mean variations is 109 sigma, relatively less than the variation in the kymograph series (previous procedure). . . . As before, no difference is disclosed between the reaction-times of the pleasant and unpleasant stimuli." [134]

It is difficult to compare these reaction-times—those secured with either the first procedure or the second—with non-hedonic reaction-times to olfactory stimuli. According to Wells, the latter vary from 207 sigma according to Moldenhauer, to 600-1000 sigma according to Zwaardemaker. If, however, one take Moldenhauer's times as the more probable because of their greater consistency with results secured in other fields, it is clear that in the case of olfactory stimuli, as in the case of visual stimuli, hedonic reaction-times are distinctly greater than are sensory ones.

Besides the problems of hedonic latent times, action-times and reaction-times, the relation of hedonic tone to the duration of stimuli involves the problem of *adaptation:* How does the hedonic tone of a phenomenon vary as the duration of the corresponding stimulus increases beyond the action-time? According to Lehmann, the early stages of this variation are in general the same for all stimuli: they involve a shift of hedonic tone in the direction of indifference. On the other hand, the later stages differ for different stimuli in that "feelings of pleasure continually decrease and finally turn into displeasure, whereas feelings of displeasure decrease at most to zero." [135] Furthermore, the rapidity of the whole process of adaptation varies from one stimulus to another. It is slower for stimuli arousing unpleasantness than for those arousing pleasantness, and slower in the case of stimuli arousing complex phenomena than in the case of those arousing simple phenomena. As to the basis of adaptation, it is always, according to Lehmann, a change in the cognitive characteristics of the phenomena experienced. This change may be due to (a) sensory adaptation, (b) addition of new sensory components due to organic changes brought about by the stimulus, (c) shift of attention.

Lehmann's account is based almost wholly on casual observation. It is consequently in great need of experimental verification. Unfortunately there is but one experiment available concerning this topic, and this single experiment is far from conclusive. In 1911, Crawford

and Washburn published a research in which they had
studied fluctuations of the hedonic tone of colors during
fixation for one minute.[136] Eighteen colored papers were
presented to 14 observers by the method of single stimuli.
"Each piece of paper was laid on a white ground before the
observer, who was asked to express her judgment as to
its pleasantness or unpleasantness by using one of the numbers from 1 to 7 in the ordinary way. The observer was
further asked to look steadily at the color for an interval
of one minute, measured by the experimenter, and to report
by means of the appropriate numbers any changes in the
affective value of the color. At the end of the period of
fixation, she was asked to give the reason for the changes
which had occurred." [137] In about $\frac{3}{4}$ of the presentations
some fluctuations in hedonic tone did occur. The causes of
these fluctuations were classified by the writers as follows:

A. Change in color itself.
   (a) Sensory adaptation.
   (b) Negative after-image.

B. Purely mental causes.
   (a) Associated ideas.
   (b) "Getting used to" and "getting tired of" colors.

Three of these four types of causes clearly involve changes
in the cognitive characteristics of the phenomenon. As to
the fourth type, it occurred very seldom. The authors
write: "Both of these last comments ('getting used to it' and
'getting tired of it') were surprisingly rare; getting used to
the color was mentioned only 6 times as a cause of increased
pleasantness, and getting tired of a color was 22 times given
as a cause of increased unpleasantness. This is in comparison with one hundred and twenty-seven cases where change
was due to the occurrence of an association." [138] As to the
direction in which hedonic tone varied in these fluctuations,
the data made it possible to determine this only in the case
of fluctuations due to association and adaptation. For these
two types of causes, the writers conclude as follows:

"Broadly speaking, the tendency of associated ideas is to raise the pleasantness of a color, and the tendency of (purely affective) adaptation is to lower it rather than raise it." [139]

This latter conclusion, however, rests upon an interpretation of the data in which not sufficient regard is given to the influence of chance-variability. The authors point out that a color whose hedonic tone is judged "7" at the outset can only decrease in value, while one judged "1" can only increase in value. "On the other hand," they write, "by far the greatest number of changes in affective value that occurred under the conditions of this experiment were changes of one place only in the scale. Therefore, if the initial value of a color were anything but 7 or 1, the chances were about equal for a rise or a fall. It ought to be sufficient, then, to correct our comparison of the number of rises in affective value produced by a given cause for a given color with the number of falls, by taking account merely of the number of maximum and minimum judgments of initial affective value made for that color." [140] But at the close of the chapter on methods I showed that the tendency for chance variability to cause a decrease in hedonic rank rather than an increase holds not only for the highest rank, but also for all ranks above the median. It follows that the mere taking into account of judgments of 7 and 1 made upon a color, by no means gives a complete picture of the direction in which chance variability will tend to change the hedonic tone of that color. From this in turn it follows that the results of Crawford and Washburn with respect to the direction and extent of hedonic fluctuations may have been due to a statistical artifact and consequently that the conclusion drawn from these results, though it may be perfectly valid, may equally well be entirely erroneous.

Insofar as the experiment of Crawford and Washburn deals with *causes* of fluctuations, its results are not subject to the source of error mentioned above. This phase of the experiment obviously supports in general Lehmann's contention that adaptation corresponds to a change in the cognitive characteristics of the phenomenon under observation.

It does not fully support this contention, however, because of the occurrence of a few cases of fluctuation ascribed by the observers to "getting tired" of the colors.

We may conclude, I think, that Lehmann's account of adaptation is reasonable, but that it must be considered as little more than a guess until further experimental data have been secured.

Temporal Form of Stimuli.—Just as completeness appears to be a very important condition for the pleasantness of *spatial* forms, so it appears to be a very important condition for the pleasantness of *temporal* forms. To take a very simple illustration, many melodic intervals are more pleasant when played in one order than the other, and this greater pleasantness is accompanied by a character of finality attached to the second tone. Concerning the fifth (2:3), for instance, Bingham writes: "If one hears it as an ascending interval, he is dissatisfied, uneasy, and under more or less tension until he hears the first tone over again. But if it is a descending fifth which he hears, there is acquiescence, satisfaction, repose, and no desire to hear the first tone a second time." [141] Again, two tones may require for finality and pleasantness not merely a specific order, but the playing of some third tone different from both the original ones. In certain experiments upon this problem, Bingham presented to five observers various successive musical intervals, asking, "Do you feel any desire to return to the first tone?" Three of the observers persistently found an additional alternative in the case of certain intervals: "the melody lacked finality, there was no desire to return, neither tone would serve as an end tone but some third tone was demanded." [142]

The same emphasis upon completeness is found in discussions of melodies. In her "Psychology of Beauty," E. D. Puffer quotes with approval the following passage by Gurney: "The melody may begin by pressing its way through a sweetly yielding resistance to a gradually foreseen climax; whence again fresh expectation is bred, perhaps for another excursion, as it were, round the same centre but with a bolder and freer sweep . . . to a point where again the motive is suspended on another temporary goal; till after a certain number of such involutions and evolutions, and of delicately poised leanings and reluctances and yieldings, the forces so accurately measured just suffice to bring it home, and the sense of potential and coming integration which has underlain all our provisional adjustments of expectation is triumphantly justified." [143] Puffer comments: "This should not be taken as a more or less practical account under the metaphor of motion. These 'leanings' are literal in the sense that one note does imply another as its natural complement and satisfaction and we seek to reach or make it. The striving is an intrinsic element, not a by-product for our understanding." [144]

Temporal completeness, like spatial completeness, is a characteristic of phenomena, not of stimuli. In the case of the latter, as in the case of the former, we are at present wholly ignorant of the corresponding physical characteristics—indeed, our only reason for assuming the existence of such characteristics is belief in the Gestalt school's contention that phenomenal configurations are largely dependent upon physical configurations.

It is difficult for me to think of any specific feature of temporal form, other than completeness, which is known to co-vary with hedonic tone. Is this not a confession of ignorance? Is not the aesthetics of music largely concerned with the pleasantness of temporal configuration? The latter question is obviously to be answered in the affirmative, but I am not so sure about the former. In the first place, works on the aesthetics of music are *justifications* of music rather than *evaluations* of music. Consider Gehring's book, "The Basis of Musical Pleasure." [145] Chapter II deals with "Form." Does it discuss the co-variation of hedonic tone and specific characteristics of auditory configurations? It does not. It discusses the formal characteristics of music, but unless one accept the dubious premise that current music is the best possible music, this discussion has no very definite bearing on the problem of the relation of hedonic tone to temporal forms. Even if, however, one accept this premise, available works on the aesthetics of musical configurations are not very illuminating. Gurney, in his classical book, "The Power of Sound," does indeed point out that rhythm must involve *small* groups of sound separated by *small* intervals of time.[146] The interpretation of small, however, is left to the reader. Indeed, when it comes to melody, one is confronted by a problem rather than a solution. In an address before the VIth International Congress of Mathematics held at Bologna in 1928, G. D. Birkhoff wrote: ". . . So far the real nature of the beauty of a simple melody remains a mystery. Helmholtz, who discovered much on the nature of harmony, made little progress in explaining the obvious facts of melody. Gurney, who studied this problem of melody from the point of view of form, was convinced that the factor of order was not essential. He believes in a special 'musical faculty' which is able to judge the 'ideal movement' constituting the soul of music, but he considers this musical faculty and this ideal movement to be beyond scientific explanation. . . . As for myself, I believe that in melody it is order alone which counts, but by order I mean hidden order as well as obvious order. At all events, there exists a mathematical problem of melody: to determine to what extent relations of order between notes constitute the effective cause of melody. . . ." [147] The solution of this problem would indeed constitute a tremendous step forward in the aesthetics of music. In the meantime the formal characteristics of melody continue to be shrouded in mystery. There is no denying that tonal configurations constitute a wonderful material for the study of the relation of hedonic tone to temporal form. Unless I am misled by ignorance, however, such a study is almost wholly a matter for the future.

Temporal Position of Stimuli (the "Hedonic Time Error") —The relation of hedonic tone to the temporal position of the stimulus has been dealt with only in connection with the problem of the hedonic time-error. K. Danzfuss, in 1923, showed that when observers are made to compare the hedonic tone corresponding to two successive tonal stimuli separated by an interval of two seconds there is a marked tendency for the second stimulus to be preferred.[148] Since that time, a number of minor experiments upon the time error have been performed at Harvard.[149] The technique of these latter experiments is very simple. All possible pairs of a set of stimuli are presented for successive comparison not merely once, but twice, each pair being presented in both possible time orders. The experimenter then determines the percentage of times that the 1st is preferred to the 2nd. As each pair is presented both in the order a b and the order b a, it is clear that for each time the first is preferred there should be a time when the second is preferred. Thus the frequency of cases in which the first is preferred should be—if there were no time-error—50%. Actually, however, the frequency of cases in which the second is preferred when the interval between stimuli is 20 seconds has been found with some observers to be as great as 70%.

The table below summarizes the results secured by Danzfuss and by experimenters at Harvard. The first column gives the interval of time between the two stimuli being compared; the second column indicates the type of stimulus

TABLE XXIX

Interval	Stim.	Predominant Time-error	Degree of Predominance	Investigator
1.5 sec.	tones	1st preferred	3/3	J. Moscovitz
2 sec.	tones	2nd preferred	1/1	J. Moscovitz
2 sec.	tones	2nd preferred	?	K. Danzfuss
20 sec.	tones	2nd preferred	3/4	J. Moscovitz
20 sec.	odors	2nd preferred	3/4	E. J. Ludvigh and J. G. Beebe-Center

employed; the third column gives the type of time-error found to predominate, i.e., the type found in the results of the greater number of observers; the fourth column gives the degree of predominance in terms of the ratio of the number of observers displaying the predominant time-error to the total number of observers; the fifth column gives the name of the experimenter. It will be seen that these results indicate a very definite relationship between the predominant time-error and the interval between stimuli. It would seem that whereas the *first* stimulus is preferred with an interval of 1.5 sec., it is the *second* which is preferred with intervals of 2 or more secs.

These results are very suggestive in view of the work of Köhler with respect to the time-error in judgments of auditory intensity.[150] He found that for intervals under 3 sec. the *first* stimulus was judged *louder* more often than it should have been, and that for intervals over 3 sec. the *second* stimulus was judged *louder* more often than it should have been. Moreover, he found that as the interval in-

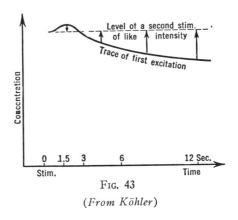

FIG. 43

(*From Köhler*)

creased beyond 3 sec. the extent of the "negative" time-error (second louder) likewise increased. He inferred that the time-error in sensory judgments was due to variation of the trace of the nervous process aroused by the first stimulus, this variation being an *increase* in its quantity from 0 to 3 sec., followed by a decrease beyond 3 sec. (cf. Fig.). It is obvious that the data available concerning the hedonic time-error are too scanty to warrant much speculation concerning their interpretation. Should further investigations, however, yield similar data, it would be natural to interpret the hedonic time-error in a fashion similar to that applied by Köhler to the intensive time-error. Such an interpretation would obviously lead to a hypothesis according to which the neural correlate of pleasantness is a *large* quantity of some central neural process aroused by sense-organ stimulation, while the basis for unpleasantness is a *small* quantity of the same process.

GENERAL HEDONIC VALUE

We have seen that variation in the qualitative, spatial, intensive or temporal characteristics of the primary stimulus determines a definite variation in the *average* hedonic tone of the corresponding phenomenon. On the other hand we have seen that this co-variation does not permit prediction of the hedonic tone corresponding to the primary stimulus in the case of any individual observer. This state of affairs obviously suggests that there is a definite relation between primary stimulus and hedonic tone, identical for all observers, but that this relation is obscured in the case of any single observer by the "chance" operation of a number of determinants of hedonic tone other than the primary stimulus. Is there any way in which we can verify this suggestion?

The best form of verification would be a positive one: actual demonstration. If there were a definite relation between primary stimulus and hedonic tone, then in an experimental situation where all determinants of hedonic tone other than the primary stimulus were held constant, variation of the primary stimulus should *in all observers* result in the same variation of hedonic tone. This form of verification, however, is far beyond our possibilities. We do not even know all the major determinants of hedonic tone, and if we did, we could not control many of them—past experience, for instance. Fortunately, positive verification, although the best, is not the only form of verification. Where positive verification fails, we can resort to negative verification in which we do not demonstrate a given relation, but demonstrate that such a relation is not inconsistent with relevant data. Is it possible to verify in this negative manner the existence of a definite relation between hedonic tone and the primary stimulus?

The first step towards a solution of this problem is to notice that it may be formulated in a different manner. If data on the co-variation of primary stimulus and hedonic tone be consistent with the existence of a definite relation between primary stimulus and hedonic tone, then such data must likewise be consistent with ascription to primary stimuli of a *general hedonic value,* in the sense of a hedonic potentiality independent of individual observers. Conversely, if it can be shown that data on the co-variation of primary stimulus and hedonic tone are consistent with ascription to primary stimuli of a general hedonic value, it must follow that these data are consistent with the existence of a definite relation between primary stimulus and hedonic tone. The problem stated above may consequently be reformulated as follows: Are data on the co-variation of primary stimulus and hedonic tone consistent with ascription to primary stimuli of a general hedonic value?

In the field of mental testing one of the most important problems has been that of ascertaining whether individuals may be considered to have a general intellectual ability which manifests itself to a greater or lesser degree in all mental tests. A method of solving this problem has been provided by Spearman. The method involves the application of the equation

$$r_{ap} \times r_{bq} - r_{aq} \times r_{bp} = 0$$

called by Spearman the *tetrad equation* and representing a particular type of intercorrelation between four abilities a, b, p, and q. Spearman writes: "Whenever the tetrad equation holds throughout any table of correlations, and *only* when it does so, then every individual measurement of every ability (or of any other variable that enters into the table) can be divided into two independent parts which possess the following momentous properties. The one part has been called the 'general factor' and denoted by the letter g; it is so named because, although varying freely from individual to individual, it remains the same for any one individual in respect of all the correlated abilities. The second part has been called the 'specific factor' and denoted by the letter s. It not only varies from individual to individual, but even for any one individual from each ability to another." [151]

Spearman points out that the application of this theorem is quite general—indeed, he states that it is not even restricted to psychology. It is consequently perfectly legitimate to extend it from the field of mental testing to that of hedonic tone, provided only that it be possible to interpret the terms involved in the theorem in such a way as to fit the data of experiments upon affection. Let us try to do so.

Let us first of all consider the judgments of an observer O_1 upon the hedonic tone of a set of stimuli S_1, S_2, S_3 . . . S_n to be measurements of the *ability* of these stimuli to please observer O_1. We can for short say that they are measurements of the ability A_{o_1} of stimuli S_1, S_2, S_3 . . . S_n. Let us likewise consider the hedonic judgments of observers O_2, O_3 . . . O_n upon S_1, S_2, S_3, . . . S_n to be measurements of abilities A_{o_2}, A_{o_3} . . . A_{o_n} of these stimuli. Clearly if we establish the hedonic rank order of stimuli S_1, S_2, S_3 . . . S_n for observers O_1, O_2, O_3 . . . O_n and intercorrelate these rank orders we can arrange the results in the form of a table which indicates the degree of correlation between any two of the abilities A_{o_1}, A_{o_2}, A_{o_3} . . . A_{o_n} (i.e., between any two of the abilities of the stimuli to please observers O_1, O_2, O_3 . . . O_n). Now according to the theorem quoted above from Spearman, if the tetrad equation holds throughout such a table and only if it does, every individual measurement of every ability can be divided into two factors, a general factor "g," and a specific factor "s," the former (g), although varying freely from individual to individual, remaining the same for any one individual in respect of all correlated abilities. But according to our conventions, "ability" is "ability to please," and the "individuals" are the stimuli. Thus if in a table of correlations arranged as indicated, the tetrad equation holds throughout, and only if it does, we may conceive that there is a general characteristic which, although varying freely from stimulus to stimulus, remains the same for any one stimulus in respect of all correlated abilities to please the different observers —that, in brief, the stimuli involved have a general hedonic value for the observers involved, in spite of the divergences of the hedonic judgments of the individual observers.

If the considerations above be legitimate, the application of Spearman's method to hedonic tone enables one not only to judge the legitimacy of assuming a general hedonic factor in the case of a given class of stimuli, but also, to ascertain the degree of generality of such a factor. This degree of generality is clearly equal to the proportion of unselected observers whose hedonic ranking of the stimuli when intercorrelated yields coefficients of correlation which satisfy the tetrad equation.[152]   Should it be found that any group of observers chosen at random satisfies these conditions, the general hedonic factor may be considered to be entirely general.

But further—provided always that our theoretical considerations be correct—the application which we are proposing for Spearman's method enables us to ascertain the degree to which the general hedonic factor is operative in the judgments of any given observer and its value in the various individual stimuli. This information can be secured very easily by applying to appropriate hedonic data the formulae proposed by Spearman for computing the correlation between a specific ability and "g," [153] and for computing the amount of "g" of a specific individual.[154]

It might be added that this line of thought suggests a ready means of distinguishing aesthetic hedonic value from non-aesthetic—hedonic value being considered aesthetic in proportion as it is general in the sense in which the term is used above. It also suggests a means of distinguishing between the aesthetically sensitive and the aesthetically dull. Given a set of aesthetic objects, i.e., objects to which there have been assigned entirely general hedonic values in the sense in which the term is used above, the aesthetic sensitivity of an individual to these objects could be considered a function of the correlation between the hedonic values assigned by him to the objects and their general hedonic values. What results are yielded by the actual application of Spearman's method to appropriate hedonic data? In the course of an experiment upon hedonic habituation carried out at Harvard in 1925-26, I had occasion to determine the hedonic rank orders of 14 olfactory substances for each of 8 observers.[155] Intercorrelation of these rank orders yielded the Spearman co-efficients given in the table below.[156]

TABLE XXX

	Ad.	Br.	Bu.	De.	Ka.	Ke.	Wa.	Zc.
Ad.		.62	.30	.40	.60	.37	—.21	.27
Br.	.62		.74	.81	.72	.69	.35	.45
Bu.	.30	.74		.66	.66	.88	.58	.38
De.	.40	.81	.66		.76	.64	.53	.66
Ka.	.60	.72	.66	.76		.73	.48	.45
Ke.	.37	.69	.88	.64	.73		.63	.54
Wa. ...	—.21	.35	.58	.53	.48	.63		.33
Ze.	.27	.45	.38	.66	.45	.54	.33	

Do these correlations indicate that olfactory substances may be considered to have a general hedonic value which determines in part the hedonic judgments of these eight observers? In order to answer this question we determine the 420 tetrad differences involved in the intercorrelation of 8 variables and compare their distribution around zero to the distribution which could be expected from errors of sampling for a set of tetrad differences equal in number and of like probable error. The tetrad differences t.d. are given by the formula

$$\text{t.d.} = r_{ap} \times r_{bq} - r_{aq} \times r_{bp},$$

in which a, b, p and q represent four abilities and r_{ap} represents the correlation between abilities a and p, r_{bq} the correlation between abilities b and q, etc.[157]   The probable error is best given, according to Spearman, by the formula

$$p.e. = \frac{1.349}{N^{\frac{1}{2}}} [r^2(1-r)^2 + (1-R)S^2]^{\frac{1}{2}}$$

in which

$$R = 3r \frac{n-4}{n-2} - 2r^2 \frac{n-6}{n-2}.$$

N is the number of individuals tested, n the number of abilities involved, r the mean of the correlations taken into

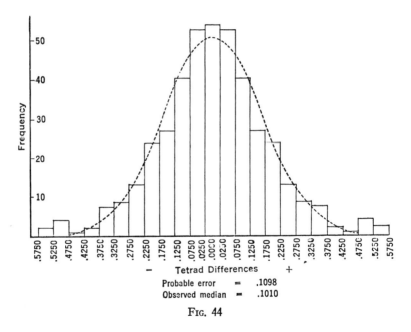

Probable error   =   .1098
Observed median   =   .1010

FIG. 44

account, and S^2 the mean squared deviation of all the correlations from their mean.[158]   In Fig. 44, the observed distribution is indicated by a continuous line; the theoretical distribution to be expected from errors of sampling alone is indicated by a broken line. The two distributions are practically identical. According to Spearman, this indicates that the table satisfies the tetrad criterion and consequently if our previous theoretical considerations be correct, we may infer the likelihood that olfactory substances may be considered to have a general hedonic value which we may call h_{olf}. I say "likelihood" because it is clear that both the number of olfactory substances and the number of observers were too small in this experiment to allow a high degree of probability in the conclusions. This deficiency, however, can easily be remedied by more extensive investigation.

The fact that our first question is answered positively at once raises two further questions: (1) To what extent does the general hedonic value h_{olf} of our olfactory substances determine the hedonic judgments of our observers; and (2) What are the general hedonic values of our olfactory substances?

The first question may be answered as follows: According to Spearman, the correlation between the general factor "g" and any ability a is given by the formula[159]

$$r_{ag} = (A^2 - A')^{\frac{1}{2}} / (T - 2A)^{\frac{1}{2}},$$

where "A is the sum of the correlations between a and every other test, A' is the sum of the squares of these correlations, and T is the total of all the correlations in the whole table." [160] But in our case "g" is the general hedonic value of the olfactory substances and a is the ability of these substances to please a given observer. This equation consequently enables us to calculate the correlation between the general hedonic value of the substances and their hedonic value to the various individual observers, and thus to ascertain the part which the general hedonic value of the substances plays in the judgments of the various observers. Application of the equation yields the following results.

TABLE XXXI

Observers	Correlation between General Hedonic Value of Olfactory Substances and their Hedonic Value to Particular Observers
De.	.89
Ke.	.89
Ka.	.88
Br.	.87
Bu.	.83
Ze.	.58
Wa.	.48
Ad.	.41

Clearly if our theoretical considerations be correct and if one disregard the fact that our data are very limited in scope, it is possible to infer that observers De. and Ke. judge olfactory substances far more in accord with their general hedonic value than do observers Wa. and Ad. From this in turn it is possible, if one accept the definition of "aesthetically sensitive" given above, to state that De. and Ke. are aesthetically more sensitive to odors than are Wa. and Ad.

The second question raised above, that concerning the general hedonic values of the olfactory substances involved in the experiment, may be answered as follows. According to Spearman, the amount of "g" for any individual x tested by a battery of tests a, b. . .z is proportional to G_x as defined by the equation

$$G_x = W_a \times M_{ax} + W_b \times M_{bx} + \cdots + W_x \times M_{zx},$$

in which M_{ax}, M_{bx} . . . M_{zx} indicate the scores of individual x in tests a, b. . .z; and W_a, W_b . . . W_z indicate optimal weights to be given to the respective scores.[161] These optimal weights in turn are best determined according to Spearman by the formula

$$W_u = r_{ug}/(1 - r^2_{ug}),$$

in which u is any one of tests a, b. . . .z.[162] But in our case "g" is the general hedonic value of odors and a, b. . .z are the abilities of these odors to please different observers. These equations consequently enable us to ascertain the closest approximation possible from our data for the general hedonic values of the different olfactory substances used by us. Application of these equations yields the following general ranks for the 14 olfactory substances used in the experiment (the measurement of the hedonic values of the odors in the experiment was by the method of paired comparison and yielded only rank orders):

TABLE XXXII

Rank	Olfactory Substances
1 (most pleasant)	Sweet Orange
2.............................	Extract of Carnation
3.............................	Oil of Jasmin
4.............................	" " Bergamot
5.............................	" " Ylang
6.............................	" " Cloves
7.............................	" " Ceylon Cinnamon
8.............................	" " White Rose (synthet.)
9.............................	" " Neroli bitter
10............................	" " Cananga
11............................	" " Petit grain
12............................	" " Thyme
13............................	" " Rosemary
14 (least pleasant)	" " Geranium

It is interesting to note that this rank order agrees very highly with that determined by the mere summing of the ranks assigned to the odors by the different observers. The correlation between the two rank orders is .98 by the Spearman formula. It is clear that the summing of ranks, whether weighted or not, introduces a large source of error when these ranks are considered to represent, as in this case, serial position with respect to an intensive continuum. The same source of error is present, however, in the use of Spearman's rank correlation formula, and this formula has nevertheless been of great value of psychology.

It is clear that application of Spearman's method to these data indicates that olfactory stimuli may be considered to have general hedonic values, makes it possible to determine these values in the case of individual odors, and shows that these values are closely approximated by the average hedonic tone of the odors. It follows, from the considerations mentioned at the beginning of this section, that the data are consistent with the existence of a general relation between olfactory substances and hedonic tone, and that this relation is approximated with considerable accuracy by the co-variation of these substances and of average hedonic tone. Whether a similar state of affairs obtains with respect to all stimuli cannot at present be decided. An as yet unpublished investigation by Mr. E. J. Ludvigh, however, shows that it does obtain in the case of colors. There is consequently some likelihood that further investigation will show the legitimacy of inferring that observed co-variations between stimulus and average hedonic tone are close approximations of general relations between such variables, and that individual divergencies from these co-variations are due to the operation of determinants of hedonic tone other than the primary stimulus.

FOOTNOTES AND REFERENCES

1 M. WERTHEIMER. Experimentelle Studien über das Sehen von Bewegung, Z. f. Psychol., 61, 1912, 253 seq.

2 M. YOKOYAMA. Affective Tendency as Conditioned by Color and Form, Amer. J. Psychol., 32, 1921, 82. Yokoyama cites the following references: W. WUNDT, Phys-Psychol., 6 Aufl., 1910, II, 351 ff; O. KÜLPE, Outlines of Psychology, trans., 3 ed., 1909, 264; W. McDOUGALL, Physiological Psychology, 1905, 80; Body and Mind, 3 ed., 1915, 313; E. B. TITCHENER, Textbook of Psychology, 1910, 258.

3 Cf. M. YOKOYAMA, op. cit., 82. Yokoyama gives a bibliography of the early works dealing incidentally with the topic.

4 L. R. GEISSLER. The Affective Tone of Color-combinations, in Studies in Psychology Contributed by Colleagues and Former Students of E. B. TITCHENER, Worcester, 1917, 150-174.

5 GEISSLER also used an alternative method of treating the data, but as its results were in general the same as those secured by the method outlined above, we shall disregard both the alternate method and its results.

6 L. R. GEISSLER, op. cit., 160.

7 Ibid., 174.

8 M. F. WASHBURN, D. HAIGHT and J. REGENSBURG. The Relation of the Pleasantness of Color Combinations to That of Colors Seen Singly, Amer. J. Psychol., 32, 1921, 145.

[9] *Ibid.*, 145-6.

[10] *Ibid.*, 146.

[11] *Ibid.*, 146.

[12] M. YOKOYAMA. Affective Tendency as Conditioned by Color and Form, *Amer. J. Psychol.*, 32, 1921, 81.

[13] *Ibid.*, 102.

[14] *Ibid.*, 103.

[15] J. COHN. Experimentelle Untersuchungen über die Gefühlsbetönung der Farben, Helligkeiten und ihrer Combinationen, *Philos. Stud.*, 10, 1894, 599.

[16] T. ZIEHEN. Leitfaden der physiologischen Psychologie, 10th Edit., 1914, 207.

[17] K. DANZFUSS. *Philos u. Psychol. Arbeiten,* 1923, No. 5, 87.

[18] *Ibid.*, 87.

[19] J. COHN. Experimentelle Untersuchungen über die Gefühlsbetönung der Farben, Helligkeiten und ihrer Combinationen, *Philos. Stud.*, 10, 1894, 562-603.

[20] *Ibid.*, 599-600.

[21] D. R. MAJOR. On the Affective Tone of Simple Sense Impressions, *Amer. J. Psychol.*, 7, 1895, 57.

[22] *Ibid.*, 76.

[23] J. COHN. Gefühlston und Sättigung der Farben, *Philos. Stud.*, 15, 1899, 279.

[24] E. J. G. BRADFORD. On the Relation and Aesthetic Value of the Perceptive Types in Color Appreciation, *Amer. J. Psychol.*, 24, 1913, 545.

[25] M. LUCKIESH. A Note on Color Preference, *Amer. J. Psychol.*, 27, 1916, 251.

[26] *Ibid.*, 255.

[27] JASTROW is said to have secured the judgments of 4500 visitors to the world's fair in Chicago upon six colors. The results are said to have been as follows: (reading from most pleasant to least pleasant) blue, red, light blue, blue-violet, red-violet, and light red-violet. The reference given —which I cannot verify—is: The Popular Aesthetics of Color, *Popular Science Monthly*, 1897, 361 ff.

[28] E. J. G. BRADFORD. *Amer. J. Psychol.*, 24, 1913, 545.

[29] M. F. WASHBURN. A note on the Affective Value of Colors, *Amer. J. Psychol.*, 22, 1911, 114.

[30] M. LUCKIESH. Color and Its Application, N. Y., 1915, 263.

[31] L. R. GEISSLER. Studies in Psychology, Titchener Memorial Volume, Worcester, 1917, 172.

[32] F. M. MERCER. The Color Preferences of One Thousand and Six Negroes, *J. Comp. Psychol.*, 5, 1925, 109. Cf. in this connection J. Dashiell, *J. of Exper. Psychol.*, 2, 1917, 466-475.

[33] G. J. v. ALLESCH. Die Ästhetische Erscheinungsweise der Farben, *Psychol. Forsch.*, 6, 1925, 281.

[34] E. J. G. BRADFORD. A Note on the Relation and Aesthetic Value of the Perceptive Types in Color Appreciation, *Amer. J. Psychol.*, 24, 1913, 545.

[35] Further details in regard to this experiment are as follows: The stimuli were 15 pieces of colored paper, rectangular in shape and about 30

inches in area. Three observers participated in the experiment. The rank orders were determined by the method of choice. The coefficients of correlation between the various rank orders were determined by the Spearman formula.

[36] M. YOKOYAMA. Affective Tendency as Conditioned by Color and Form, *Amer. J. Psychol.*, 32, 1921, 81.

[37] Further details of this experiment are as follows: Stimuli: 7 squares, 5 x 5 cm., cut from Milton-Bradley pigment-papers. Method: paired comparisons, with repetition of the series in reverse spatial order. Statistics: the method of calculating the degree of agreement between rank orders was a slight modification of that used by Foster and Roese.

[38] In Yokoyama's article a single table gives the results of two series of experiments, one on color, the other on form. Above there is reproduced only that part of the table which deals with color. The results on form will be treated infra. Furthermore, there is omitted from the table "revised" figures for observer B.

[39] M. YOKOYAMA, *Op. cit.*, 81.

[40] R. M. DORCUS. Color Preferences and Color Associations, *Pedag. Sem.*, 33, 1926, 432.

[41] No information is given by Bradford concerning the training of his observers in this respect. One of them, however, is symbolized by the initials E. B., which are those of Bradford himself. As to Yokoyama's observers, he tells us that "All but M were highly trained observers and had had experience in observation under the conditions of the experiment." (M. YOKOYAMA, *Op. cit.*, 82.)

[42] J. COHN. *Philos Stud.*, 10, 1894, 599-600.

[43] *Ibid.*, 603.

[44] E. S. BAKER. Experiments on the Aesthetic of Light and Color: On Combinations of Two Colors, *Univ. of Toronto Studies, Psychol. Series,* Vol. I, 1900, 248.

[45] E. S. BAKER. Spectrally Pure Colors in Binary Combinations, *Univ. of Toronto Studies, Psychol. Series,* Vol. II, 1907, 43.

[46] F. L. BARBER. Combinations of Colors With Tints and With Shades, *Univ. of Toronto Studies, Psychol. Series,* Vol. II, 1907, 179.

[47] L. R. GEISSLER. Studies in Psychol. contr. by Colleagues and Former Students of E. B. TITCHENER, 1917, 164.

[48] J. T. METCALF. The Pleasantness of Brightness Combinations, *Amer. J. Psychol.*, 38, 1927, 607.

[49] E. S. BAKER. *Univ. of Toronto Studies, Psychol. Series,* Vol. II, 1907, 42.

[50] E. S. BAKER. *Univ. of Toronto Studies, Psychol. Series,* Vol. I, 1900, 248.

[51] S. A. CHOWN. Combinations of Colours and Uncoloured Lights, *Univ. of Toronto Studies, Psychol. Series,* Vol. II, 1907, 97.

[52] F. L. BARBER. Combinations of Colors, Tints and Shades, *Univ of Toronto Studies, Psychol. Series,* Vol. II, 1907, 45-46.

[53] K. GORDON. A Study of Aesthetic Judgments, *J. of Exper. Psychol.*, 6, 1923, 36.

[54] *Ibid.*, 37-38.

[55] *Ibid.*, 39.

[56] D. R. Major. On the Affective Tone of Simple Sense Impressions, *Amer. J. Psychol.*, 7, 1895, 57.

[57] *Ibid.*, 72.

[58] T. Ziehen. Leitfaden der physiologischen Psychologie, 10th Edit., 1914, 206.

[59] C. W. Valentine. The Aesthetic Appreciation of Musical Intervals Among School Children and Adults, *Brit. J. Psychol.*, 6, 1913, 190.

[60] *Ibid.*, 195.

[61] *Ibid.*, 196. The existence of individual differences is also shown by a comparison of the rank order of clangs established by Valentine to the following rank order reproduced by Ziehen from Krueger (Ziehen, Leitfaden der Psychologie, 207). The most pleasant intervals are at the top.
Octave (1:2) ; Fifth (2:3)
Maj. Third (4:5)
Min. Third (5:6) ; Fourth (3:4)
Maj. Sixth (3:5)
Min. Sixth (5:8)
Tritone (5:7)
Maj. Second (8:9)
Maj. Seventh (8:15)
Min. Second (15:16)

[62] C. C. Pratt. Some Qualitative Aspects of Bitonal Complexes, *Amer. J. Psychol.*, 32, 1921, 490.

[63] A. M. Brues. The Fusion of Non-musical Intervals, *Amer. J. Psychol.*, 38, 1927, 624-638.

[64] *Ibid.*, 628.

[65] The most striking feature of this experiment—with no direct bearing upon our problem—was that the non-musical intervals were by no means antagonistic to fusion—indeed, "If we recognize the fact that there are degrees of fusion, we find that the most non-musical intervals are as well fused as the most musical intervals, including the perfect fifth." (*Ibid.*, 638.)

[66] C. P. Heinlein. The Affective Characters of the Major and Minor Modes in Music, *J. Comp. Psychol.*, 8, 1928, 101-102.

[67] *Ibid.*, 138-140.

[68] D. R. Major. *Amer. J. Psychol.*, 7, 1895, 72.

[69] A. Wohlgemuth. On the Feelings and Their Neural Correlate, with an examination of the nature of pain, *Brit. J. Psychol.*, 8, 1917, 450.

[70] R. Engel. Experimentelle Untersuchungen über die Abhängigkeit der Lust und Unlust von der Reizstärke beim Geschmacksinn, *Arch. f. d. ges. Psychol.*, 64, 1928, 1.

[71] H. Henning. Der Geruch, Leipzig, 1916, 168-183.

[72] *Ibid.*, 178. This preference may be connected with the fact that camphor is said to keep away certain worms which destroy Bamboo, a wood much used in Japan.

[73] *Ibid.*, 181-182.

[74] A. E. Findley. Further Studies of Henning's System of Olfactory Qualities, *Amer. J. Psychol.*, 35, 1924, 444.

[75] P. T. Young. Constancy of Affective Judgments to Odors, *J. of Exper. Psychol.*, 6, 1923, 182.

212   RELATION TO PRIMARY STIMULI

76 *Ibid.,* 191.

77 P. T. YOUNG. *Amer. J. Psychol.,* 40, 1928, 399.

78 KATE GORDON. The Recollection of Pleasant and of Unpleasant Odors, *J. Exper. Psychol.,* 8, 1925, 225.

79 J. H. KENNETH. A Few Odor Preferences and Their Constancy, *J. Exper. Psychol.,* 11, 1928, 56.

80 The discussion of variability which follows has already been published in the *J. Exper. Psychol.,* 14, 1931, 91.

81 The significance of the differences involved is so obvious from mere inspection that statistical proof of it has been omitted.

82 The averages being compared are averages of only eight coefficients. The P. E.'s of their differences are consequently of low reliability.

83 By means of Spearman's statistical technique I recently demonstrated that the relative hedonic judgments upon any one stimulus in Series I of the experiment described above could be considered to involve a "general factor" common to the judgments of all eight observers and "special factors" peculiar to the judgment of each individual observer. (Cf. J. G. BEEBE-CENTER, General Affective Value, *Psychol. Rev.,* 36, 1929, 472.) The conclusion above obviously implies that such "general factors" depend primarily upon the like constitution of the observers, while the "special factors" depend primarily upon their different past experience.

84 M. BABBITT, M. WOODS and M. F. WASHBURN. Affective Sensitiveness to Colors, Tone Intervals and Articulate Sounds, *Amer. J. Psychol.,* 26, 1915, 289-290.

85 *Ibid.,* 290.

86 D. CLARK, M. S. GOODELL and M. F. WASHBURN. The Effect of Area on the Pleasantness of Colors, *Amer. J. Psychol.,* 22, 1911, 578-579.

87 *Ibid.,* 579.

88 *Ibid.,* 579.

89 G. T. FECHNER. Vorschule der Aesthetik, Part I, 2nd Edit., Leipzig, 1897, 195.

90 L. WITMER. Zur Experimentellen Aesthetik Einfacher Räumlicher Formverhältnisse, *Philos. Stud.,* 9, 1893, 209-263.

91 R. P. ANGIER. The Aesthetics of Unequal Division, *Psychol. Rev.,* Monogr. Suppl., 4, 1903, 546.

92 E. L. THORNDIKE. Individual Differences in Judgments of the Beauty of Simple Forms, *Psychol. Rev.,* 24, 1917, 147-153.

93 *Ibid.,* 153.

94 F. H. LUND and A. ANASTASI. An Interpretation of Aesthetic Experience, *Amer. J. Psychol.,* 40, 1928, 434.

95 The experiment has not been published.

96 Cf. W. KÖHLER. Die Physischen Gestalten in Ruhe und im Stationären Zustand, Braunschweig, 1920, esp. Part IV, Ch. I, entitled "Denn was innen, das ist aussen."

97 G. D. BIRKHOFF. Quelques Eléments Mathématiques de l'art, Atti del Congresso Internationale dei Matematici, Bologna, 1929, 315.

98 HOBSON. Chinese Art, New York, 1927.

99 R. P. ANGIER. *Psychol. Rev.,* Monogr. Suppl., 4, 1903, 549.

100 E. L. THORNDIKE. *Psychol. Rev.,* 24, 1917, 149-150.

101 M. YOKOYAMA. Affective Tendency as Conditioned by Color and Form, *Amer. J. Psychol.,* 32, 1921, 107.

[102] T. Ziehen. Leitfaden der physiologischen Psychologie, 10th Edit., 1914, 199.

[103] In a footnote, Ziehen adds that "Das obige Gesetz ist übrigens wohl zuerst von Meyer (Beschreibung des ganzen menschlichen Körpers, Bd. VI, 1794, 247) ausgesprochen worden. Der allgemeine Verlauf der Kurve wurde schon von Hartley und Priestley (Introd. Essays to Hartley's theory of the Human Mind, London, 1775, XVI), richtig angegeben." (Ibid., 199.)

[104] W. Wundt. Grundzüge der physiologischen Psychologie, 5th Ed., Vol., II, Leipzig, 1902, 311-312.

[105] F. Kiesow. Sur la méthode pour étudier les sentiments simples, Arch. Ital. de Biol., 1899, 32, 159-164. Same paper in Italian in Rendic. d. R. Acad. dei. Lincei, Roma, 1899, Series 5, Vol. VIII, 469-473.

[106] Ibid. (Arch. Ital. de Biol.), 161, 163.

[107] A. Lehmann. Hauptgesetze des menschlichen Gefühlslebens, Leipzig, 1914, 190.

[108] A. Saidullah. Experimentelle Untersuchungen über den Geschmacksinn, Arch. f. d. ges. Psychol., 69, 1927, 475.

[109] R. Engel. Experimentelle Untersuchungen über die Abhängigkeit der Lust und Unlust von der Reizstärke beim Geschmacksinn, Arch. f. d. ges. Psychol. 64, 1928, 1.

[110] In connection with this possibility, Cf. V. Henri, L'année psychologique, 1, 1894, 444-5; J. Larguier des Bancels, L'année psychologique, 6, 1899, 168; C. Lalo, L'esthétique expérimentale contemporaine, Paris, 1908, 155.

[111] R. Engel. Arch. f. d. ges. Psychol., 64, 1928, 28.

[112] Daniel Bernouilli was born in 1700 in Groningen, Holland, the son of Johann Bernouilli, a professor of mathematics. He taught at St. Petersburg and later at Basel. He died in 1782.

[113] D. Bernouilli. Specimen theoriæ novæ de mensura sortis, Commentarii academiæ scientiarum imperialis Petropolitanæ, Tomus V, Petrop., 1738, 175-192. Transl. by A. Pringsheim, Leipzig, 1896.

[114] Ibid. (transl. by Pringsheim), 27-28.

[115] Cf. note by Pringsheim, Ibid., 34-35.

[116] Laplace. French mathematician and astronomer, born in 1749, died in 1827.

[117] Pierre Simon, Marquis de Laplace. Théorie analytique des probabilités, 3rd Edit., Paris, 1820.

[118] Ibid., 187.

[119] Ibid., 432.

[120] G. T. Fechner. Elemente der Psychophysik, 2nd Edit., Leipzig, 1889, 236.

[121] E. B. Titchener. A Textbook of Psychology, New York, 1928 (1909), 259.

[122] Ibid., 260.

[123] T. Nakashima. Time Relations of the Affective Processes, Psychol. Rev., 16, 1909, 303.

[124] Ibid., 308-309.

[125] Ibid., 311.

[126] Ibid., 320.

214   RELATION TO PRIMARY STIMULI

[127] *Ibid.*, 316.

[128] H. M. POTTER, R. TUTTLE and M. F. WASHBURN. The Speed of Affective Judgments, *Amer. J. Psychol.*, 25, 1914, 288.

[129] *Ibid.*, 289.

[130] F. L. WELLS. Reactions to Visual Stimuli in Affective Settings, *J. Exper. Psychol.*, 8, 1925, 64-76.

[131] *Ibid.*, 76.

[132] F. L. WELLS. Reaction-Times to Affects Accompanying Smell Stimuli, *Amer. J. Psychol.*, 41, 1929, 83-86.

[133] *Ibid.*, 84.

[134] *Ibid.*, 85.

[135] A. LEHMANN. Hauptgesetze des menschlichen Gefühlslebens, Leipzig, 1914, 207-208.

[136] D. CRAWFORD and M. F. WASHBURN. Fluctuations in the Affective Value of Colors During Fixation for One Minute, *Amer. J. Psychol.*, 22, 1911, 579-582.

[137] *Ibid.*, 579.

[138] *Ibid.*, 580.

[139] *Ibid.*, 582.

[140] *Ibid.*, 581.

[141] W. V. D. BINGHAM. Studies in Melody, *Psychol. Monogr.*, 12, 1910, No. 3, 10.

[142] *Ibid.*, 34.

[143] E. D. PUFFER. The Psychology of Beauty, Boston, 1905, 183.

[144] *Ibid.*, 183-184.

[145] A. GEHRING. The Basis of Musical Pleasure, New York, 1910.

[146] E. GURNEY. The Power of Sound, London, 1880, 127.

[147] G. D. BIRKHOFF. Quelques elements mathematiques de l'art, Atti del congresso internationale dei matematici, Tomo I, Bologna, 1929, 332.

[148] K. DANZFUSS. Die Gefühlsbetönung einiger unanalysierter Zweiklänge, Zweitonfolgen, Akkorde und Akkordfolgen bei Erwachsenen und Kindern, *Phil. u. Psychol. Arbeiten,* 1923, 5, 18 ff.

[149] None of these experiments has been published.

[150] W. KÖHLER. Zur Theorie des Sukzessivvergleichs und der Zeitfehler, *Psychol. Forsch.*, 1923, 4, 115.

[151] C. SPEARMAN. The Abilities of Man, New York, 1927, 74-75.

[152] Provided that account be taken of the influence of overlap of specific factors. Cf. Spearman, *Op. cit.*, 150 ff. and Appendix, VII-VIII.

[153] C. SPEARMAN. *Op. cit.*, Appendix, XVI.

[154] *Ibid.*, Appendix, XVII.

[155] The method was that of paired comparison. The stimuli were the substances listed in Table XXXII.

[156] These coefficients, calculated by the method of rank differences, are treated below as though they had been calculated by the product-moment method, although it has been shown that coefficients calculated from the same data by the two methods are not necessarily the same. (Cf. K. Pearson, On Further Methods of Determining Correlation, *Draper's Company Research Memoirs, Biometric Series,* IV., 1907, 9 ff.) The difference involved is so slight, however, that it has not been thought necessary to take it into account in computations which are merely for illustrative purposes.

[157] C. SPEARMAN, *Op. cit.*, 73.

[158] *Ibid.*, Appendix, XI.

[159] This formula holds only when all the correlations throughout a table obey the tetrad equation.

[160] C. SPEARMAN. *Op. cit.*, Appendix, XVII.

[161] *Ibid.*, Appendix, XVIII.

[162] *Ibid.*, Appendix, XIX.

Chapter V

Hedonic Tone in Relation to Secondary External Stimuli

As was pointed out at the beginning of the preceding chapter, phenomena are dependent not only upon the stimuli which they represent cognitively, upon *primary stimuli,* but upon a variety of other stimuli, both present and past, upon *secondary stimuli.* It is my purpose in the present chapter to discuss the relation of hedonic tone to such secondary stimuli.

SIMULTANEOUS SECONDARY STIMULI

Although the work of the Gestalt school makes it quite likely that a phenomenon depends upon the entire constellation of physiologically effective stimuli, and consequently upon all secondary stimuli, it is clear that the *degree* of dependence may vary markedly from one secondary stimulus to another. For clarity of exposition I shall distinguish between secondary stimuli known to affect the sensory characteristics of a phenomenon (e.g., stimuli inducing contrast), and secondary stimuli not known to have such an effect on a phenomenon.

Concerning the relation between hedonic tone and secondary stimuli of the former type, our information is limited to data secured by v. Allesch. Among the experiments described in his important article on the "Appearance of colors" is one in which colors were presented for aesthetic description on 24 different grey backgrounds.[1] The contrast effect of the background with respect to brilliance was in each case compensated by an appropriate addition of black or white to the primary stimulus. Von Allesch found that descriptions of a color varied greatly

216

as the background was changed. Thus a yellowish green was described as "thin and uncouth" with one background, "fresh and cool" with another, "brilliant" with a third, and "heavy" with a fourth. The observer also reported differences in hue. With one background the color was yellowish, with another greenish. As to hedonic tone, v. Allesch unfortunately did not instruct his observers to report it. In the case of certain backgrounds, however, reference was made to hedonic tone and these references showed marked variation of hedonic tone with variation of background. With one background, the observer reported, "The favorable impression is even stronger," with another, "Now the color is expressionless, indifferent, but also cold and repelling," with a third the color was said to have become "almost repulsive." It seems clear that if the experiment were repeated—as it most certainly ought to be—with specific instructions to report in terms of hedonic tone, the results would demonstrate a marked dependence of hedonic tone upon secondary stimuli which affect the sensory characteristics of the focal phenomenon.

With respect to the relation of hedonic tone to secondary stimuli affecting but little—if at all—the sensory characteristics of the focal phenomenon, the most important source of evidence is the work on the relation of hedonic tone to attention. In his "Psychologie des sentiments" Ribot wrote: "It is certain that an intense mono-ideaism, a profound concentration of attention, a fanatical exaltation, can produce a temporary or permanent analgesia. Many soldiers, in the fire of battle, have not felt their wounds. Pascal, deep in his problems, escaped neuralgia. The Aissaouas, the Fakirs, certain Lamas of Thibet, tear and wound themselves, proof against pain by their delirium, and one cannot doubt that many of the martyrs in the midst of tortures have felt only a state of rapture. In certain forms of mental alienation (maniacal excitation, melancholia, idiocy, etc.), this spontaneous analgesia is frequent and is produced under extraordinary forms. One finds numerous examples of these in special works. One person chews glass in his mouth for a half hour without feeling any ill result. Another, in a quarrel, breaks a leg, a fragment of the tibia is pushed through the outside skin; he does not cease to pursue the object of his anger, then he seats himself at table to eat, while his face does not reveal the slightest suffering. Very numerous are those who by intention or by accident plunge an arm into boiling water, lean on a red hot stove; the skin falls in pieces while they do not appear to be upset. An enumeration of analogous facts would be endless." [2] This passage obviously suggests a close relationship between hedonic tone and attention. It does not, however, prove this close relationship. The cases mentioned might well have involved not *marginal* pain, but lack of pain due to a form of inhibition similar to that found in hysterical anaesthesis. In order to secure reliable evidence concerning the relation of hedonic tone to attention it is necessary to turn to the experimental literature.

A certain amount of relevant evidence was secured by Yokoyama in the experiment mentioned in Chapter 3 in connection with hedonic summation. [3] In a first part of the experiment, Yokoyama arranged 49 color forms (7 colors combined with 7 forms) into 7 series, in each of which color varied and form was constant. In the case of each series he determined the hedonic rank order of the 7 colors by the method of paired comparison, instructing his observers to attend to the *colors*. He then compared, in the case of each observer, the rank orders of the colors in the 7 series. The results showed that these rank orders were extremely similar for all 7 series, i.e., for all 7 forms. Stated in terms of percentage of agreement, according to which 100 represents complete agreement and — 100 complete disagreement, the rank orders showed an average agreement of 87.9%, with an M.V. of 3.9. In a second part of the experiment, Yokoyama followed exactly the same procedure except that the 7 series of stimuli were so constituted that in each series color was constant while form varied. The observers, furthermore, were instructed to attend to *form*. The results showed in the case of the various observers a high agreement between the rank orders of the forms in all 7 series. The average agreement, stated in percentage of agreement, was 88.1%, with an M.V. of 3.7. Yokoyama concluded as follows: "When color-forms are presented for affective comparison of colors only, the forms have practically no influence upon the preferential order of these colors, provided the observer's attitude remains constant throughout the task, and color similarly has practically no effect upon form." [4]

Yokoyama's results certainly point to a dependence of hedonic tone upon attention, but they are not conclusive because they do not allow direct comparison of the hedonic values of colors or forms when "attended to" with their values when "attended from." In an experiment published in 1923, M. Meenes sought to carry out such direct comparison in the case of colors.[5] Using the method of paired comparison he determined for each of three observers the relative hedonic values of 21 binary combinations of 6 colors (all possible combinations including those of each color with itself) in each of 3 distinct sets of observations. In all 3 sets of observations, the pairs of binary combinations were presented for comparison with one binary combination above the other. In one set of observations, the observers were instructed to attend to the left members of each binary combination, in another set of observations to the right members of each binary combination; in a third set of observations, to both members. The table below shows for each of the three observers the m.v.'s of the averages of the frequencies of preference of the 6 binary combinations into which each of the 6 colors entered (a) when these colors were "attended to," (b) when they were "attended from," and (c) when they were attended to in conjunction with the other color of the binary combination. Thus in the case of colors "attended to," the table indicates the m.v. of the 6 averages constituted by averaging in the case of each color "attended to" the 6 frequencies with which were preferred the 6 binary combinations involving this "attended to" color.

TABLE XXXIII

Observer	For color "attended to"	For color "attended from"	For color when both colors of combination are attended to
Ba	7.37	1.23	4.09
Y	6.65	2.07	6.38
Bi	8.89	0.43	5.58

It will be noticed that the m.v.'s are for all observers greatest for colors "attended to" and least for colors "attended from." This implies that the averages of the frequencies of preference of the 6 binary combinations involving a given "attended to" color show the greatest dispersion; those of the binary combinations involving a given "attended from" color the least dispersion. It follows clearly that the effect of colors upon the frequency of preference of the binary combinations into which they enter is greatest when these colors are "attended to" and least when they are "attended from." Meenes consequently concluded: "In paired comparisons of colors affective judgments are conditioned predominantly upon the colors attended to. Colors attended from, but presented with the colors attended to, have at most but slight effect upon the judgments." [6]

How far may this conclusion be generalized? Apparently not far beyond the field of color-pairs. In 1906, Keith published an investigation of the mutual influence, with respect to hedonic tone, of simultaneous stimulation of different classes of sense-organs.[7] For each of two observers he determined by the method of single stimuli (scale of 1 to 7) the hedonic values of 28 colors, 27 tone-combinations, 14 touch-stimuli applied by the experimenter (passive), and the same 14 touch-stimuli applied by the observer (active), under two different conditions, namely when presented singly and when presented in pairs consisting of members affecting different sense organs. Thus, for instance, the hedonic value of the 28 colors was determined when they were presented alone, and also when paired with tones, active touches and passive touches. The results of this experiment are given in the table below, copied from Keith.

TABLE XXXIV

Obs. F	Avg. Stand- ard	% of judgments			Av. + or — influ- ence on each	
		Raised	Lowered	Not affected		
1 Colors	4.35	28	59.6	11.9	(Colors)	— .26
Tones	4.33	16	77	6	(Tones)	— .74
2 Colors	4.35	32	53	13	(Colors)	— .13
A. Touches ...	4.55	34	62	3	(A.T.)	— .38
3 Colors	4.35	57	25	16	(Colors)	+ .40
P. Touches ...	4.56	51	23	25	(P.T.)	+ .30
4 Tones	4.33	68	24	7	(Tones)	+ .45
A. Touches ...	4.55	64	32	3	(A.T.)	+ .23
5 Tones	4.33	72	17	10	(Tones)	+ .52
P. Touches ...	4.56	42	34	23	(P.T.)	+ .14
Obs. M						
1 Colors	4.44	23	59	17	(Colors)	— .29
Tones	4.20	12	81	6	(Tones)	— 1.08
2 Colors	4.44	58	24	17	(Colors)	+ .43
A. Touches ...	4.24	54	43	1.8	(A.T.)	+ .17
3 Colors	4.44	71	13	15	(Colors)	+ .72
P. Touches ...	5.14	43	17	39	(P.T.)	+ .26
4 Tones	4.20	99	.2	.5	(Tones)	+ 1.71
A. Touches ...	4.24	63	36	.2	(A.T.)	+ .31

The numerals in the first column refer to various combinations of two classes of stimuli. Thus No. 1 refers to the combination of tones and colors. In the case of each numeral the column marked "average standard" gives the average hedonic value of each of the two classes of stimuli when each stimulus was presented *singly*. The last column gives the change in hedonic value of each of these classes when the stimuli were paired with members of the other class. The three intermediate columns give for each class the percentage of judgments raised, lowered and unchanged from the first mode of presentation to the second. It is unfortunate that the author does not give us data to evaluate the significance of the shifts in hedonic value. In many cases, however, the shifts are so marked that they can hardly be ascribed to chance factors. It seems reasonable, therefore, to accept the author's conclusion that "our appreciation of each of several stimuli in combination is different from our appreciation of the same stimuli when taken separately." [8]

This conclusion in turn points to a further conclusion more clearly related to our problem. Keith's account of his experiment is very sketchy, and he does not mention the attentive attitude of his observers. It seems obvious, however, that when an observer was judging one of two stimuli in combination, he was attending to the one judged, and not to the other. The other stimulus, then, must have been "attended from"—secondary. This other stimulus, however, was clearly operative as a partial determinant of the hedonic value of the primary stimulus. It follows that the hedonic value of a stimulus "attended to" is in some cases altered by the presence of a stimulus "attended from," and consequently that the conclusion of Meenes will not bear complete generalization.

It is obvious that further work is required on the relation of hedonic tone to simultaneous secondary stimuli. The data above, however, make it possible even now to describe this relationship in very general terms. The hedonic tone of a phenomenon is markedly dependent upon secondary stimuli which affect its sensory characteristics (v. Allesch). In the case of secondary stimuli which do not have such a sensory effect, hedonic tone is sometimes markedly dependent upon the secondary stimuli (Keith), sometimes little if at all (Yokoyama, Meenes).

Past Secondary Stimuli

Successive Contrast. —The problem of successive hedonic contrast has in the past given rise to much disagreement. For Fechner, such contrast was a special case of a more general law applying to both simultaneous and successive events. This general law was as follows: "That which gives pleasure gives more pleasure the more it enters into contrast with sources of displeasure or of lesser pleasure; and a corresponding proposition holds for that which gives displeasure." [9] For this law to hold, however, certain conditions had to be fulfilled: (a) the experiences involved had to be appreciably different with respect to hedonic value; (b) the two factors had to bear a certain resemblance to each other; (c) in the case of successive impressions, only the second could be affected by contrast. Fechner ascribed to the non-satisfaction of condition b the fact that contrast did not hold between experiences of different modalities. Lehmann,[10] one of the eminent authorities on feeling in the early 1900's, accepted Fechner's law insofar as it related to successive contrast. In his treatise on feeling he wrote: "The feeling aroused by a given stimulus is dependent upon previous conditions inasmuch as the feeling either becomes weaker or changes into its opposite when a stronger feeling of the same type has preceded it." As early as 1895, on the other hand, Marshall—also an authority on feeling—denied the validity of Fechner's law of contrast. He wrote: "I am not able to follow Fechner and other thinkers of authority in holding that there is a law of contrast for pleasure and pain *per se* apart from the contents to which the algedonic qualities are attached." [11] Three years later the same view was put forth by W. Wirth. "Perceptual contrast," he said, "is the result of a discrepancy between an apperception and the (unchanged) sensation upon which it is based. Feelings cannot 'seem' to be weaker or stronger, since there is no substratum with which to compare them. However, when perceptions contrast, the feeling is different from what it would have been without contrast. When our attention is on the objects, we speak of perceptual contrast; when contrasting objects are so related as to arouse strong feelings of opposed quality, we speak of affective contrast." [12]

In spite of this disagreement it was not until 1914, with the publication of a research by Bacon, Rood and Washburn, that experimental data became available concerning the problem of hedonic contrast.[13] These investigators first made each of 84 observers pick from 90 Bradley colors 6 which were extremely disagreeable, and 6 which were extremely pleasant. The investigators then chose from the remaining colors 18, including an equal number of saturated colors, tints and shades. "These eighteen colors were shown to the observer, one at a time, on a white ground. Between the showing of each color and that of the next, one of the pleasant colors selected by the observer was shown. As each color was presented, the observer was asked to express her judgment of its pleasantness or unpleasantness by using one of the numbers from 1 to 7 in the usual way. When all of the eighteen colors had been shown, each preceded by one of the very pleasant colors, the experiment was continued without pause and the same eighteen colors were again presented in a different order, each this time preceded by one of the very unpleasant colors chosen by the observer. . . . In order to equalize fatigue conditions, with other observers the colors were first presented, preceded by the unpleasant colors and later preceded by the pleasant ones." [14]

One group of observers, 47 in number, worked with knowledge of the problem. Of this group, there were 30 to whom the unpleasant stimuli were given first. For these observers the investigators point out, hedonic contrast, if operative, should have brought about a *lowering* of the hedonic values of the colors on their second presentation. The results showed that of these 30 observers, 14 had more judgments lowered on the second presentation than were raised, 5 of the 14 having more judgments lowered than were either unchanged or raised. Eleven of the observers, on the other hand, had more judgments raised on the second presentation than were lowered, 5 of these 11 having more lowered than were either unchanged or raised. The investigators concluded that in the case of the observers working *with* knowledge, no contrast-effect is demonstrated by the results.

Another group of observers, 37 in number, worked without knowledge. In the case of this group, 11 of 12 observers to whom the unpleasant stimuli were given first and for whom contrast should consequently have lowered hedonic values on the second presentation, showed more hedonic values lowered on the second presentation than were either raised or left unchanged. The individual results for these observers are given below:

TABLE XXXV

Observer	Lowered	No. of Judgments Raised	Unchanged
1	12	2	4
2	12	0	6
3	11	1	6
4	16	0	2
5	15	0	3
6	8	2	8
7	11	0	7
8	11	0	7
9	18	0	0
10	13	0	5
11	13	0	5
12	16	0	2

Twenty-five of the observers working without knowledge were shown the pleasant inducing stimuli first. In this case, the effect of contrast should have been to raise the values of the colors on the second presentation. Twenty-three of these twenty-five observers had more hedonic values raised on the second presentation than lowered, and of these twenty-three, twelve had more hedonic values raised on the second presentation than were either lowered or left unchanged. Two of the twenty-five observers had more hedonic values lowered than were either raised or left unchanged. The investigators concluded that in the case of observers working *without* knowledge, the results demonstrate with certainty the influence of hedonic contrast. They formulated the law of hedonic contrast as follows: "The pleasure of an agreeable experience is heightened, if it is preceded by a disagreeable experience, and an impression in itself unpleasant may be felt as pleasant if a more unpleasant state has been its antecedent. In like manner unpleasantness may be heightened or even created through contrast with a preceding agreeable affective state." [15]

The law of contrast formulated by Miss Washburn—as

indeed all preceding laws of contr. st—makes the hedonic tone corresponding to a stimulus depend upon the hedonic tone corresponding to the immediately preceding stimulus. It is a law of "individual contrast." In 1914, it was natural to consider such a law as the only possible description of the facts. With the rise of the Gestalt school, however, this situation became altered. In his article on hedonic contrast published in 1929, A. J. Harris pointed out that Miss Washburn's results could be equally well described by two very different laws, her own law of individual contrast or a law of "mass contrast" in which the hedonic tone corresponding to a primary stimulus is considered to depend upon the hedonic tone corresponding to *all* preceding stimuli subjectively related to the primary stimulus.[16] In order to establish which of these laws is the more adequate, he sought to find out whether or not "in an experiment involving a contrast effect, the different judgments upon a single stimulus vary in a definite way with the affective value of the immediately preceding experience." [17] Harris' technique was very similar to that of Miss Washburn. Ninety Milton-Bradley colors were first shown each observer with the request that he select the 10 most pleasant and the 10 least pleasant. This gave a P (pleasant) *determining* series and an U (unpleasant) *determining* series for each observer. From the colors which had not been selected by any of the observers Harris chose a *test* series consisting of 20 colors. The experiment was divided into two parts, separated by three weeks. For two observers (Se and Ki) Part I involved presentation of the test series mingled with the U determining series, while Part II involved presentation of the test series mingled with the P determining series. For the other two observers (Ob and Tu) the test series was mingled with the P determining series in Part I, with the U determining series in Part II. In both parts the order of presentation was such that every determining stimulus was followed once by each of the test stimuli. The instructions to the observers called for absolute judgments of hedonic

tone in terms of a scale running from — 3 (very unpleasant)
to + 3 (very pleasant).

"The results from each O were treated separately.
From the judgments made on the determiners the average
affective value of each determiner was found, and the determiners were arranged in rank order of pleasantness. Every
test stimulus was presented once after each of the determiners, so the average affective value of the test stimuli following a determining stimulus could be made the basis for
comparing the effect of various determiners on the affective
value of the test stimuli. The results for each O in Part I
are shown in Fig. 45. If contrast is an individual effect,

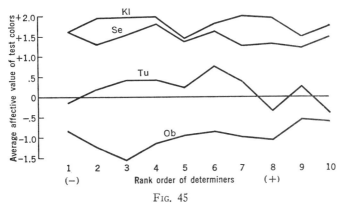

Fig. 45

Average Value of the Test Colors Following the Different Determiners
(*From Harris*)

in the sense of depending solely on the immediately preceding experience, the average value of the test colors following the least pleasant determiners, those on the left,
should be higher than the average value following the most
pleasant determiners, those on the right. The results show
no such tendency." [18] Similar treatment of the results in
Part II likewise failed to show evidence of contrast-effects
by individual determining stimuli. When, on the other hand,
the average hedonic tone corresponding to the test colors
for the whole of Part I was compared to that for the whole
of Part II, it was found that the average was distinctly

higher when the test colors were combined with an U determining series than when they were combined with a P determining series. (Cf. table below.)

TABLE XXXVI

Showing the Difference in the Average Value of the Test Colors
When the Determining Colors are Changed

O	Test average after P determining series	Test average after U determining series
Tu	0.15	0.50
Ob	— 0.97	0.02
Ki	0.69	1.73
Se	0.01	1.42

It was further found that the shift of the average in the case of the different observers was practically proportional to the difference between the average hedonic tone corresponding to the two determining series for these observers (cf. Fig. below).

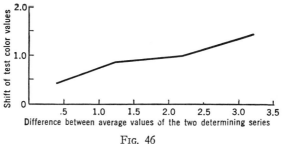

FIG. 46

(*From Harris*)

It is clear from these results that hedonic contrast is not a relation between the hedonic tone corresponding to a present stimulus and that corresponding to an immediately preceding stimulus, but one which involves the hedonic tone corresponding to a whole group of preceding stimuli. As Harris has aptly put it, there is no *individual* hedonic contrast, but only *mass* hedonic contrast. This mass contrast seems best described for the present by the following law: *The hedonic tone corresponding to a present stimulus varies conversely with the sum of hedonic tone corresponding to those past stimuli whose phenomenal correlates constitute with the phenomenal correlate of the present stimulus a unitary temporal group.*[19]

This formulation of the law of contrast, though more accurate than earlier formulations, is still rather equivocal. What determines that a given set of phenomena shall constitute a "unitary temporal group"? A complete answer to this question must wait upon further experimentation. Although it would be of great practical importance to know the effect of instructions and of "attitudes" on the constitution of "unitary temporal groups," such information is completely lacking. A partial answer to the question, however, is even now possible. In the first place, the experiment of Harris shows that a series of odors experienced under the same general conditions—in the same room, at the same hour of the day, in the presence of the same experimenter and under the same instructions—does indeed constitute such a unitary group. In the second place, a further experiment by Mr. Harris throws considerable light on membership in a single modality as a condition of membership in a "unitary temporal group." The technique in this second experiment was much the same as in the first. The observers gave absolute hedonic judgments on a test series of 20 colors under two different sets of conditions. In one case the colors were intermingled with nine pleasant odors; in the other they were intermingled with nine unpleasant odors. In the case of a few observers the average hedonic tone corresponding to the colors shifted significantly in the direction of contrast; in the case of a few it shifted significantly in the opposite direction, which we may term that of assimilation. For the majority of observers, finally, there was no shift which could be considered statistically significant. These results are unfortunately not clear-cut, as were those of the experiment described above. They certainly warrant the conclusion, however, that "affective contrast does not generally occur between experiences as different as visual and olfactory experiences." [20] It follows that membership in a single sense-modality is a condition favorable, though not absolutely necessary, to the constitution of a "unitary temporal group" in the sense in which this expression is used in the law of contrast.

My own work, finally, throws light on *temporal proximity* as a possible condition of membership in a "unitary temporal group." [21] In a first experiment I ascertained the difference in the hedonic tone corresponding to a set of 21 olfactory stimuli under two different conditions: First, after frequent stimulation with the 10 *least* pleasant members of the set, and then after frequent stimulation with the 10 *most* pleasant members of the set. The procedure, in the case of each of three observers, was essentially as follows: For five experimental hours, distributed over two weeks, the observer was made to judge the hedonic tone of the 10 odors which, on the basis of past information, were known to be the least pleasant to him (U determining series). The method of presentation was that of paired comparison, but the observer was required not only to state which odor of each pair was the more pleasant, but also whether each odor was pleasant, indifferent or unpleasant. As the purpose of this part of the experiment, which I shall call Part 1, was merely to influence the *subsequent* judgments of the observer, no use was made of the data. Part 2, which began two days after the close of Part 1, was similar to the latter, except that all 21 stimuli (Test Series) were presented for judgment. In treating the data from Part 2, the relative judgments were disregarded. From the absolute judgments there was computed for each stimulus a "percentage of pleasantness" P, defined by the equation $P = 100 \, (p + i/2) \, / \, (p + i + u)$, in which p stands for the number of "pleasant" judgments elicited by the stimulus, i for the number of indifferent judgments, and u for the number of unpleasant judgments. Part 3, which followed Part 2 after an interval of about two weeks, was identical with Part 1, except that the 10 stimuli presented in order to influence the subsequent judgments of the observer were the 10 known to be most pleasant to him (P Determining Series). Part 4, which began two days after the close of Part 3, was identical with Part 2. The chronological distribution of the experimental hours during this experiment is indicated in the figure below for one of the observers. The distribution for the two other observers was practically identical.

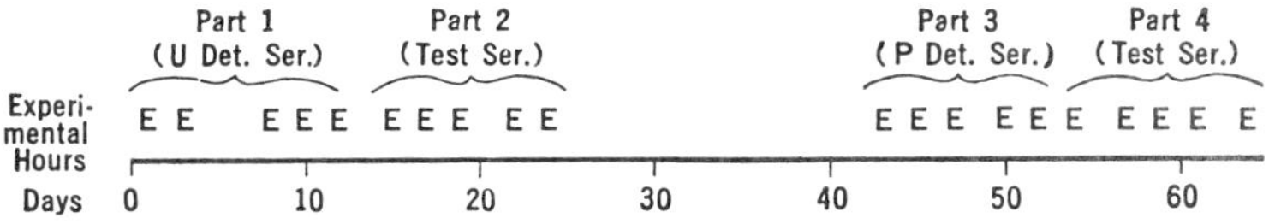

	Part 1 (U Det. Ser.)	Part 2 (Test Ser.)		Part 3 (P Det. Ser.)	Part 4 (Test Ser.)
Experimental Hours	E E E E E	E E E E E		E E E E E E	E E E E
Days	0 10	20 30	40	50	60

Fig. 47

The results of this experiment are shown in the table and figure below. The table gives for each observer the

TABLE XXXVII

O	Part 2 (After Unpleasant Determination)	Part 4 (After Pleasant Determination)
Bu	82%	73%
De	33%	14%
Ka	65%	38%

average of the percentages of pleasantness of the 21 stimuli in Part 2 and the corresponding average for Part 4. The figure gives for the three observers the percentages of pleasantness of the individual stimuli in Parts 2 and 4. The abscissae represent ranks of the stimuli as determined by their respective percentages of pleasantness in Part 2. The ordinates represent percentages of pleasantness. It is clear from both the tables and the figure that the hedonic tone of the 21 olfactory stimuli was greater—more pleasant— two days after the close of the U determining series than it was two days after the close of the P determining series.

The shift in hedonic tone of the 21 olfactory stimuli in the experiment above conforms to the law of contrast.

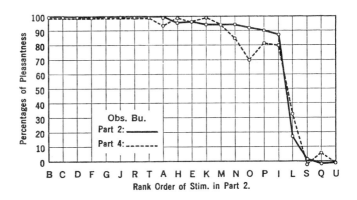

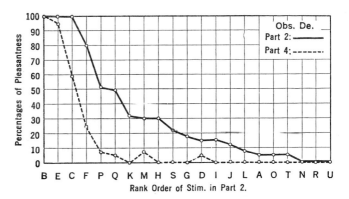

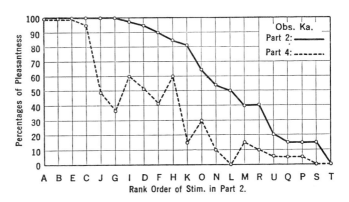

Fig. 48

This conformity, however, might be misleading, for the shift might be due wholly to a tendency for stimuli to become *less pleasant upon repetition*. In order to guard against this possibility, a second experiment was performed. The hedonic tone of 21 olfactory stimuli was determined for three new observers as in Part 2 of the experiment above. The observers were then stimulated for five experimental hours with the 10 least pleasant of these olfactory stimuli. Two days later the hedonic tone of the 21 olfactory stimuli was again determined. The results are indicated in the table below. It is clear that here there is for all observers

TABLE XXXVIII

Observer	Part 1 (No previous Determination)	Part 3 (Previous Determination with U stimuli)
Mc	32%	44%
Vo	53%	58%
Ze	49%	58%

a shift in the hedonic tone of the 21 olfactory stimuli— of the "Test" stimuli—which is in an opposite direction from that observed in the first experiment, but which again conforms with the law of contrast. It is safe to infer that the shifts in both experiments are instances of hedonic contrast.

This being so, it is clear that the experiments throw light on the relation of temporal proximity to membership in a "unitary temporal group." In both experiments the stimuli inducing contrast were not intermingled with the stimuli of the Test Series, but were presented from two to fourteen days earlier. The experiments show, therefore, that past phenomena may enter into a "unitary temporal group" with a present phenomenon even though they have preceded it by two days, and perhaps even though they have preceded it by as much as fourteen days. Temporal proximity, then, is not a condition for membership in a "unitary temporal group." Indeed, if we consider the results above in the light of what we know of the curve of forgetting, it seems likely that the mere interval of time between past and present phenomena is in no way a factor in determining membership in a "unitary temporal group," but that such membership persists indefinitely until broken up by contrary phenomenal groupings. Before asserting this latter proposition, however, it will be necessary to have evidence from experiments involving time-intervals of a month or more.

The law of hedonic contrast, in the form in which it has been stated above, accounts for a number of hitherto unrelated facts in the psychology of hedonic tone. A first such fact is the relativity of so-called "absolute" hedonic judgments. So obvious is this relativity that Titchener uses, for the method involving such judgments, the name Serial Method, and warns the reader that, "if the method is to be valid, O must keep in mind the serial nature of the impressions . . . the affective curve in this case is no more absolute than are the curves of the preceding experiment (by the Method of Paired Comparisons)." [22] Not only does the law of contrast imply such a relativity; it further implies the particular form which this relativity will take. A second fact which can be considered as a consequence of the law of contrast is that almost all sensory modalties —indeed, the only possible exception seems to be pain— involve both pleasant and unpleasant qualities.[23] This fact, so familiar as usually to escape mention, clearly follows from the law of contrast in view of the introspective unitariness of modalities.[24] A third fact which can be subsumed under the law of contrast, finally, is the circumstance that experiments with absolute hedonic judgments never seem to involve pleasantness alone or unpleasantness alone, but both these qualities in comparable proportions.[25]   G. B. Phelan, for instance, in an experiment involving a very large number of stimuli belonging to several modalities, found that, of the total number of feelings reported, 55% were pleasant and 45% were unpleasant.[26]   Phelan attributes this distribution to the selection of stimuli: "These percentages," he writes, "do not express a general rule; it is merely a situation of fact. The different frequencies evidently depend upon the stimuli chosen for the experiments.[27] Although I should never venture to question the importance of the stimulus as a partial determinant of hedonic tone, I am inclined to see in results such as these the operation not only of the stimulus, but of the law of hedonic contrast.

Before leaving the topic of hedonic contrast I should like to point out that laws formally identical with that of hedonic contrast are applicable to many other psychological variables. Wever and Zener, for instance, have shown that, when observers are made to judge a set of weights in terms of the categories "heavy," "medium" and "light," they soon distribute the categories fairly evenly over the scale, calling the heavier weights "heavy" and the lighter weights "light."[28] Truman and Wever have shown that, with a shift of the range of stimulation, there occurs a shift in the application of the categories "high," "medium" and "low" to sets of auditory stimuli.[29] Volkmann, using auditory intensities and lengths of lines as stimulus-variables, has shown that judgments in terms of various sets of absolute categories distribute fairly evenly over the range of stimuli which happens to be in use.[30] These findings have been interpreted by the experimenters as indicating the dependence of absolute judgments on what Wever and Zener have called an "absolute series," i. e., "the mental formation which represents the O's conception of the stimuli as a series—the O's organized body of knowledge about the arrangement of stimulus-magnitudes."[31] If emphasis be less methodological, if the judgments be considered not as ends in themselves, but as means of measuring psychological variables, all of these findings may equally well be interpreted as instances of laws formally identical with the law of hedonic contrast. This fact suggests that hedonic tone is closely akin to other psychological variables, such as length, loudness and weight, and that the physiological basis of hedonic tone is probably of the same general type as the physiological basis of these other variables.

Successive Assimilation.—In discussing the law of contrast I mentioned that Harris, presenting to his observers a series of colors intermingled with a series of odors, found in certain cases that the hedonic tone of the colors was significantly shifted by the odors in a direction opposite to that of contrast—in the direction of *assimilation*. The colors were judged more pleasant when mingled with pleasant odors than when mingled with unpleasant odors. Such assimilative shifts had been observed before—witness Ziehen's doctrine of hedonic "irradiation" [32]—but observation had been too casual to yield data on their conditions. In Harris' experiment, however, the observers were required to give detailed introspective reports, and these reports shed considerable light on the conditions of hedonic assimilation. Of the six observers who yielded assimilative shifts which were statistically significant, five reported that the odors aroused definite "general states" or moods. In the case of the sixth, the difference between pleasant and unpleasant odors was greater than for any other observer, a fact which suggested that his negative report concerning moods might have been in error. Harris concluded tentatively that hedonic assimilation occurs when stimuli of one modality are judged during the prevalence of a definitely pleasant or unpleasant mood aroused by hedonically extreme stimuli of a different modality. [33]

This conclusion is well in accord with an incidental observation of P. T. Young. [34] In an experiment on the constancy of hedonic judgments, Young required his observers to judge the hedonic value of 33 olfactory stimuli on 12 successive days. The judgments were in terms of an absolute scale, extending from -5 (very great displeasure) to $+5$ (very great pleasure). On the fourth day one of the observers was "distinctly in a U mood. She was dull, cross, and her general behavior corresponded to the verbal report of mood." On this day the algebraic sum of her hedonic judgments on the 33 stimuli was -78, whereas on all the 11 other days it varied from -58 to -20, with a mean at -35. Young concludes: "The writer hesitates to interpret the result, but the fact is clear that a distinctly

U mood on day 4 coincided with a decided swing toward U affective judgments." [35]

It seems likely, then, that Harris' conclusion is, in the main, correct. His conclusion cannot, however, be considered a definite statement of the conditions of hedonic assimilation. The concept mood is too ill-defined to be used in formulating a psychological law. There is need of further experimentation in order to establish the conditions of hedonic assimilation in terms of stimuli and instructions.

Sensitization and Adaptation with Consecutive Repetition.—In discussing the relation of hedonic tone to stimulation, Fechner equated consecutive repetition to duration. Continuous stimulation, he pointed out, resulted in an increase of pleasantness or of unpleasantness to a maximum, followed by a gradual decrease and ultimately by a change of pleasantness to unpleasantness or of unpleasantness to pleasantness. This variation of hedonic tone, however, could also be produced by repeated stimulation, provided only that the intervals between applications of the stimulus were not long enough to allow complete recovery from the effects of previous stimulation.[36]

The dependence of hedonic sensitization and adaptation upon consecutive repetition receives a certain support from two recent experiments. The first, performed by M. F. Washburn, M. S. Child and T. M. Abel, involved repetition of musical themes five times in rapid succession.[37] The duration of the themes was about one minute, and the interval between successive presentations was 30 seconds. After each audition the observers—there were 220 in all —recorded the hedonic tone of their experience in terms of an absolute scale of 5 degrees. Four types of themes were used, namely "severely classical," "serious popular classical," "easy popular classical" and "popular." Two themes of each type were used with each observer. The results are shown below in graphical form (the graph was drawn by the writer from data in the article under consideration). In the case of each of the four types of themes there is shown, for each audition, the number of observers who experienced at that audition the greatest degree of enjoyment from either of the two themes.[38] It is clear that

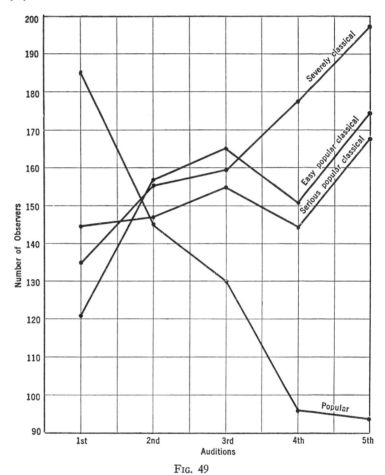

Fig. 49

(*Data from Washburn, Child and Abel*)

these results may be interpreted to show hedonic sensitization followed by adaptation, provided that one assume that for classical themes more repetition is needed to reach maximal pleasantness than for popular music.

The second experiment which supports the view of Fechner concerning the effects of consecutive repetition, is by E. M. Verveer, H. Barry, Jr., and W. A. Bousfield.[39] In this experiment the observers (26 in all) were given ten consecutive auditions of jazz records. Auditions 1 to 4 and 6 to 9 were of one record (fatigue record) ; auditions 5 to 10 were of another record (control record). After a week's interval the same procedure was repeated with the same observers. Immediately after each audition the observers rated their enjoyment of the experience on a scale of — 10 (maximal unpleasantness) to + 10 (maximal pleas-

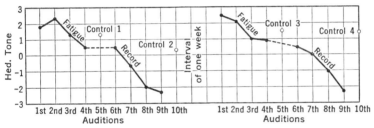

Fig. 50

(*From Verveer, Barry and Bousfield*)

antness). The results for all 26 observers are indicated on the graph above, in which abscissae represent successive auditions, and ordinates average degrees of hedonic tone. It will be seen that the hedonic value of the control record does not vary appreciably, while that of the fatigue record at each sitting varies through a maximum and then decreases below indifference in complete accord with the view propounded by Fechner.

An experiment by A. Karsten, however, indicates that, no matter how frequent the occurrence of sensitization and adaptation with consecutive repetition, the former cannot be considered to depend directly upon the latter.[40] The stimuli in Karsten's experiment were *actions* ("Handlungen"), performed by the observers themselves. The observers were made to repeat consecutively certain simple tasks (e. g., drawing parallel strokes in sets of 3 and 5, drawing figures, reading brief poems) until they were so *satiated* with the tasks that they refused to continue repeating them in accordance with the instructions. In some cases repetition was continued for several hours. The hedonic tone of the tasks at the various stages of the experiment was ascertained only in a rough way from the spontaneous remarks of the observers and from their answers to questions put them by the experimenter. The data were sufficient, however, to bring out two important facts. In the first place, when satiation occurred, its development was accompanied by increase of unpleasantness of the tasks. In the second place—and this is the important point—satiation did not always occur. Among the observers was a group of unemployed who were being paid for their work by the hour. These men displayed no sign of satiation even after repetition lasting as much as four hours. Karsten draws the obvious conclusion that satiation, of which loss of pleasantness is an important feature, although it often accompanies consecutive repetition, is not a direct function of such repetition.

If Karsten's data are not due to some experimental artifact—and there is no reason to believe that they are—it is clear that Fechner's view is wrong, that consecutive repetion does not, like continuous stimulation, determine a stage of sensitization followed by a stage of adaptation. Acceptance of this conclusion, however, at once raises the further problem of explaining the frequent occurrence of sensitization and adaptation with consecutive repetition. Concerning sensitization, a suggestion is afforded by the protocols of the observers in Miss Washburn's experiment. When asked to account for increases in the pleasantness of musical themes with repetition, these observers alleged the following causes with the frequencies named :[41]

TABLE XXXIX

Reasons	Frequencies (in 0/0)	
	Musical Observers	Unmusical Observers
Agreeable imagery	29.3	27.9
Increased comprehension of the composition	13.8	11.6
Greater attention to melody	12.3	6.9
Increased familiarity	9.3	13.8
Greater attention to rhythm	9.3	15.1
"Getting used to it" (where original pleasantness was low: affective adaptation)	6.1	11.6
Better adjustment of mood to that of composition	6.1	3.4
Greater attention to harmony	4.6	
Associations	3.	2.3
"Improves with hearing" (no explanation)		4.6
Greater attention to piano		2.3

As to adaptation, its occurrence with consecutive repetition is explained by Miss Washburn's observers as due to fatigue.[42] Karstens, however, finds no evidence of such dependence.[43] He believes rather that loss of pleasantness with consecutive repetition is in some cases due to "marking time"—to being obliged to continue an activity without making any progress—and in others due to difficulty in maintaining constant a single attentive field.[44] It is clear from these tentative explanations, however, that much remains to be done before we can satisfactorily account for hedonic sensitization and adaptation with consecutive repetition.

Habituation.—According to a number of psychologists, intermittent repetition—"familiarization"—determines a change of hedonic tone towards indifference.[45] This change may best be termed hedonic *habituation,* because of its dependence upon familiarization rather than upon continuity or frequency of stimulation. It is my purpose, in the present section, to examine the evidence which bears upon such hedonic habituation. I shall deal first with the evidence concerning *relative* hedonic habituation, concerning shifts towards indifference, in consequence of intermittent repetition, of the hedonic value of a stimulus *relative* to other similar stimuli. I shall then discuss the evidence bearing upon *absolute* hedonic habituation, upon shifts of the *absolute* hedonic value of a stimulus towards indifference as a function of intermittent repetition.

The evidence on relative hedonic habituation is very meagre. Indeed, there have been, to the best of my knowledge, but two experiments which bear at all directly upon the problem, one by S. C. Pepper[46] and one by myself.[47]

In Pepper's experiment the observers, 7 in number, were first made to judge, on a scale of 15 points (A + to E —), the hedonic tone of 66 paired combinations of 12 Bradley colors. From the data thus secured, Pepper calculated the "average consistency" of judgment of each observer, i. e., the average of the sum of the differences between the two judgments of an observer upon the same stimulus.[48] Six of the color combinations mentioned above were then presented to each observer for four experimental hours (one hour per week) with instructions to observe but not judge them, and during a fifth experimental hour with instructions to judge their hedonic tone. This procedure was repeated until the end of the year, four hours of exposure alternating with one hour of hedonic judgments. With respect to changes in hedonic value of individual stimuli, Pepper found that: "More than one-third of the judgments showed a change of appreciation at the end of the experiment over the beginning exceeding the average consistency of the subject, this change on the whole being toward neutrality." [49] The total number of points gained or lost for each grade is indicated in Table XL below:

TABLE XL

Grade	A	B	C	D	E
Points gained	0	2	1	21	9
Points lost	13	20	3	9	0
Points gained minus points lost.	— 13	— 18	— 2	12	9

Pepper concludes: "While there is some evidence of a change in individual aesthetic judgment, the results are not sufficient to warrant a definite conclusion or more detailed analysis." [50] Even this conclusion, however, is too definite. In Chapter 2, it was pointed out that, when the hedonic value of a set of stimuli is measured upon two separate occasions, the operation of chance factors tends to cause stimuli having high hedonic value on one occasion to have lower hedonic value on the other occasion, and stimuli having low hedonic value on one occasion to have higher hedonic value on the other occasion. The shift noted by Pepper may consequently be due not to repetition, but to the operation of chance factors. It follows that Pepper's results do not allow any conclusions whatever concerning relative hedonic habituation.

In my own experiment the hedonic rank of 14 olfactory substances was determined by paired comparison for eight observers on two different occasions, separated by two weeks. During these two weeks the observers were subjected to intensive familiarization with respect to one or two of the 14 stimuli. The familiarization-stimuli were not the same in the case of all observers; for each observer one (or two) stimuli were selected which were "moderately pleasant" to that particular observer. The familiarization-stimuli were presented in fairly continuous fashion during six experimental hours. At each experimental hour the observers being familiarized with a single stimulus were made to sniff it a total of 210 times, the sniffs being distributed in 15 groups of 1 to 50 sniffs, and the observers being familiarized with two stimuli were made to sniff each a total of 155 times, distributed in 6 groups of 1 to 50 sniffs. Absolute hedonic judgments were required of the observers at the end of each group of sniffs.

The results of this experiment are shown in the table below. Column 1 gives the observers in arbitrary order; column 2, the familiarization-stimuli for the various observers; column 3, the ranks of the familiarization-stimuli prior to familiarization; column 4, their rank after familiarization; column 5, the difference between these two ranks, and column 6, the average of the differences between ranks of all 14 stimuli, as determined before and after familiarization with the familiarization-stimuli. The differences in column 5 were computed by subtracting rank after familiarization from rank before familiarization, and consequently a positive difference indicates that rank after familiarization was higher—nearer the pleasant end of the series—and a negative difference indicates that rank after familiarization was lower—nearer the unpleasant end. As the familiarization-stimuli were all at the outset pleasant, a positive difference indicates a shift in hedonic value away from indifference and contrary to hedonic habituation, whereas a negative difference indicates a shift towards indifference, and consequently in accord with hedonic habituation.

TABLE XLI

1	2	3	4	5	6
Obs.	Fam.—Stim.	Rank before Fam.	Rank after Fam.	Change of Fam.—Stim.	Av. Change of all Stim.
Ad.	Oil of Sw. Orange ... 2.5		3.5	— 1.	1.92
Br.	Oil of Sw. Orange ... 3.5		3.	.5	1.38
Wa.	Oil of Sw. Orange ... 2.5		5.	— 2.5	1.50
Ke.	Ex. Carn. ... 3.		2.	1.	2.43
	Oil Cloves ... 6.		8.	— 2.	
Ze.	Ex. Carn. ... 2.		5.	— 3.	1.17
	Oil Cloves ... 6.		8.	0.	
Bu.	Oil Ylang ... 3.		2.	1.	.58
	Oil Berg. ... 6.		6.	0.	
De.	Oil Ylang ... 4.		4.	0.	2.25
	Oil Berg. ... 2.		2.	0.	
Ka.	Oil Ylang ... 7.		7.	0.	2.32
	Oil Berg. ... 3.		2.	1.	
Arithmetical average .. 3.88			4.26	.92	1.69
Algebraic average............... —.38					

Inspection of column 5 shows that 4 of the values in this column are negative, 4 positive and 5 zero. This indicates that the rank of the familiarization-stimulus after repetition was in 4 cases lower than before repetition, in 4 cases higher and in 5 cases unchanged. It follows that habituation, if at all operative under the conditions of this experiment, is operative only in a very slight degree.

In view of this fact, it is necessary to resort to statistical procedure and to deal with averages rather than individual values. In respect to such averages, inspection of the table shows that: (a) the arithmetical average of the changes in rank of the familiarization-stimuli for all observers (.92 ranks) is but 54% of the arithmetical average of the changes in rank of all stimuli for all observers (1.69 ranks); (b) the algebraic average of the changes in rank of the habituation stimuli for all observers is — .38. In Chapter II, however, we saw that the degree and direction of change in rank of a stimulus, from one series to another, is a definite function of the position of that stimulus in the first series. Before drawing inferences from the facts stated above, therefore, it is necessary to inquire into the degree and direction of change in rank which is to be expected of the familiarization-stimuli in consequence of their original ranks. In Chapter II, it was found that the extent of the change will tend to be maximal for stimuli occupying positions near the quartiles of the series, and minimal for those occupying the first, median, and last positions. Assuming that this relationship is a function whose graphic representation is a smooth curve, we may divide a series of 14 members into "regions of extent of change," as indicated in Figure 51, below. If now we indicate in this figure the number of adaptation stimuli of each rank by appropriate ordinates, we may, by comparing the number of habituation stimuli in regions of maximal change to that in regions of minimal change, ascertain in a rough way the proportion which the average extent of change in rank of the habituation stimuli should bear to the average extent of change in rank of all stimuli according to the relationship stated above.

Inspection of this figure shows that the number of

habituation stimuli in regions of minimal change (ranks 1-2, 6-9) is 7, while the number in regions of maximal change (ranks 3-5) is 6. From this it follows that the average of the extent of change in rank of the familiarization-stimuli should, according to the relationship between rank and extent of change stated above, have been slightly less than the average of the extent of change in rank of all stimuli. Thus the fact that the former average was actually found to be 54% of the latter average is no evidence at all of relative hedonic habituation. We further saw in Chapter II that the direction of change in rank will tend to be downward for stimuli whose position is above the median,

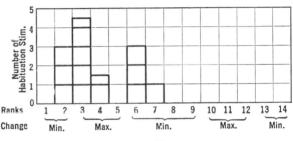

FIG. 51

and upward for those whose position is below the median. As the average rank of the familiarization-stimuli was before familiarization 3.88, and as none of these stimuli had a rank lower than 7, it follows that without any reference to habituation the change in rank of the familiarization-stimuli should have turned out to be negative. Thus the fact that the change actually was negative on the average is no proof whatever of hedonic habituation.

My own experiment, then, yields no evidence of relative hedonic habituation. As the only other relevant experiment, that of Pepper, is completely inconclusive, we must obviously conclude that there is at present no evidence whatever of relative hedonic habituation.

When we turn to absolute hedonic habituation, to the

shift of absolute hedonic value towards indifference as a function of intermittent repetition, we find a wealth of data at our disposal. Unfortunately, these data are far from univocal. On the one hand, there are a number of experiments in which intermittent repetition has been accompanied not by a shift of absolute hedonic value towards indifference, but by a shift in the opposite direction. Thus Max Meyer found the aesthetic value of quartertone [51] music to increase with intermittent repetition; A. R. Gilliland and H. T. Moore observed a similar [52] increase in the enjoyment of musical selections; J. E. Downey and G. E. Knapp likewise,[53] and L. J. Martin found that intermittent repetition of pictures was accompanied by an increase in the enjoyment which they yielded.[54] These experiments agree with the frequently voiced contention that familiarity with a work of art is a prerequisite to its full enjoyment.

Certain other experiments, however, indicate that intermittent repetition is indeed accompanied by a shift of hedonic value towards indifference. In an investigation of the constancy of hedonic judgments, P. T. Young had 4 observers judge the absolute hedonic value of 8 odors 15 times in the course of 5 weeks.[55] The judgments, originally in verbal terms (very unpleasant to very pleasant), were transmuted by Young into judgments on a numerical scale extending from -3 to $+3$. Fig. 52, next page, shows the average, for all observers, of the arithmetical sum of the numerical hedonic values of the eight odors at each of the 15 trials. It will be seen that, although this average increases from trial 1 to trial 5, it decreases thereafter in fairly steady fashion until, at the last trial, its value is distinctly lower than it was for the first trial. As a decrease of the arithmetical sum of the hedonic values of the 8 stimuli indicates convergence of their hedonic values towards indifference, this experiment clearly shows a shift which may be interpreted as absolute hedonic habituation. More recently J. P. Herrig presented to 14 children in the first grade one of the following taste-substances: Honey, chocolate, salt, egg-white and vinegar.[56] "Each child came daily and tasted one and only one substance for weeks, some tasting chocolate, some salt, etc." [57] The liking or disliking evidenced by a child on each occasion was measured by means of estimates by two adult observers trained in such judgments. The estimates were stated in terms of a number-series, extending from — 30 (extreme disliking) through O to + 30 (extreme liking). In the case of

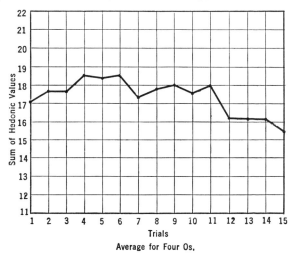

Fig. 52

(*Data from Young*)

every child the liking or disliking for the particular substance concerned decreased in amount, i. e., tended towards zero of the scale mentioned above. The experiment was continued for all the children 19 days, and for some—who continued to show decrease on the 19th day—as long as 32 days. The averages of the likes (in terms of estimates by 2 judges on a — 30 to + 30 scale) displayed by 4 children for honey and by 3 for chocolate are indicated for the different days on the graph opposite. The averages of the dislikes displayed by 4 children for egg-white, by 2 children for vinegar and by one for salt are likewise indicated on the graph. It will be seen that the two curves definitely converge towards zero. Consideration of individual data further showed that in no case did repetition determine a change from liking to disliking, or vice-versa, and that the more a substance was initially liked or disliked, the greater was the resultant change. These experiments obviously support the idea that "familiarity breeds contempt."

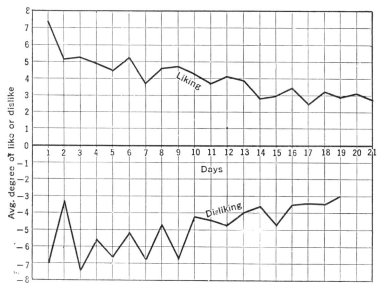

FIG. 53

(*After Herrig*)

In certain other experiments, finally, intermittent repetition has not been accompanied by any significant change in hedonic value. Valentine had 5 observers give absolute hedonic judgments upon the 12 musical intervals 33 times in the course of "one or two" weeks.[58] Comparison of the hedonic values of the intervals at the beginning and at the end of the experiment showed no appreciable change in the case of two observers; no change except the shift of one discord (the major second) from unpleasant to pleasant in the case of one observer, and for the two other observers no change of the consonant intervals, but a shift of three discords from unpleasant to pleasant. The figure below illustrates the results for one of the latter observers (abscissae: successive presentations; ordinates: algebraic average. of hedonic values). It is clear that this experiment fails to show any general shift of hedonic value as a function of repetition: two observers show no shift at all; three show only shifts confined to certain specific stimuli (discords). Similar results

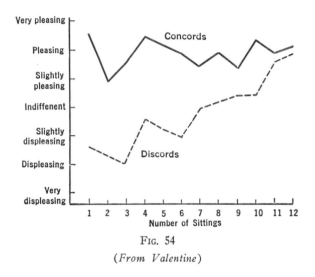

Fig. 54

(*From Valentine*)

were yielded by an experiment of my own in which 10 stimuli were presented to three observers 43 times over a period of 4½ months. The observers were made to judge the absolute hedonic value of the stimuli on a scale of — 3 to + 3 at the first and second presentations, at the sixteenth and at each presentation from the thirtieth to the forty-third. Fig. 55, opposite, shows the average of the arithmetical sum of the hedonic values of all stimuli for the three observers upon each occasion when judgment was required. It will be noted that the total hedonic value (either positive or negative) for the three observers remained fairly constant throughout the experiment. Here, again, then, we find no general shift in the sense of a shift distributed over all stimuli and occurring for all observers. This constancy of the group results naturally covers up shifts in the results for individual observers and for individual stimuli, but the fact that these particular shifts offset each other indicates that they do not constitute evidence of a general shift as a function of intermittent repetition.[59]

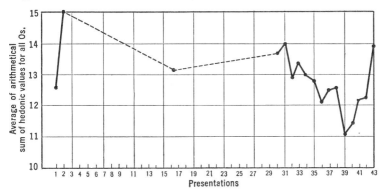

FIG. 55

What may we conclude concerning absolute hedonic habituation? Some experiments yield evidence of such a process, but others yield no such evidence, and yet others yield evidence of a contrary nature. It is clear that absolute hedonic habituation, like relative, lacks experimental substantiation.

There is, then, no generally valid law of hedonic habituation: it is not true that hedonic value shifts towards indifference *as a function* of intermittent repetition. Both with respect to relative and to absolute habituation, however, we saw that intermittent repetition is sometimes *accompanied* by a shift of hedonic value towards indifference. In discussing relative habituation we saw that some, at least, of such pseudo-habituative shifts are best to be described as regressions towards the mean due to errors of measurement. As to absolute pseudo-habituative shifts, various classes of them are likewise implied by a number of well-established psychological and physiological laws. One such law is the law of hedonic contrast. Let us assume that a single hedonic stimulus be presented to an observer repeatedly, and that these presentations determine a series of phenomena constituting a unitary temporal group. According to the law of hedonic contrast, the second phenomenon of such a series will tend to have an hedonic tone such as to compensate the hedonic tone of the first, the third an hedonic tone such as to compensate the combined hedonic tones of both the first and the second, and the nth phenomenon an hedonic tone such as to compensate the combined hedonic tone of the n — 1 preceding phenomena. With a sufficient number of repetitions, the total hedonic tone to be compensated will increase to such a degree that the hedonic tone corresponding to the stimulus will be brought to indifference. A further group of such laws is that dealing with motor habituation. Dodge, for instance, has been able to demonstrate decrease of nystagmus with intermittent repetition of rotation,[60] the work of Blatz indicates habituation of fear-responses in man,[61] and the Peckhams [62] and Wasmann [63] have observed the habituation of emotional responses in insects. In cases where unpleasantness is in part dependent upon responses thus subject to habituation, it is clear that intermittent repetition must be accompanied by decreased unpleasantness. Hedonic pseudohabituation is likewise implied by the laws of acclimatization and of pharmacological habituation. Davenport and Castle, for instance, demonstrated many years ago that tadpoles, reared at a temperature of 25° C., will not display "heat rigor" (complete cessation of motion) until the temperature has been raised to 43° C., while comparable tadpoles reared at 15° C. display "heat rigor" at 40° C.[64] Again Davenport and Neal showed that "stentor reared for 2 days in a culture solution, containing .00005% $HgCl_2$, resists a killing solution of 0.001% $HgCl_2$ nearly 4 times as long as those reared in water." [65] The effect of such physiological habituation upon the hedonic value of stimuli is well shown in Ruckmick's study of learning to smoke.[66] "While the physiological eliminating processes were under way, organic and kinaesthetic sensations were prominent and somewhat unpleasant. . . . The unpleasant features of the experience were practically removed after the third attempt."[67] The obvious connection, finally, between pleasantness and the satisfaction of drives—a connection to be discussed in detail in the next chapter—implies that in so far as drives are subject to permanent satisfaction, as is true of certain curiosities, the hedonic value of stimuli arousing these drives will decrease with intermittent repetition.

FOOTNOTES AND REFERENCES

[1] G. J. v. ALLESCH, Die Aesthetische Erscheinungsweisen der Farben, *Psychol. Forsch.*, 6, 1925, 255 ff.

[2] TH. RIBOT. La Psychologie des Sentiments, 11th Edit., Paris, 1922, 33-34.

[3] M. YOKOYAMA. Affective Tendency Conditioned by Color and Form, *Amer. J. Psychol.*, 32, 1921, 81.

[4] *Ibid.*, 90.

[5] M. MEENES. Attention as a Condition of Affection, *Amer. J. Psychol.*, 34, 1923, 117-122.

[6] *Ibid.*, 122.

[7] J. A. H. KEITH. The Mutual Influence of Feelings, *Harvard Psychol. Studies*, 2, 1906, 141.

[8] *Ibid.*, 157.

[9] FECHNER. Vorschule der Aesthetik, II, 2nd Edit., Leipzig, 1898, 232.

[10] A. LEHMANN. Hauptgesetze des menschlichen Gefühlslebens, 2nd Edit., Leipzig, 1914, 251.

[11] H. T. MARSHALL. Pleasure and Aesthetics, London and New York, 1894, 326.

[12] A. J. HARRIS. Studies in Affective Contrast, Thesis, Harvard University, 1930, 4.

[13] M. M. BACON, E. A. ROOD and M. F. WASHBURN. A Study of Affective Contrast, *Amer. J. Psychol.*, 25, 1914, 290-291.

[14] *Ibid.*, 291.

[15] *Ibid.*, 290.

[16] A. J. HARRIS. An Experiment on Affective Contrast. *Amer. J. Psychol.*, 41, 1929, 617-624.

[17] *Ibid.*, 618.

[18] *Ibid.*, 620.

[19] This law was originally proposed by me in a slightly different connection under the name "law of affective equilibrium." My original formulation was as follows: "The affective value of the experimental correlate of a stimulus varies conversely with the sum of the affective values of

those experiences preceding this correlate which constitute with it a unitary temporal group." As Harris has demonstrated that it describes the facts of hedonic contrast, I feel that it no longer needs a special name, but should merely be considered as a formulation of the law of hedonic contrast.

[20] A. J. HARRIS. Studies of Affective Contrast, Thesis, Harvard University, 1930, 116.

[21] J. G. BEEBE-CENTER. The Law of Affective Equilibrium, *Amer. J. Psychol.*, 41, 1929, 64.

[22] E. B. TITCHENER. Experimental Psychology, I, pt. ii, 1901, 157.

[23] "Every O, except A, reported both P and U sensations from every sense department. A reported them with sensations of smell, taste and touch. . . . A left the University before the completion of her series, and had no opportunity to observe with visual and auditory stimuli." (J. P. NAFE. An Experimental Study of the Affective Qualities, *Amer. J. Psychol.*, 35, 1924, 540.)

[24] "Introspection leaves no doubt that the sensations, regarded as qualitative processes, fall into a number of separate groups. All color sensations, for instance, go together; all tonal sensations go together." (TITCHENER, Textbook of Psychology, 1910, 55.)

[25] In comparable, but not in equal proportions. J. C. Flügel has shown that when Os record their feelings over long periods of time there is a noticeable predominance of pleasantness over unpleasantness. *Cf.* J. C. FLÜGEL, *Brit J. Psychol.*, 15, 1925, 327ff. These results are in harmony with those of a large number of other experiments. *Cf.* the findings of G. B. PHELAN mentioned in the text above; *cf.* also A. E. FINDLEY, *Amer. J. Psychol.*, 35, 1924, 444, and C. W. VALENTINE, *Brit. J. Psychol.*, 6, 1913, 190. I suggest that this preponderance of pleasantness may be ascribed to the effects of tradition and learning, which eliminate situations conducive to unpleasantness (e. g., extremes of temperature, lack of food, putrid odors) and bring about situations conducive to pleasantness (e. g., physiologically favorable temperature, regular meals, perfumes).

[26] G. B. PHELAN. Feeling Experience and Its Modalities, 1925, 112.

[27] *Ibid.*, 113.

[28] E. G. WEVER and K. E. ZENER. The Method of Absolute Judgment in Psychophysics, *Psychol. Rev.*, 35, 1928, 466.

[29] S. R. TRUMAN and E. G. WEVER. The Judgment of Pitch as a Function of the Series, *Univ. Calif. Publ. Psychol.*, 3, 1928, 215.

[30] J. VOLKMANN. Absolute Impression as a Psychophysical Method, Thesis, Harvard University, 1931.

[31] *Ibid.*, 8.

[32] TH. ZIEHEN. Leitfaden der Physiologischen Psychologie, Jena, 1914, 272-273.

[33] A. J. HARRIS. Studies of Affective Contrast, Thesis, Harvard University, 1930, 116.

[34] P. T. YOUNG. Studies in Affective Psychology, VIII, The Scale of Values Method, *Amer. J. Psychol.*, 42, 1930, 17.

[35] *Ibid.*, 26.

[36] G. T. FECHNER. Vorschule der Aesthetik, II, 2nd Edit., Leipzig, 1898, 240-246.

[37] M. F. WASHBURN, M. S. CHILD and T. M. ABEL. The Effects of Immediate Repetition on the Pleasantness or Unpleasantness of Music, in "The Effects of Music," edited by M. Schoen, New York, 1927, 199-210.

[38] When an observer reported maximal enjoyment of a piece at more than one presentation, a maximum was credited to *both* presentations.

[39] E. M. VERVEER, H. BARRY, JR., and W. A. BOUSFIELD. Change in Affectivity with Repetition, to be published in *Amer. J. Psychol.*

[40] A. KARSTEN. Psychische Sättigung, Untersuchungen zur Handlungs —und Affektpsychologie, edited by K. Lewin, *Psychol. Forsch,* 10, 1928, 148-254.

[41] M. F. WASHBURN, M. S. CHILD and T. M. ABEL, *op. cit.,* 206.

[42] *Ibid.,* 206.

[43] KARSTENS. *Op. cit.,* 194 seq.

[44] *Ibid.,* 253-254.

[45] *Cf.* O. KÜLPE. Grundriss der Psychologie, Leipzig, 1893, 269; E. B. TITCHENER, A Textbook of Psychology, New York, 1909, 229; B. B. BREESE, Psychology, New York, 1917, 361.

[46] S. C. PEPPER. Changes in Appreciation for Color Combinations, *Psychol. Rev.,* 26, 1919, 389-396.

[47] J. G. BEEBE-CENTER. Affective Habituation, Thesis, Harvard University, 1926.

[48] The data, originally secured in alphabetical form, were transposed into numerical form according to the following system of correspondencies:

A +	A	A —	B +	B	B —	C +	C	C —	D +	D	D —	E +	E	E —
1	2	3	4	5	6	7	8	9	10	11	12	13	14	15

From the transposed data Pepper computed for each observer a value which he termed the "average consistency" of the observer and which is defined by the following equation:

$$A. C. = \frac{\Sigma(J_1 - J_2)}{n},$$

in which A. C. represents "average consistency," J_1 and J_2 the two judgments upon a single stimulus, and n the number of stimuli in the experiment.

[49] *Ibid.,* 393.

[50] *Ibid.,* 393.

[51] M. MEYER. Experimental Studies in the Psychology of Music, *Amer. J. Psychol.,* 14, 1903, 207-214.

[52] A. R. GILLILAND and H. T. MOORE. The Immediate and Long-Time Effects of Classical and Popular Phonograph Selections, *J. Appl. Psychol.,* 8, 1924, 309-323.

[53] J. E. DOWNEY and G. E. KNAPP. The Effects on a Musical Programme of Familiarity and of Sequence of Selections, in "The Effects of Music," edited by M. Schoen, New York, 1927, 223-243.

[54] L. J. MARTIN. An Experimental Study of Fechner's Principles of Aesthetics, *Psychol. Rev.,* 13, 1906, 175-179.

[55] P. T. YOUNG. Constancy of Affective Judgments to Odors, *J. Exper. Psychol.,* 6, 1923, 182-191.

[56] J. P. HERRIG. The Measurement of Liking and Disliking, *J. Educ. Psychol.,* 21, 1930, 159-196.

[57] *Ibid.,* 176.

[58] C. W. VALENTINE. The Method of Comparison in Experiments with Musical Intervals and the Effect of Practice on the Appreciation of Discords, *Brit. J. Psychol.*, 7, 1914, 118.

[59] For details of this experiment, *cf.* J. G. BEEBE-CENTER, Affective Habituation, Thesis, Harvard University, 1926.

[60] R. DODGE. Habituation to Rotation, *J. Exper. Psychol.*, 6, 1923, 1-34.

[61] W. E. BLATZ. The Cardiac, Respiratory and Electrical Phenomena Involved in the Emotion of Fear, *J. Exper. Psychol.*, 8, 1925, 109-132.

[62] G. W. and E. G. PECKHAM. Some Observations on the Mental Powers of Spiders, *J. of Morphology*, I, 1887, 393-395.

[63] E. WASMANN. Die Psychischen Fähigkeiten der Ameisen, *Zoologica*, Heft 26, 1899, 35 seq.

[64] C. B. DAVENPORT and W. E. CASTLE. Studies in Morphologenesis, III, On the Acclimatization of Organisms to High Temperatures, *Arch. f. Entwickelungsmechanik der Organismen*, 2, 1895, 227-249.

[65] C. B. DAVENPORT and H. V. NEAL. Studies in Morphologenesis, V, Acclimatization of Organisms to Poisonous Chemical Substances, *Arch. f. Entwickelungsmechanik der Organismen*, 2, 1896, 581.

[66] C. A. RUCKMICK. Experiences During Learning to Smoke, *Amer. J. Psychol.*, 35, 1924, 402-406.

[67] *Ibid.*, 406.

Chapter VI

Hedonic Tone in Relation to Motivating Factors

Common sense recognizes relationships of hedonic tone not only to physiological motivating factors such as bodily needs, but to so-called psychological motivating factors, such as wishes and dispositions. The day will doubtless come when relationships of the latter type will be dropped from psychology. Psychological motivating factors are at present but vague concepts, defined not with respect to spatio-temporal localization and physico-chemical nature, but only in terms of remote antecedents and consequents. It is likely that they will remain vague, for there is little chance that individual factors correspond to simple physiological processes and thus are capable of ultimate definition in physico-chemical terms. For the time being, however, psychology cannot afford to omit relationships involving psychological motivating factors, for the knowledge which they provide cannot be stated in any other terms. The present chapter, therefore, will be devoted to the relations between hedonic tones and motivating factors of both types, namely, *cognitive dispositions, evaluative dispositions, needs* and *wishes.*

HEDONIC TONE IN RELATION TO COGNITIVE DISPOSITIONS

The existence of a relationship between hedonic judgments and cognitive dispositions was first demonstrated by J. Segal in 1906.[1] Whereas the interest of Fechner and of his immediate followers had lain in establishing the average aesthetic value of stimuli for large groups of observers, the interest of Segal lay in studying the conditions determining individual aesthetic judgments. His observers were shown a variety of figures with instructions not only to judge the figures hedonically, but to describe the general impressions produced by the figures. The results showed that one and the same stimulus might give rise to very different phenomena in different observers, or in the same observer at different times, and that such phenomenal differences were correlated with marked differences in hedonic tone. Thus a particular line was seen by an observer on one occasion as an ill-drawn horizontal line, arousing dislike; on another occasion as an arrow, rousing marked liking; and on a third occasion as an ill-drawn vertical, again arousing dislike. The results of Segal were confirmed in an experiment by L. W. Legowski, published in 1908.[2] Legowski had his observers judge figures hedonically under two different instructions, the first requiring judgment upon immediate impression, the second requiring judgment upon the figures as features of objects of specific types, such as arches or visiting cards. Legowski found marked differences between hedonic values ascribed to the same objects under the two different instructions.

In 1908, E. Bullough published a very extensive experiment upon the relation of initial perception to hedonic judgment—the "perceptive problem" of aesthetics, as he called it—in the particular case of colors.[3] Thirty-five observers were shown thirty-five colored papers singly, with instructions first to judge whether the colors were pleasant, indifferent or unpleasant, and secondly to give introspective reports explaining their judgments. A special effort was made to impress upon the observers that it was less their opinion of the colors which was desired than the reasons that prompted their judgments—how each color appeared to them, and by reason of what special features they liked or disliked it.

The results showed marked differences in the types of experiences involved. The various experiences, according to Bullough, represented four main "aspects of color," i. e., four main types of color experience, and consequently indicated the occurrence of four main cognitive dispositions in the observers. The four main "aspects of color" were named and characterized as follows by the author:

1. *The objective aspect,* involving such phenomenal characteristics as purity, goodness, brightness and their converses.

2. *The physiological aspect,* involving characteristics which produce effects on the observer, such as stimulation, soothing and temperature effects.

3. *The associative aspect,* involving phenomena suggested (or "associated") with the color. Examples of such concomitant phenomena are: sunsets, moonlight, trees, seasons, dress materials, etc.

4. *The character aspect,* involving characteristics which, if predicated of a human being, would be included under the terms mood, character and temperament. Such characteristics of color are: cheerfulness, affectionateness, impetuousness, etc.

The four main perceptive attitudes are represented, according to Bullough, by four perceptive types, these types being collective terms for a number of individuals who tend to the perception of one aspect, or group of aspects, rather than to another. The four main perceptive types were characterized by the author as follows:

1. *The objective type* is inclined to intellectual appreciation rather than emotional. It is apt to involve absence of any definite color preference in the abstract.

2. *The physiological type* is particularly sensitive to the "physiological" effects of color. Statements such as "the color is glaring," "trying to the eyes," "fatiguing to look at" are always indicative of the physiological type.

3. *The associative type* is characterized by Bullough chiefly by its tendency to experience the associative aspect of color.

4. *The character type* is characterized by a tendency to exteriorize physiological aspects, such as strength, temperature, etc., into the color itself. It may, according to Bul-

lough, be considered as a development from the physiological type.

An examination of the hedonic tone reported for the various aspects of color showed that certain aspects were hedonically more effective than others. The objective aspect, in particular, was found to involve but little hedonic tone, while the physiological aspect and the character aspect (supposedly developed from the former by exteriorization) showed marked hedonic tone. Thus, according to Bullough, the variability of hedonic judgments upon a single stimulus is, in part, due to the facts that this stimulus may give rise to very different types of cognitive contents because of different cognitive dispositions on the part of the observers, and that these various types of cognitive contents have very different hedonic effectiveness.

It should be added that Bullough, an aesthetician, ascribes very different aesthetic worth to his four perceptive types. For him "the agreeable" is to be distinguished from "the beautiful": . . . "Agreeableness is the consciousness of our being pleasantly affected by a thing, whereas beauty appears to the unsophisticated mind—and even to the sophisticated one, while the impression lasts—as an attribute of the thing itself. That we are affected in both cases and that both agreeableness and beauty involve a relation between *ourself* and the thing is, of course, undeniable, but the point of difference lies in the different emphasis which we give to either term of the relation, either to the self or to the thing. This amounts to saying that the distinction consists in the difference of position which the object occupies in our consciousness. If we call it 'agreeable,' *we* occupy the centre; the pleasantness, *our* pleasure, is the rationale of the whole situation. The thing itself lingers somewhere on the confines of our consciousness, and may even fade into a merely inducing factor, a mere source of pleasure. Thus a warm bath: The bath itself is not the point of stress in my consciousness, but I myself, with all the delightful sensations of coolness, of softness and of gentle relaxation, and my pleasure, not *identified with,* but only *derived from* the bath, represent the pivot of the experience. But in the case of beautiful objects, it is the object which stands in the focus of my attention. *My own* affections drop out of its range, sometimes so completely that the question of liking or dislike, even pleasantness, appears almost absurd to the subject. However subjective the 'beauty' may be as to its original source, it appears as an objective quality of the thing, precisely because the self which invested it with it has faded out of consciousness." [4]

Granting this distinction, it is clear that mere hedonic effectiveness is not equivalent to aesthetic worth. According to Bullough, in aesthetic evaluation of his four perceptive types, the physiological type, which experiences agreeableness, but not beauty, ranks lowest from the point of view of aesthetics. The character type, on the other hand, which exteriorizes all of the orginally "subjective affections" of the physiological type and thus experiences them not as agreeableness, but as beauty, holds the highest aesthetic rank.

The dependence of hedonic tone upon cognitive disposition, demonstrated for optical figures by Segal and Legowski, and for colors by Bullough, has more recently been shown to hold for musical intervals by C. C. Pratt.[5] In the course of an experiment on fusion, Pratt ascertained the hedonic values of the 12 musical intervals for 5 observers by the method of paired comparison. It was found that there were marked individual differences, and that these individual differences indicated the existence of two types of observers, the types differing markedly from each other, but being very homogenous within themselves. One type, involving 2 observers, preferred the octave to all other intervals, and ranked the major third in sixth place. The other type, including 3 observers, preferred the major third and ranked the octave in fifth place. Examination of the introspective reports of the observers showed that to the two types there corresponded very different cognitive contents for a single stimulus and, consequently, that these types were essentially distinguished by their cognitive dis-

position. Both observers representing the type which preferred the octave were found to be judging hedonic value
on the basis of "smoothness-roughness," while the three observers representing the type which preferred the major
third were found to be judging hedonic value on the basis
of musical meanings.

The specifically original part of Bullough's contribution
to the "perceptive problem" in aesthetics—namely, his doctrine that there are four main perceptive aspects corresponding to four perceptive types—has not fared any too well
at the hands of subsequent investigators. In an experiment
with tones and bichords (pairs of simultaneous tones), published in 1914, Myers and Valentine were forced by their
data to alter two of Bullough's four aspects.[6] The objective
aspect was extended to include "a passive regard of the
sound as having meaning or use as an independent object," [7] and the physiological aspect (rechristened "intra-
subjective") was extended to include "the experiences of
self-activity which the sounds may produce in the subject." [8]
On the basis of further data secured with music, Myers
later subdivided Bullough's objective aspect into two aspects, the objective (purity, pitch, etc.) and the pragmatic
(use and meaning as an object).[9] J. Downey, finally, from
data secured with words as stimuli, added to the list a symbolization aspect, which included word-coloration, visual
patterning of auditory content and time-of-day connota-
tion.[10]

As to perceptive types, their fate has been much the
same as that of imaginal types. In the experiment mentioned above, Myers and Valentine found in the first place
that "pure" types were very rare. In order to explain the
difference between this finding and the observations of Bullough, they compared results for observers given Bullough's
instructions (requiring statement of like or dislike and reason for this) and given their own (requiring description
"of what came into the observer's mind, how he was affected, etc., by the sound"). They found that observers who
reported in terms of *one* aspect under Bullough's instructions

would frequently report in terms of *several* aspects under their own instructions. Myers and Valentine found in the second place that certain observers shift from one type to another with variation of conditions. Of fourteen observers who had taken part in both their experiment and that of Bullough, five failed to maintain their type completely and "one subject, K, who, for colors, is strictly of the character type and showed no associations, proves very strongly of the associative type for tones." [11] In the third place, Myers and Valentine found that the frequency with which a single set of observers reported the four main aspects differed for different types stimuli (cf., the table below indicating the percentage of reports belonging to the four main aspects for three types of stimuli). All of these findings are clearly contrary to Bullough's doctrine of perceptive types. Fur-

TABLE XLII

	Intra-subj.	Obj.	Char.	Assoc.
Single Tones	24	35	13	28 per cent
Single Bichords	17	47	8	28 " "
Pairs of Bichords	23	56	7	14 " "

thermore, in the subsequent investigation upon aesthetic reactions to music by Myers alone, pure types turned out to be even more rare for music than for tones and bichords. Myers wrote: "Hardly any subject shows himself absolutely pure to one type, to the complete exclusion of all others." [12] It would seem, then, that Bullough's perceptive types, like imaginal types, are nothing more than ideal reference points for approximate and temporary classification. To say that an individual belongs to the objective perceptive type is merely to say that under current conditions he will recognize predominantly the objective aspects of phenomena.

It has been my purpose in the present work to deal with the establishment of facts rather than with their application. I cannot refrain, however, from pointing out the effectiveness of the relation of hedonic tone to cognitive dispositions as a tool for the control of likes and dislikes.

In a Lowell Lecture delivered in 192ɔ, Paul Hazard pointed out that before the eighteenth century the French had little, if any appreciation for the beauties of nature. "To be sure, the French had always been fond of what they called 'voyages en campagne'—journeys into the country. But, in truth, what were these trips? If one investigates the matter one will find that in reality a 'voyage en campagne' meant simply that one traveled to some chateau in the provinces, where one's comfort was extremely well served, and where the company shut itself up in the rooms of the chateau for conversation and drawing-room diversions, broken only by walks in the garden. No one seems to have gone into the country to enjoy the rural scene for itself, or to have taken much note of the country's beauty." [14] As to the mountains, they were considered "simply as ugly, forbidding waste-land, which was infertile and produced no good. . . . Even so intelligent a man as Montesquieu limited his whole description (1729) of a trip from Rome to Munich to this statement: 'I made a very painful journey, half of the way in excessive heat, the other half in mortal cold, in the month of August, in the mountains of the Tyrol.' All the grandeur of these mountains, and the beauty of Lake Constance among them, meant to him nothing." [15]

Then came Rousseau, the lover of nature. M. F. Maury wrote: "All of nature, the Alps, the Jura, the rocks of La Meillerie, the vines of Clarens, the blue of the lake, lend their marvelous framework to the joys and sorrows of Saint-Preux (one of Rousseau's characters). Thus the author brings back to us that secret harmony between the soul and the outer world, which Vergil had known, but which for us had become lost." [16] The effect upon educated French people was not long in showing itself. Many of Rousseau's readers "set out on pilgrimages into Switzerland to 'make the trip Rousseau had made.' " [17] Marie Antoinette gave herself up to rural life at the Petit Trianon, and great ladies assumed the role of shepherdesses. In literature, Bernardin de Saint-Pierre and André Chénier were opening the way to romanticism. France had become conscious of nature and of its beauties.

Radically different in its nature, but leading to the same conclusion, is the evidence afforded by an experiment of Washburn and Grose on the voluntary control of likes and dislikes.[18] The main purpose of the experiment was to test the validity of the Stoic maxim, "Everything is opinion, and opinion is in our power" in so far as it relates to judgments. The observers were shown single colors with the request to judge their hedonic value in terms of a scale of 1 to 7. As soon as they had made such a judgment, the experimenter said: "Now I want to see if you can dislike that color," if the judgment has been favorable, or "I want to see if you can like that color," if the judgment had been unfavorable. If the observer were able to alter her judgment, the new judgment was recorded and the observer was asked to state how the change had been made. It was found that a change in hedonic value was brought about in all but 6.3% of the trials. Of chief interest to us in the present connection, however, is the fact that in 46.1% of all the trials the change was brought about either by means of an imaginary context, i. e., by thinking of the colors in a context different from the actual ones, or by means of shifts of attention to marginal associates. It is clear that nature and the laboratory are at one in proving the effectiveness of cognitive dispositions in the control of likes and dislikes.

Hedonic Tone in Relation to Evaluative Dispositions

Hedonic Disposition.—Indirect evidence of a relationship between hedonic tone and a specific disposition to make hedonic judgments has been in existence for a number of years. In an experiment upon choice published in 1920,[19] R. H. Wheeler found that "when the observer sat completely relaxed he was unable to choose." [20] Wheeler interprets this fact as indicating that an essential feature of choosing is the making of a motor adjustment towards the alternative. If we consider that some of his choices were between musical selections, it seems likely that the attitude of passivity not only precluded actual choice, but likewise preference. Again, in his experiment upon the "affective qualities," published in 1924, J. P. Nafe found that a prerequisite for "an observable affective experience (i. e., a bright or dull pressure) was a 'psychological, non-perceptive attitude.'" [21] Young verified this finding when, in a repetition of Nafe's experiment, the only observer to report bright and dull pressures was one who had observed for Nafe at Cornell.[22] In view of the high correlation between bright and dull pressure and pleasantness and unpleasantness, these results obviously suggest that hedonic tone also depends upon a non-perceptive attitude on the part of the observer. As in the case of Wheeler's experiment, however, such a conclusion is merely suggested.

The first experiment to yield direct evidence on the problem at issue is one published by E. F. Wells in 1930. Wells, working at Cornell, presented a number of normally pleasant or unpleasant stimuli to 4 observers, with a general instruction "requiring a description of the total experience from the moment preceding the presentation of the stimulus (initial attitude) to the termination of the affection." [23] The reports of the observers showed that their initial attitudes varied considerably, but could all be considered to belong to one of three main types. These types were: (a) *the critical affective attitude,* "a set to react affectively to the stimulus and to observe critically the total experience. . . . Under this set the O is predisposed towards affective experience, more specifically towards affective *content* rather than affective significance"; [24] (b) *the critical perceptive attitude,* "a set to observe the stimulus-experience critically without reacting affectively to it"; [25] (c) *the common-sense attitude,* "a set with which we take experience in everyday life as opposed to the critical laboratory set." [26] Miss Wells then presented stimuli to her observers with specific instructions requiring them to assume some one of these typical attitudes. The resulting reports, together with those secured in the first part of the experiment, showed the influence of these attitudes to be as follows: Under the critical affective attitude, "Experience usually develops as an affective pattern in which qualitative content predominates. This pattern is typically a total fusion without clear-cut division into focus and background or specific localization. . . . The content of the affective pattern usually includes diffuse pressure-like experience; affective stuff, which diffuses through the total; bright and lively in P; dull, dead and heavy in U." [27] Under the critical perceptive attitude, "Affective experience does not occur. Experience develops as a perceptual pattern, sharply divided into a clear focus and an obscure background. . . . When an affective reaction occurs under instructions for a critical perceptive attitude, there is always a shift away from the perceptive attitude." [28] Under the common-sense attitude, "Affective experience occurs as a patterned reaction, in which the content aspect is too obscure to be observed in detail and the meaning or significance of the reaction dominates. Bodily experience comes as vague, undeveloped stuff. There is nothing as specific as bright pressure or dull pressure in it." [29] The following is an example of report under this attitude: " . . . That was a P smell. Again, I didn't notice any bodily change when experience became affective. It was simply that the smell was P, that I liked it." [30]

The results secured by Wells have been partly confirmed by F. W. Hazzard in an experiment on the olfactory qualities, performed at Cornell.[31] Hazzard's purpose was to test the adequacy of Henning's classification. She presented her observers the following odorous substances, with instructions to maintain a passive attitude and to describe the course of experience—heliotropin, geranium oil, tonka bean, coumarin, tar, amyl alcohol, carbon disulfide, pyridine, hydrogen sulfide, benzol, apiol, sweet orange oil, cedarwood oil, cinnamon oil. Almost all of these substances constitute excellent hedonic stimuli. Nevertheless, Hazzard writes:

"The experiences, on the whole, were not taken affectively. This aspect drops out entirely with the advent of the third series (there were four series of observations in all), and does not, under the conditions of this experiment, correlate with stimulus. We can neither affirm nor deny the relation that Henning and Findley have determined." [32] An experiment by K. W. Oberlin, finally, likewise points to the importance of a hedonic attitude in determining hedonic tone.[33] Oberlin first had his observers judge the relative *brilliance* of heterochromatic pairs of colors presented for one second. Occasionally he would ask the observers, immediately after an exposure, to judge the stimuli with respect to one of the following characteristics: Hue, saturation, extensity, shape and hedonic tone. The "postdetermined" judgments of hedonic tone appeared to be more mediate than the other post-determined judgments. One observer invariably judged hedonic tone from surrogates. Another did likewise, but the surrogates were frequently associatively aroused. A third also judged hedonic tone from surrogates, and stated that "affection does not come unless asked for" and that then "it builds up very slowly." The fourth observer invariably judged hedonic tone associatively. This observer described her post-determined judgments (including those on hedonic tone) as follows: "I am always looking for brilliance and not conscious of looking for anything else until asked for it. After being asked, sometimes I can answer right away, but am not conscious of knowing that before. If the answer does not come at once, then I try to look back or recall a surrogate." [34] In a second part of his experiment, Oberlin presented the same stimuli to four new observers with different instructions. The observers were told: "You will be presented with two stimuli simultaneously for one second. You are to tell me the difference between the two—any difference. Try to be passive in this experiment and do not look for any particular difference. Report as quickly as possible. In the introspection, report on the basis of the

judgment and the process of the judgment." [35] Three observers gave a good many reports of hedonic differences,
although for two the hedonic judgments seemed indirect in
the sense of coming last in a temporal series or of involving
associated content or surrogates. Of the fourth observer,
however, Oberlin wrote: "The data from Ch. indicated
that, in order to experience affection, this O required a
special affective determination. He gave no judgments of
differences in affection until the first third of the material
had been presented. Then in his introspective report we
find: 'It occurred to me at this point for the first time that
perhaps I could find differences in P and U between the
stimuli—as far as I can recall, none of them has appealed
to me as P or as U—perhaps that is determined by the set.'
For the remaining stimuli, however, he gave judgments of
difference in affection in more than 40% of the cases." [36]

What conclusions may be drawn from these results? It
seems quite clear that for the phenomenal correlates of
many stimuli characterization with respect to hedonic tone
requires a special disposition on the part of the observer.
This is true not only of overt characterization by means of
report, but of covert characterization, of the mere awareness that a phenomenal entity is pleasant or unpleasant.
Is lack of hedonic characteristization, however, equivalent
to absence of hedonic characteristics, or, as I should prefer
to put it, to hedonic indeterminateness? If by phenomenal
entity be meant an ultimate reality, not necessarily known
or even knowable to science, answer to this question will
depend upon philosophical affiliations. On the other hand,
if phenomenal entity be taken to mean an entity constructed
or inferred from available data—the only scientific meaning of the term, it seems to me—the answer fortunately is
dictated by facts. To the best of my knowledge the data
upon which are based such inferences are at present of two
main types. First, there are the data of stimulus-constancy,
which show that the characteristization of the phenomenal
correlate of a stimulus with respect to a certain attribute,

secured by appropriate determination, will usually vary within narrow limits. It is from these data that Titchener explicitly inferred the sensation in his well-known reply to Rahn.[37] Second, there are the data which may be grouped under the term phenomenon-constancy, which show that in the case of a durable phenomenal process considered by the observer to remain self-identical, characterization with respect to a certain attribute, secured by proper determination, usually varies within narrow limits. It is from these latter data that the Gestalt school, rejecting the data of stimulus-constancy because of their limitations, infer phenomenal configurations—albeit the inference is always implicit. It is from these data also that common sense infers "perceptions" and "ideas." Indeed, it is a question in my mind whether the data of phenomenon-constancy are more than tautologies, whether phenomenal self-identity has for an observer any other meaning than constancy of characterization. If now phenomenal entities are inferred on the basis of stimulus-constancy or of phenomenon-constancy, or of both, it is clearly impossible to have a hedonically determinate phenomenal entity, for the facts of contrast preclude hedonic stimulus constancy, and hedonic phenomenon-constancy is precluded by frequent report of phenomena becoming more or less pleasant.[38] From this in turn it seems to follow that lack of hedonic characterization, whether overt or covert, must be considered as *prima facie* evidence of hedonic indeterminateness. As the data reviewed above constitute the only relevant evidence, it is clearly reasonable to conclude—very tentatively, because of the paucity of data and of the complexity of their interpretation—that, in the case of many stimuli—possibly of all—hedonic tone depends upon a specific evaluative disposition which we may call a hedonic disposition.

Moods.—The close relationship of hedonic tone to moods is an obvious fact to the layman. A common statement is: "So-and-so is in such a mood today that nothing would be pleasant to him." This relationship is also stressed by many psychological works. Thus Lehmann, in his well-known monograph, writes: "As every mood (Stimmung) may be conceived as the perseveration (Nachbild) of an emotion, there are as many different moods as there are emotions. They fall, however, into two main groups, according to whether pleasantness or unpleasantness predominate. These groups are called in daily life good or bad frames of mind (Launen). If one is in a good frame of mind, sensitivity to unpleasantness is strongly decreased, minor bothers are either entirely overlooked or throw but very passing shadows on the joyful condition to which they must quickly again make way. Entirely analagous is the manifestation of a bad frame of mind, of dejection (Verstimmtheit). In this condition all impressions normally provocative of joy are usually devoid of any effect or, at most, produce only a momentary cheerfulness." [39]

These assertions may well be true, but they rest for the most part on mere casual observation. In discussing assimilation (Chapter V), we saw that, in an experiment by Young on the constancy of hedonic judgments, an observer in a very depressed mood judged a whole set of stimuli to be far more unpleasant than usual; [40] we also saw that, in an experiment by Harris on the effect of odors upon the hedonic tone of colors, assimilative shifts in the hedonic tone of the colors seemed dependent on the arousal of moods by the odors. [41] This evidence, however, is very incidental. In neither case was any attempt made to vary mood systematically and to study the corresponding variations of hedonic tone. There is indeed another source of experimental evidence, namely, a study by Powelson and Washburn of the effect of verbal suggestion on the hedonic tone of colors, [42] but in this case the evidence is distinctly indirect. Powelson and Washburn had 35 observers give absolute hedonic judgments (scale of 1 to 7) on each of 90 Bradley colors on two different occasions. In the case of all but 18 colors, the judgments on both occasions were made under identical conditions. In the case of 18 colors, however, the presentation of each color was on one occasion accompanied by a verbal suggestion that the color was agreeable, whereas on the other occasion it was accompanied by the verbal suggestion that the color was disagreeable. In the case of each observer the change in the average hedonic value of these 18 colors was computed and compared to the change in the average hedonic value of the colors presented without suggestion. The difference between these two changes was considered to represent the amount of alteration of the hedonic judgment by suggestion. Twenty-five of the thirty-five observers gave results indicating a positive effect of suggestion. In eight cases the amount of alteration was more than 1; in six, of more than .50, and in five, the amount, though less than .50, was nevertheless appreciable. Ten observers gave results indicating a negative effect of suggestion, but in the case of only one did the amount of alteration exceed 1, and in the case of five it was negligible. As to the average of the amounts of alteration for each of the two groups of observers mentioned above, it was .64 for those showing a positive effect of suggestion and only .38 for those showing a negative effect. The writers conclude that: "Direct verbal suggestion regarding the pleasantness or unpleasantness of a color has a fairly decided positive effect on the judgment of observers of the type and under the conditions found in our investigation." [43] In so far as the verbal suggestions in this experiment may be considered as inducing moods, the results may be interpreted as evidence that moods influence hedonic tone. The need of this assumption, however, makes this evidence distinctly indirect.

What conclusion shall we draw? The only obvious conclusion is that direct experimentation is sorely needed upon the variation of the hedonic value of stimuli as a function of systematic variation in mood. Pending such experimentation, we can only state that casual observation and a modicum of experimental evidence make it likely that a pleasant mood is accompanied by an increase in the hedonic value of stimuli, an unpleasant mood by a corresponding decrease.

Hedonic Tone in Relation to Physiological Needs

A close relationship between hedonic tone and physiological needs—shortages of definite substances in the organism—is implied directly or indirectly by many theories of hedonic tone. Thus A. Lehmann considers hedonic tone to be wholly dependent upon the ratio of assimilation to dissimulation in cerebral tissues,[44] and McDougall believes it to depend entirely on the satisfaction or non-satisfaction of instincts.[45] This relationship has been sorely neglected by experimental psychologists, interested primarily in variations of the stimulus. Excepting the experimental work of E. G. Boring and of Boring and A. Luce on various appetites, direct evidence concerning the relation of hedonic tone to physiological needs is limited to the results of fairly casual observation. Fortunately, this direct evidence is supplemented by a considerable body of indirect evidence. A good deal of information is to be found in physiological and medical journals concerning cravings and their relation to physiological needs. This information does not bear directly upon the problem of interest to us here, for it usually makes no mention whatever of hedonic tone. Casual observation, however, although it does not warrant the view that there is a strict co-variation between hedonic tone and cravings, does show conclusively that there is some correlation between these variables. Thus any correspondence or lack of correspondence which may have been established between cravings and physiological needs is *prima facie* evidence for or against a correlation—though not necessarily a high correlation—between the latter and hedonic tone.

Need of Water.—There is no question but that deficiency of water in the organism is frequently accompanied by extreme unpleasantness and its removal by extreme pleasantness. In his Croonian lecture on thirst, Cannon writes: "McGee, an American geologist of large experience in desert regions, who made numerous observations on sufferers from extreme thirst, has distinguished five stages through which men pass on their way to death from lack of water. In the first stage there is a feeling of dryness in the mouth and throat, accompanied by a craving for liquid. This is the common experience of normal thirst. The condition may be alleviated, as everyday practice demonstrates, by a moderate quantity of water, or through exciting a flow of saliva by taking into the mouth fruit acids, such as lemon or tomato juice, or by chewing insoluble substances. In the second stage the saliva and mucus in the mouth and throat become scant and sticky. There is a feeling of dry deadness of the mucous membrane. The inbreathed air feels hot. The tongue clings to the teeth or cleaves to the roof of the mouth. A lump seems to rise in the throat, and starts endless swallowing motions to dislodge it. Water and wetness are then exalted as the end of all excellence. Even in this stage the distress can be alleviated by repeatedly sipping and sniffling a few drops of water at a time. 'Many prospectors,' McGee states, 'become artists in mouth moistening, and carry canteens only for this purpose, depending on draughts in camp to supply the general needs of the system.' The last three stages described by McGee, in which the eyelids stiffen over eyeballs set in a sightless state, the distal tongue hardens to dull weight and the wretched victim has illusions of lakes and running streams, are too pathological for our present interest." [46]

This concomitance, however, seems far from invariable. Cannon has shown conclusively that the thirst experience is but remotely—indirectly—dependent upon a *general* lack of water in the organism. In the lecture referred to above, Cannon first points out that the osmotic pressure of the blood does not change in conjunction with thirst. He then turns to the close connection between thirst and dryness of the mouth and throat. Why is it, he asks, that this dryness occurs when the body is short of water? Why is it in particular that lack of water produces a dryness in this special part of the body? Because of decreased flow of saliva. Thus he found that chewing tasteless gum determined the occurrence of thirst, and that the degree of thirst was roughly inversely proportional to the amount of saliva secreted per unit of time (the amount being measured by the amount of saliva produced in chewing gum for five minutes).

He further found that excessive perspiration, known to determine thirst, also determined a marked decrease of salivary flow. "In one instance the loss in about one hour of approximately 500 c.c. of body fluid as sweat was accompanied by a reduction in the salivary output of almost 50%." [47] Cannon also showed that checking of salivary flow by atropine produced thirst, although the general water content of the body was unchanged, and that this thirst was accompanied by marked decrease in salivary flow. "Before the injection, the amount secreted during five minutes by chewing averaged 13.5 c.c. After the full effect of the drug was manifest, the amount fell to 1 c.c. All the feelings that were noted in ordinary thirst—the sense of dry surfaces, the stickiness of the moving parts, the difficulties of speaking and swallowing—all were present." [48] From this and other evidence, Cannon concludes as follows: "On the basis of the foregoing evidence I would explain thirst as due directly to what it seems to be due to—a relative drying of the mucosa of the mouth and pharynx. This may result either from excessive use of this passage for breathing, as in prolonged speaking or singing, or it may result from deficient salivary secretion. In the latter case 'true thirst' exists, but it is not to be distinguished, so far as sensation is concerned, from 'false thirst.' True thirst is dependent on the fact that the salivary glands, which keep the buccal and pharyngeal mucosa moist, require water for their action. According to the observations and inferences of Wettendorff, the osmotic pressure of the blood is maintained, in spite of deprivation of water, by the withdrawal of water from the tissues. The salivary glands are included under 'tissues,' and they appear to suffer in a way which would support Wettendorff's view, for in the presence of a general need for water in the body, they fail to maintain the normal amount and quality of secretion. The same is doubtless true of other glands. The importance of this failure of action of the salivary glands, however, to the mechanism of the water supply of the body, lies in the strategic position of these glands in relation to a surface which tends to become dry by the passage of air over it. If this surface is not kept moist, discomfort arises and with it an impulse to seek well-tried means of relief. Thus the diminishing activity of the salivary glands becomes a delicate indicator of the bodily demand for fluid." [49]

But even the dependence of thirst upon dryness of the mucosa of the mouth and pharynx does not seem to be direct. In an attempt to analyze the experience of thirst, E. G. Boring made his observers go without water for periods of 32 to 50 hours and record the resulting experiences.[50] One observer wrote the following report after going without drink for 37 hours: "Very thirsty. Mouth getting actually dry. Lips have to be moistened constantly. Impulse to get water very strong. Chief symptom is general weakness and lassitude. Going upstairs tires me out. I tried experiment of putting cracked ice in a thin rubber bag in my mouth. Just as good as a drink. However, pleasant cold in mouth sets up impulse to swallow. If I swallow it as far as my throat, the cold in the throat is even more pleasant than that in the mouth. This surprises me because I have very few thirst sensations in my throat and ordinarily do not notice my throat. It is perhaps barely dry and aches a little, but I have no desire for water there until I put the bag of ice water in my mouth. The thirst disappeared entirely as long as the bag was in my mouth. The bag even felt wet, although it was actually dry. I could not keep it in long, however, because my mouth soon ached from the cold. On removing it the thirst returned immediately. As soon as the ice in the bag had melted, it ceased to be effective." [51] Here we obviously find not only need for water present in the organism without the occurrence of thirst, but physiological dryness of the mouth without concomitant thirst. It follows that thirst, though due indirectly in most cases to dryness of the mouth and throat, cannot possibly be considered to be an invariable concomitant of such dryness.

The lack of invariable concomitance between thirst and need for water clearly suggests that there is no invariable concomitance between the latter and unpleasantness. This suggestion is strongly supported by the reference to pleasantness and unpleasantness in the quotation from Boring above. The observer does not say in so many words that the cold bag removed the unpleasantness previously accompanying need for water; he does imply this, however, and he states explicitly that the cold in the mouth and throat were pleasant. It would obviously be well to have further experimentation on this point. For the present, however, we may conclude tentatively that there is indeed a definite relation between hedonic tone and need for water, but that this relation is indirect. A general need for water determines as a rule a physiological dryness of the mouth and pharynx; this in turn constitutes a stimulus which, if operating alone and under proper attitudinal conditions, determines an unpleasant experience of thirst, but when operating in conjunction with other stimulation (e. g., that produced by ice), determines experiences other than thirst, which may not be unpleasant and indeed may be markedly pleasant.

Need of Food.—There is no question but that in the case of need of food, as in that of need of water, the need itself is frequently accompanied by unpleasantness and its removal by pleasantness. It is by no means obvious, however, whether this concomitance is invariable, or whether, as in the case of need of water, it is subject to marked exceptions. Data concerning this problem come from two very different sources, from investigations of the *food-appetite,* "a food-seeking attitude or meaning, a reaching out after food" [52] and from investigations of *hunger,* "a peculiar dull ache . . . referred to the epigastrium," which may "grow into a highly uncomfortable pang or gnawing, less definitely localized as it becomes more intense." [53] I shall deal separately with the data from these two sources.

In their investigation of the food-appetite, E. G. Boring and A. Luce had observers eat an experimental meal after giving each a notebook with the following instructions: "You are to write in this book successive reports which shall deal with the 'attitude' and mental processes immediately involved in eating this meal. You should report all *attitudes* or *meanings* that pertain to food-taking (e. g., hunger, desire for food, revulsion, etc.) and all *mental processes* (particularly those sensations which are referred to the mouth, throat, oesophagus and stomach) which underlie these 'attitudes' or meanings. You are to make a report whenever there is a marked change in the 'attitude' or in the sensory complex referred to the alimentary canal. It is suggested that you will probably wish to make at least three reports: One before the meal, one after taking a little food and one toward the end of the meal." [54] With respect to hedonic tone, the results showed clearly that appetite need not be unpleasant and may indeed be pleasant. One observer reported: "Appetite loses the unpleasant accompaniment of hunger," and on another occasion, again with reference to appetite: "I get a sort of squirming pressure in the pit of the stomach; it is a light, bright, half-pleasant experience." [55] Another observer described "gastric appetite" as a "bright lively ache, brighter and livelier than hunger, with a different temporal-spatial pattern from hunger (small, fixed, constantly persisting) and pleasant. 'This pleasantness seems to hang right into the quality in just the way that the pleasantness in the ache of stretching does.'" [56] In the case of appetite, then, it seems that need of food is frequently, perhaps habitually, accompanied by pleasantness rather than unpleasantness.

Investigations of hunger have sought the physiological basis of its sensory features and have totally disregarded its hedonic tone. In consequence, their results, though bearing upon the relation of hedonic tone to lack of foods, do so only in an indirect manner. The starting point of these investigations was the opposition between the two main types of theories, the general theories relating hunger to a widespread condition of the organism, and the local theories relating the phenomenon to a condition in some one part of the body. Their outcóme has been distinctly in favor of a local theory. In a recent treatment of the subject, W. B. Cannon cites the following evidence against theories of the general type: "1. Careful studies of the blood have shown that there are no changes in it which are associated with actual bodily need. . . . 2. The cells of the brain are relatively insensitive to chemical stimulation; indeed, they are insensitive to most forms of stimulation except deprivation of oxygen. . . . 3. In certain times of great general bodily need, as, for example, during fever, when food is not relished, when it is commonly not taken in considerable amounts and may be ill-digested, when there is actual wasting of the body—when, in short, hunger as a general sensation should be most intense—it is in fact usually absent.   4. The swallowing of indigestible materials, such as scraps of leather, bits of moss, or even clay, has been reported as a means of stopping the sensation of hunger." [57] 5. The theories do not account for the quick onset nor for the periodicity of hunger. 6. The theories do not account for the reference of hunger to the epigastrium. In place of the general theories of hunger, Cannon advocates a local theory which makes hunger a sensation aroused by certain specific contractions of the empty stomach, usually termed "hunger contractions." This theory is based primarily upon the results of an experiment by Cannon and Washburn in 1911. An observer was made to swallow a rubber balloon, connected by a tube with a tambour in such a fashion that any contractions of the stomach were recorded by kymograph. It was found that when the stomach was empty there occurred contractions of the stomach lasting about 30 seconds and recurring at intervals of from 30 to 90 seconds. It was further found that at the height of each such contraction the observer reported hunger pangs, and that in the absence of such contractions he did not report hunger pangs.

The theory is supported by a variety of evidence secured by Carlson and other investigators. Thus it is found that hunger usually begins with occasional weak contractions of the empty stomach. These gradually become more vigorous and more closely spaced until an acme of activity is reached which may end in a true spasm of the gastric muscle. After the acme the stomach usually relaxes for a while, and then the cycle of contractions starts again. The contractions occur periodically during sleep. They are stopped by chewing, by strong emotional states, alcoholic beverages and strong exercise. Tightening of the belt will stop them for a time. Tobacco weakens them. Some physiologists, it is true, still refuse to accept Cannon's local theory. In a recent article, for instance, F. Hoelzel argues that hunger really depends upon lack of nutrition in the blood; that this, in turn, causes hunger contractions which result in hunger pangs.[58] Such a view clearly involves a definition of hunger different from that of Cannon, for whom hunger and hunger pangs are synonymous. If one follow Cannon and Boring—and modern psychological usage—in distinguishing between appetite and hunger, it seems impossible to escape the conclusion reached by Cannon, namely, that hunger is due to contractions of the stomach-wall rather than to a general condition of the organism. The bearing of this conclusion upon the relation of hedonic tone to lack of food is quite plain. In the case of the unpleasantness of hunger, this relation seems to be of the following indirect type: Need of food may determine at intervals contractions of the stomach; these constitute stimuli to visceral sense organs, and the stimulation of these sense-organs determines hunger and its characteristic unpleasantness.

We have seen that in the case of appetite need of food is frequently—perhaps even habitually—accompanied by pleasantness rather than unpleasantness. We have also seen that hunger with its usual unpleasantness is not determined directly by need of food, but indirectly, through the induction of hunger contractions which in turn stimulate visceral sense organs. This evidence is not enough to warrant a definite conclusion. It strongly suggests, however, that the relationship between hedonic tone and need of food, like that between hedonic tone and need of water, is an indirect one: that need of food under certain conditions determines rhythmic contractions of the stomach, which constitute a stimulus for unpleasant hunger pangs, and under other conditions (which may undoubtedly include olfactory and gustatory stimulation) arouses the frequently pleasant experience called appetite.

Specific Needs.—The physiological literature throws light not only on the organic basis of general cravings, such as thirst and food-appetite, but also on that of cravings for specific materials or substances. A number of years ago, there broke out in certain South African cattle herds a disease known as "Lecksucht," a fatal disease which took its name from the fact that cattle suffering from it licked all objects indiscriminately. Certain specialists sent out to investigate this disease found that it occurred only in herds exhibiting osteophagia, an inordinate desire to eat bones, and further found that the disease was indirectly caused by osteophagia in that it developed in animals whose craving for bones went so far as to make them eat bones covered with putrified flesh. The specialists consequently turned to an investigation of osteophagia, with the hope of learning how to control this craving and thus indirectly to control "Lecksucht." This investigation definitely showed that osteophagia was determined by a deficiency of phosphorous in the animals exhibiting it.[59] It was found in the first place, that the food-stuffs eaten by cattle displaying osteophagia were deficient in phosphorous, as compared to the usual run of foodstuffs. But, further, it was found that "administration of any phosphorous compound utilizable by the animals leads to rapid disappearance of the perverted appetite; within a few weeks, if the supply is large enough."[60]

Another specific craving frequently found in animals is

the craving for salt. The effectiveness of this craving in determining the behaviour of animals was well known to the early settlers of the West, who used to lie in wait for game at the so-called "salt-licks," i.e. saline areas where animals would satisfy their salt craving by licking the ground. According to H. H. Green, "Mountain climbers and Alpine hunters tell of mountain sheep which show salt hunger so markedly that they press irresistibly in the way of oncoming men, and greedily lick their clothes saturated with saltish perspiration." [61] Data concerning animals are not sufficient to warrant ascription of this craving to a physiological deficiency in salt, although such an explanation seems very reasonable in view of the fact that salt craving seems always to occur in inland and mountain regions where salt is found only in a few places. Fortunately our knowledge from animals is here supplemented by knowledge from human beings. R. Turro, in dealing with salt craving, writes: "To determine what it (salt craving) indicates, it is necessary to submit the individual to the regime of dechlorination, to which doctors so often have recourse in the treatment of oedemas. There is seen to appear then a violent and a single desire, that for salt. An epileptic woman, strictly committed to this regime for the purpose of saturating her with bromine, felt such a pressing need for salt that she took it by handfuls when she could escape surveillance." [62]

The same writer refers also to the chalk craving of birds whose manifestation at the time of laying eggs suggests its dependence upon a chalk deficiency in the organism. He writes: "Towards the laying-time the hens seek in the soil or in the walls of the courtyard the calcareous elements of which they have need. This need is not overlooked by breeders of pigeons. Thus they procure for them powdered egg shells so that they may satisfy it. In the case of male birds this sensation is not noticed. . . ." [63]

Sugar craving is a frequent phenomenon in normal adults, and the fact that it arises when the individual has for some reason or other decreased his usual consumption of sugar suggests that this craving also depends upon a physiological lack of the craved substance. A friend of mine once undertook a cure which completely excluded sweets. One day his sugar craving became too much for him and he ate a two-pound box of chocolates at a single sitting. But definite proof of the dependence of sugar craving upon a physiological lack of sugar content is not available. In this connection I might suggest that diabetic patients, whose blood sugar content is known to their physicians, would constitute a fertile field for investigation. Although definite proof of the dependence of sugar craving upon physiological lack of sugar is not available, certain considerations of R. Turro make it very likely that such a dependence exists. Children, Turro points out, display a much greater desire for sugar than do adults. But children likewise need sugar physiologically for three reasons: "First, there is growth: besides the quantity of food which must furnish the material for growth, another quantity of food must furnish the energy sufficient to raise the potential of the food to the potential of the living material. The second reason is the mobility of the child; the third is a greater thermic loss, for in its case the surface of irradiation is greater comparatively for the volume. That is why its food budget is proportionately higher than that of the adult, that is why in particular its appetite is directed to the substances which yield their energy more easily." [64]

The relationship between craving for sour substances and the physiological condition of the organism has been studied in connection with a form of anaemia called chlorosis. It is a characteristic symptom of chlorosis that the patient shows a marked craving for a great variety of sour foodstuffs. O. Rosenbach, an authority in this field, ascribes this craving not to an anomaly of the digestive juices, but to an excessive alkalinity of the blood. He writes as follows: "According to our observations, acetic acid and foodstuffs prepared with vinegar (salad, herring), plant acids, citric acid, and fresh fruit, are eaten with relish in great quantities by those patients whose appetite and digestion subsequently show a marked improvement. It is consequently reasonable to assume that the hydrochloric acid does not—or at least does not only—operate to counteract hypo-acidity of the stomach, but rather that the craving for it corresponds to a real acid-need of the organism, i.e. is probably to be ascribed to excessive alkalinity of the blood. Indeed, careful observers have established such an increased alkalinity of the blood in both light and severe cases of chlorosis, and consequently confirmed a view which had been advanced by us earlier on the basis of clinical observations." [65] Von Noorden, another authority in this field, although he does not deny the possibility of a dependence of the sour craving of chlorosis upon hypoacidity of the blood, definitely rejects its dependence upon hypoacidity of the stomach. He repeatedly determined the acidity of the stomach contents of six patients suffering from chlorosis, who displayed the usual craving for sour substances to a particularly marked degree. Instead of finding hypoacidity, he found in all cases an excess of hydrochloric acid, this hyperacidity varying from a minimum of 0.28% of hydrochloric acid to a maximum of 0.37%. Indeed, he gave two of his patients instead of sour substances frequent doses of calcium carbonate, whereupon the craving for sour substances at once disappeared.[66] As to the dependence of sour craving upon excessive alkalinity of the blood, Von Noorden does not consider the available evidence to be conclusive. In his book written in collaboration with Von Jagic, he points to the contradictory results of various researches on this question and ascribes this situation to the inadequacy of the methods used. The only writer, however, whose method he considers adequate, namely A. Loewy, found, in the only case of chlorosis upon which he worked, a marked increase in the alkalinity of the blood.[67]

The evidence which we have reviewed relating cravings to physiological lacks is strikingly supplemented by the results of a recent experiment on the selection of foodstuffs by children. C. M. Davis let 13 newly weaned infants eat what they chose and as much as they chose from a large selection of simple unmixed foods.[68] At the time of publication three of the children had been thus selecting their food for six months, and the others for periods of one to three and one-half years. The selection of foods comprised "a full range of edible meat products, seafish, eggs, nine vegetables, five cereals, six fruits, milk, sweet and sour (that is, fermented lactic) and sea salt." Three meals a day were served, each "consisting of eight to eleven articles, the articles involved in any one meal were served simultaneously on a large tray, and the child either helped itself, or (when too young) was fed the articles for which it reached." With respect to the relation of cravings to needs the main results were as follows: The individual meals of the children seemed to indicate arbitrary choices. "But if their food records are studied month by month as expressed in protein, carbohydrate, fat, calories, acidity and alkalinity, instead of as beef, bananas, and so forth, law and order begin to appear out of the chaos. The relation between these different food elements and the relation of calories to weight are found to have some similarity." [69] Furthermore, the choices were quite obviously affected by climatic conditions: on hot, humid days the infants drank more orange juice—frequently as much as 16 ounces at a meal—and their food represented less calories than usual; on cold winter days the infants consumed more meat, potatoes and cereals than usual, and the number of calories ingested was greater. Clearly, these results suggest that the relation of cravings to physiological needs is not limited to a few substances, but is a very general relationship.

A number of specific cravings, then, have definitely been related to specific physiological lacks, and there is evidence clearly suggesting that these relations are special cases of a general rule. From what is known of the pleasantness and unpleasantness of cravings in general, it is reasonable to infer that in some cases at least the pleasantness or unpleasantness of a substance is a function of the excess or lack of this specific substance in the organism. Is this relationship more direct than is that of hedonic tone to general lacks such as lack of food or water? Evidence on this question is woefully scanty, but what little there is points to a negative answer. Any inveterate smoker who has given up the habit will agree that lack of nicotine, though very disagreeable at certain times, has no appreciable influence on hedonic tone so long as attention is strongly directed to external events. Again, L. T. Troland has pointed out that "the breathing of air which is low in oxygen may result in a syncope without respiratory distress." [70] It seems likely, therefore, that the concomitance between the hedonic tone of materials or substances and lack of these substances in the organism is by no means invariable, and consequently that the relationship at the basis of this concomitance is by no means direct.

Conclusion.—Far more information on the relationship of hedonic tone to physiological needs is needed before we can hope to formulate this relationship with any degree of finality. The facts which we have reviewed, however, warrant a number of tentative conclusions. In the first place, all of the evidence indicates that hedonic tone is markedly influenced by physiological needs, persistence of the need being usually accompanied by unpleasantness and its removal by pleasantness. In the second place, the frequent exceptions to this general rule indicate that the relationship is not a direct one. The study of thirst and hunger, finally, strongly suggests that a necessary link in the indirect relationship is the stimulation of internal sense organs. It would seem, therefore, that the part played by physiological needs in the determination of hedonic tone is not essentially different from that played by alterations of the external environment, and that explanation in the former case, as in the latter, is essentially a matter of explaining the relation of hedonic tone to the stimulation of sense-organs.

HEDONIC TONE IN RELATION TO WISHES

The term wish is here interpreted in the wide sense favored by K. Lewin, namely as "an inner pressure, with a definite direction . . . , which tends towards the accomplishment of the resolution." [71] I shall deal with the relation of hedonic tone to three types of wishes (in the sense defined above), namely wishes artificially aroused under laboratory conditions, wishes aroused under natural conditions in normal individuals, and wishes aroused naturally in psychotic individuals.

Artificial Wishes.—The outstanding investigation of volition under laboratory conditions is that of N. Ach, published in book form in 1910.[72] Ach's procedure was in general as follows: First, the observers were made to read a list of non-sense syllables a specified number of times, thus— to follow Ach—establishing between the syllables bonds whose strength could be estimated in terms of the number of readings. Then the observers were instructed to respond to stimulation by means of one of these syllables in a way different from that favored by the established bonds. In some cases the observers were to transpose the first and third letter of the syllable presented, and in others to give a syllable rhyming with it. The purpose of this instruction was to arouse what Ach called a *"determination,"* and defined as "that peculiar after-effect of the will which brings about a development of mental process in accordance with intention, resolution, etc." [73] As a check the observers were also instructed now and then to respond with the first syllable which occurred to them. After the observer had received his instructions, certain members of the previously learned list of non-sense syllables were presented, the response of the observer and his reaction time were recorded, and introspective reports were taken. The general aim of this procedure, which Ach called the "combination procedure" (Kombiniertes Verfahren) was to cause artificially established habits to be broken down by the operation of the will and thus to arouse "acts of will" artificially and to render them amenable to analysis. An interesting feature of this procedure is that it allows measuring the strength of the wish or "determination" aroused by the instructions in terms of its *associative equivalent,* i.e. of the "number of repetitions of a list of syllables which must just be exceeded in order that the association established, and not the determination, shall condition the development of the occurrence." [74]

The results of this experiment which have reference to the relation of hedonic tone to wishes are discussed by Ach in a special chapter. The introspections of the observers, Ach states, frequently revealed the occurrence of feelings which depended on the operation of the "determination." These feelings he calls "determined feelings." The hedonic tone of these feelings was found to be related to the "determination" according to the following laws:

"1. If realization occurs in accordance with the determination, there results as a rule a pleasant feeling.

"2. If, on the other hand, the realization does not occur in accordance with the determination, i.e. if a failure is experienced, there usually results an unpleasant feeling. . . .

"3. The stronger the determination, the stronger are as a rule the resulting feelings. . . .

"4. The stronger the resistances which oppose the determination, the more intense the resulting feelings." [75]

5. The more complete and accurate the realization of the end set by the "determination," the more pleasant the hedonic tone.

6. Previous pleasantness or unpleasantness has a contrasting effect upon "determined feelings" if it has been of brief duration, an assimilative effect if of long duration.

7. The operation of a further "determination" prevents the full development of a "determined feeling." Thus if immediately after a wrong response the right syllable is spoken, the development of an unpleasant feeling is hindered.

8. "Determined feelings" tend to weaken the increased automatization of the activity required by the "determination."

9. "Determined feelings" occurring in sequence may summate.

It is clear from Ach's definition of "determination" that this motivating factor is a wish in the sense favored by

Lewin and adopted by us. Thus Ach's laws relating hedonic tone to determination may be translated into laws relating hedonic tone to wishes by mere substitution of wish for "determination." In view of the importance of these laws not only to psychology, but to the conduct of life, it is very unfortunate that they have never been subjected to systematic verification. What meagre experimental evidence there is, however, is in general favorable to Ach's laws. In a study by F. Grossart upon misreading, in which words were presented tachistoscopically, so as to make them hard to read, the introspections of the observers showed that pleasantness frequently occurred "when a reading fitted well the impression, when the word snapped smoothly into perception," whereas unpleasantness occurred "when, despite frequent presentations at a favorable distance that which was seen was not correctly cognized and would not develop into an appropriate word." [76] H. R. Crossland, in an investigation of forgetting, found that "the appearing of any datum, whether correct or incorrect, just at the moment when the observer's efforts to recall were most active, contributed to the feeling of pleasantness: this occurred very frequently and most frequently after forgetting had made an extensive headway. The failure of the observer to 'get started' upon a recall, or his failure to remember any datum in a recall, usually contributed to the feeling of unpleasantness and this experience of unpleasantness was the more intensive the greater the observer's efforts in attempting to recall."[77]

These findings verify Ach's first four laws, but the phrase "whether correct or incorrect" in the excerpt from Crossland is implicitly at odds with the fifth law. It is to be hoped that further experimentation will soon be forthcoming which will either establish Ach's laws on the firm foundation of independent verification, or bring to light any errors which may exist in their formulation.

Normal Natural Wishes.—The best data on the relation of hedonic tone to wishes aroused under natural conditions are to be found, in my opinion, in R. Katz's study of loss of appetite in children.[78] Around his fourth year, Julius, one of Mrs. Katz's children, began to refuse foodstuffs of all sorts, and consequently started to lose weight. Convinced from the results of a physical examination that the basis for this loss of appetite was primarily psychological, Mrs. Katz adopted the plan of letting the child order his own meals beforehand, impressing upon him that a meal which had been ordered must naturally be eaten. This procedure was completely successful. Whatever the child had ordered, he would eat without the slightest sign of loss of appetite. The first day, he ordered for his main meal potatoes, soup, meat, carrots, vanilla dessert with vanilla sauce. His meal was prepared accordingly, care being taken that the amounts of each food be not too large in order to facilitate the accomplishment of his undertaking. He ate everything without the slightest resistance. The next day he ordered the same meal over again, and again ate it without sign of lack of appetite. On the third day, he ordered the same meal except that vanilla sauce was changed to chocolate sauce, and he ate the entire meal with apparent enjoyment. Incidentally, the writer here points out the interesting fact that children require much less variety in their meals than do adults—babies requiring no variety at all, but being satisfied with milk. But to return to Julius. On the fourth day he ordered meat, potatoes, carrots, semolina and ice cream with vanilla sauce—and again ate everything. And so, day after day, the ordered meal was consumed without any sign of rejection. Clearly these results suggest that by making the child order his own meal there was established in him a wish tending towards the eating of this meal, and that this wish manifested itself in making the child not only eat, but eat with relish the very same foodstuffs which previously he had rejected.

The same suggestion arises from the success of a slightly different procedure used by Mrs. Katz to overcome temporary losses of appetite. In certain cases her children would unexpectedly refuse to eat the meal being placed before them. Clearly the former procedure was of no avail;

the problem required solution without delay. In such cases the children were told that they could prepare any dish they cared to from the foodstuffs on the table or from those in the kitchen, or eat these foodstuffs in any sequence that appealed to them. This procedure was entirely successful in that it made the children eat a meal with apparent relish, even though many of the combinations of foods and sequences of foods seemed to the father and mother to be anything but palatable. A few reports on such individual meals follows: "June 16, 1927, lunch. Chocolate and lard are cut up and put in a plate of bean soup. This is a mixture the very appearance of which is unpleasant to us adults, and which we would never have been able to eat. Julius, however, eats the mixture with the greatest relish and it agrees with him perfectly. . . . September 17, 1927, supper. Here it is the order of the foodstuffs which is particularly striking. 1. Meat and bread with butter; 2, bread with honey; 3, ice (ice cream?); 4, honey eaten with a spoon directly from the plate; 5, meat eaten with the hand; 6, honey with a spoon; and 7, as a conclusion, meat eaten by hand. . . . October 4, 1927, supper. Potatoes, sauce made of fat and onions fried brown, and sugar, all mixed together in a plate and eaten with a spoon. This mixture is supposed to have been especially delicious." [79] It is obvious that these data do not *prove* a specific relationship between hedonic tone and the wishes of every-day life. They do make it likely, however, that patient observation of children—or of adults, if they could be kept ignorant of the problem at issue—would show that the pleasantness of one and the same object or activity is as a rule greater when a wish has been aroused for it than otherwise.

Another source of information on the relation of hedonic tone to natural wishes is the study of religious enjoyment. Unfortunately this evidence rests to a large extent upon interpretation. It is a well known fact that religion is to many human beings a source of great enjoyment. Upon what does this enjoyment rest? The most reasonable answer seems to be that of William James, namely that religious enjoyment rests essentially upon an acceptance of the universe which is not grudging and partial, but whole-hearted and complete. In his "Varieties of Religious Experience," he wrote: " 'I accept the universe,' is reported to have been a favorite utterance of our New England transcendentalist, Margaret Fuller; and when some one repeated this phrase to Thomas Carlyle, his sardonic comment is said to have been: 'Gad! she'd better!' At bottom the whole concern of both morality and religion is with the manner of our acceptance of the universe. Do we accept it only in part and grudgingly, or heartily and altogether? Shall our protests against certain things in it be radical and unforgiving, or shall we think that, even with evil, there are ways of living that must lead to good? If we accept the whole, shall we do so as if stunned into submission,—as Carlyle would have us—'Gad! we'd better!'—or shall we do so with enthusiastic consent? Morality pure and simple accepts the law of the whole which it finds reigning, so far as to acknowledge and obey it, but it may obey it with the heaviest and coldest heart, and never cease to feel it as a yoke. But for religion, in its strong and fully developed manifestations, the service of the highest never is felt as a yoke. Dull submission is left far behind, and a mood of welcome, which may fill any place on the scale between cheerful serenity and enthusiastic gladness, has taken its place." [80] But if religious enjoyment is essentially dependent upon acceptance of the universe, it is essentially dependent upon the satisfaction of wishes, for what is acceptance of the universe other than the agreement of the individual's wishes with whatever befalls him? This conclusion is strikingly verified in the writings of mystics.[81] Saint Theresa, for instance, thanks God for everything. her "Life" opens with the sentence: "The joy of having virtuous and God-fearing parents, as well as the gifts with which I was favored by God, should have been sufficient to keep me on the right path, had I not been so unfaithful." [82] After reviewing her years of spiritual darkness, she writes: "O Lord of my soul, what language will suffice to depict the gifts showered upon me during those years, to state how, at the time when I most offended you, you suddenly disposed me, by vivid repentance, to taste your sweetness and your divine caress?" [83] For her new life, with its ecstasies, she naturally feels unbounded gratefulness to God: " . . . To see you accord such sovereign gifts to souls that have offended you—that is what confounds my understanding." [84] Indeed, the very writing of the life is due to God's assistance. "Blessed be the Lord, who thus favors the ignorant. . . . God illuminated my understanding . . . His divine Majesty wishes, as I see it, to say Himself, in the case of this oration as in the case of the preceding one, that which I am incapable of understanding and of writing." [85]

Pathological Wishes.—There is no question but that morbid anxiety is essentially unpleasant. Consider the following characterization given by E. Jones: "In the mental manifestations the emotional element is naturally the most prominent. It consists in a curious admixture of dread, panic, terror, anguish and apprehension. It varies greatly from, on the one extreme, a slight abashment, awkwardness, embarrassment, or confusion to, on the other, a degree of indescribable dread that may even rob the sufferer of consciousness. Common to all degrees is a sense of something impending, of anxious expectation of something harmful or awful." [86] What is at the basis of morbid anxiety? There is marked concensus of opinion that this anxiety depends upon frustrated wishes, although the nature of the wishes is a matter of controversy. For Jones, a follower of Freud, "morbid anxiety means unsatisfied love"; [87] for McDougall, it depends upon interference with the instinct of flight; [88] for T. V. Moore, it depends upon an apparently irreconcilable conflict between incompatible desires. [89] The latter psychiatrist gives a very good general description of such a conflict: "The soldier, for instance, cannot be sure of saving his life if he risks it. If he tries to save it he runs into the danger of being called a coward. It was this conflict that lay at the basis of the anxiety neuroses of the war.

These neuroses differed from the other war neuroses in that the patients from one point of view desired, and from another point of view did not desire both horns of their dilemma. They wanted to make good, but they did not want to be killed. They wanted to escape danger, but they did not want to be called cowards." . . . "A similar conflict exists in those whose conflict proceeds from difficulties of the moral life. They want to keep the moral law, and maintain an appearance of respectability in the eyes of others, and also in the form of their own conscience; and at the same time they feel a craving for pleasures that are prohibited by the moral law. This craving is suppressed with more or less success. If unsuccessful, so that the craving is at times indulged, the anxiety remains associated with the desire that causes it. If successfully, so that the craving is never indulged, and the patient does not even admit to himself that he has it, the anxiety is likely to attach itself to other things in which the patient does not scruple to admit his interest." [90]

Clearly, the modern conception of anxiety strongly corroborates the view that thwarting of wishes is usually accompanied by unpleasantness.

Conclusion. —Investigation of the relation of hedonic tone to wishes has obviously yielded positive results. The study of wishes aroused in the laboratory has allowed the tentative formulation of a number of laws, the more important of which are brought together in the following proposition: *hedonic tone is definitely related to wishes; fulfillment of a wish as a rule determines pleasantness, the degree increasing with the completeness of the fulfillment; thwarting of a wish as a rule determines unpleasantness; the degree of pleasantness or unpleasantness increases both with the strength of the wish and the strength of the resistance which it encounters.* Furthermore, the study of natural wishes, both normal and abnormal, confirms the laws established under laboratory conditions.

These results, however, are not wholly satisfactory. It will be noted that the main affirmations, in the proposition above, are qualified by the terms "as a rule." This is because the laws established by Ach, which underlie these affirmations, are likewise so qualified. Does this mean that the relationship between hedonic tone and wishes is an indirect one, as seems to be that between hedonic tone and physiological needs, or does it mean that we do not know the relationship well enough to warrant an unqualified affirmation? A well-motivated answer to this important question is impossible until Ach's experiment has been repeated in such a manner as to yield quantitative results. All that can be done at present is to point out that Lewin's work on wishes makes it rather likely that the relationship between hedonic tone and wishes will turn out to be indirect. In his "Resolution, Will and Need," Lewin adduces much evidence of the fundamental similarity between wishes and needs.[91] Both wishes and needs "require" certain definite situations and tend towards certain definite ends. Corresponding to both are classes of objects or events which "draw" the organism, which have an "arousal value" (Aufforderungscharakter). In both cases these classes of objects having "arousal value" *extend* with an increase in the strength of the wish or need, are subject to *contraction* through habit (thus yielding "fixation,") and cease to exist when satisfaction is achieved. Both wishes and needs, finally, are subject to *vicarious satisfaction*. So great, indeed, is the similarity that Lewin uses the term "quasi-need" in referring to wishes. Clearly, if wishes have a good deal in common with needs, it is likely that the relation of the former to hedonic tone will be of the same type as the relation of the latter to hedonic tone, namely indirect.

FOOTNOTES AND REFERENCES

[1] J. Segal. Ueber die Wohlgefälligkeit Einfacher Räumlicher Formen, *Arch. f. d. ges. Psychol.,* 7, 1906, 53-124.

[2] L. W. Legowski. Beiträge zur Experimentellen Aesthetik, *Arch. f. d. ges. Psychol.,* 12, 1908, 237-311.

[3] E. Bullough. The Perceptive Problem in the Aesthetic Appreciation of Single Colors, *Brit. J. Psychol.,* 2, 1908, 406-463.

[4] *Ibid.,* 460. Concerning this distinction, Bullough added: "It is the

296 RELATION TO MOTIVATING FACTORS

same point at which Witasek aims from the point of view of pleasure, when he observes that in aesthetic objects the *cause* and the *object* of pleasure coincide, while in other cases they are referred to different things (in the case of the bath, for instance, the *cause* is the bath, but the *object* my sensations)." (*Ibid.*, 461.) *Cf.*, according to Bullough: S. WITASEK, Zur Psychologischen Analyse der Aesthetischen Einfühlung, *Z. f. Psychol. u. Physiol. d. Sinnesorgane*, XXV, pp. 12, 13; Grundzüge der Allgemeinen Aesthetik, Leipzig, 1904, pp. 19-21.

5 C. C. PRATT. Some Qualitative Aspects of Bi-tonal Complexes, *Am. J. Psychol.*, 32, 1921, 490.

6 C. S. MYERS and C. W. VALENTINE. A Study of Individual Differences in Attitude Towards Tones, *Brit. J. Psychol.*, 7, 1914, 68-112.

7 *Ibid.*, 72.

8 *Ibid.*, 72.

9 C. S. MYERS. Individual Differences in Listening to Music, *Brit. J. Psychol.*, 13, 1922, 52-71.

10 J. E. DOWNEY. Individual Differences in Reaction to the Word in Itself, *Amer. J. Psychol.*, 39, 1927, 323-342.

11 C. S. MYERS and C. W. VALENTINE. *Brit. J. Psychol*, 7, 1914, 89.

12 C. S. MYERS. *Brit. J. Psychol.*, 13, 1922, 57.

13 J. E. DOWNEY. *Amer J. Psychol.*, 39, 1927, 342.

14 Report of lecture by PAUL HAZARD. *Boston Evening Transcript*, Nov. 10th, 1928.

15 *Ibid.*

16 M. F. MAURY. In Histoire de la Langue et de la Littérature Francaise, edited by L. *Petit de Julleville*, VI, Paris, 1909, 490.

17 Report on lecture by PAUL HAZARD. *Boston Evening Transcript*, Nov. 10th, 1928.

18 M. F. WASHBURN and S. L. GROSE. Voluntary Control of Likes and Dislikes; the Effects of an Attempt Voluntarily to Change the Affective Value of Colors, *Amer. J. Psychol.*, 32, 1921, 284.

19 R. H. WHEELER. An Experimental Investigation of the Process of Choosing, *Univ. of Oregon Publications*, 1920, Vol. No. 2.

20 R. H. WHEELER. The Science of Psychology, N. Y., 1929, 333.

21 J. P. NAFE. *Amer. J. Psychol.*, 35, 1924, 540.

22 P. T. YOUNG. *Amer. J. Psychol.*, 38, 1927, 167-185.

23 E. F. WELLS. The Effect of Attitude Upon Feeling, *Amer. J. Psychol.*, 42, 1930, 573-580.

24 *Ibid.*, 575 and 580.

25 *Ibid.*, 580.

26 *Ibid.*, 580.

27 *Ibid.*, 580.

28 *Ibid.*, 580.

29 *Ibid.*, 580.

30 *Ibid.*, 579.

31 F. W. HAZZARD. A Descriptive Account of Odors, *J. Exper. Psychol.*, 13, 1930, 297-331.

32 *Ibid.*, 311-312.

33 K. W. OBERLIN. The Relative Immediacy of Sensory, Perceptual and Affective Characteristics, *Amer. J. Psychol.*, 42, 1930, 621-627.

34 *Ibid., 624.*

35 *Ibid., 624.*

36 *Ibid., 624.*

37 E. B. Titchener, Sensation and System, *Amer. J. Psychol.,* 26, 1915, 258-267.

38 "Wr said that a very pleasant odor tended to make the color less unpleasant, and that the unpleasant odors made the colors less pleasant." (A. J. Harris. Studies of Affective Contrast, Thesis, Harvard University, 1930, 106.) In the same experiment another observer reported: "I would recognize a pleasant color while feeling unpleasant from the odor, and would have to wait a second before the pleasantness came in." (*Ibid.,* 123.)

39 A. Lehmann. Die Hauptgesetze des Menschlichen Gefühlslebens, 2nd Edit., Leipzig, 1914, 243.

40 P. T. Young. *Amer. J. Psychol.,* 42, 1930, 26.

41 A. J. Harris. Studies in Affective Contrast, Thesis, Harvard University, 1930, 116.

42 I. Powelson and M. F. Washburn. The Effect of Verbal Suggestion on Judgment of the Affective Value of Colors, *Amer. J. Psychol.,* 24, 1913, 267.

43 *Ibid.,* 269.

44 A. Lehmann. Die Hauptgesetze des Menschlichen Gefühlslebens, 2nd Edit., Leipzig, 1914, 163-168.

45 W. McDougall. Outline of Psychology, N. Y., 1928, 269.

46 W. B. Cannon. The Physiological Basis of Thirst, *Proc. of the Royal Society of London,* Ser. B., 90, 1919, 286-287.

47 *Ibid., 297.*

48 *Ibid., 298.*

49 *Ibid., 299-300.*

50 E. G. Boring. Processes Referred to the Alimentary and Urinary Tracts: A Qualitative Analysis, *Psychol. Rev.,* 22, 1915, 306-331.

51 *Ibid.,* 308-9.

52 E. G. Boring and A. Luce. The Psychological Basis of Appetite, *Amer. J. Psychol.,* 28, 1917, 452.

53 W. B. Cannon. Bodily Changes in Pain, Hunger, Fear and Rage, 2nd Edit., 1929, 271.

54 E. G. Boring and A. Luce. *Amer. J. Psychol.,* 28, 1917, 446. The instructions given for the first experimental meal differed slightly from those quoted above.

55 *Ibid.,* 446-447.

56 *Ibid., 449.*

57 W. B. Cannon. Hunger and Thirst, in Foundations of Experimental Psychology, Worcester, 1929, 435-436.

58 F. Hoelzel. Central Factors in Hunger, *Amer. J. Physiol.,* 82, 1927, 665-671.

59 H. H. Green. Perverted Appetites, *Physiol. Rev.,* 5, 1925, 339.

60 *Ibid., 344.*

61 *Ibid.,* 339. Cf. Hutyra-Marek. Spezielle Pathologie und Therapie der Haustiere, 6th Edit., Fischer, Jena, 1922.

62 R. Turro. Psychophysiologie de la Faim, II, *Journal de Psychologie,* 7, 1910, 409.

[63] *Ibid.*, 414.

[64] *Ibid.*, 414-415.

[65] O. ROSENBACH. Entstehung und Hygienische Behandlung der Bleichsucht, Leipzig, 1893, 76.

[66] C. H. VON NORDEN and N. VON JAGIC. Die Bleichsucht, Wien, 1912, 95.

[67] *Ibid.*, 62-63.

[68] C. M. DAVIS. What Infants on the Self Selected Diet Experiment Eat; *Transactions of the Section on Diseases of Children, American Medical Association,* Chicago, 1930, 137-144.

[69] *Ibid.*, 142-143.

[70] L. T. TROLAND. Psychophysiology, Vol. II, N. Y., 1930, 368.

[71] K. LEWIN. Vorsatz, Wille und Bedurfnis, *Psychol. Forsch,* 7, 1926, 348.

[72] N. ACH. Ueber den Willensakt und das Temperament, Leipzig, 1910.

[73] *Ibid.*, 4.

[74] *Ibid.*, 43.

[75] *Ibid.*, 308-309.

[76] F. GROSSART. Das Tachistoscopische Verlesen unter Besondere Berücksichtigung des Einflusses und der Frage des Objektiven und Subjektiven Typus, *Arch. f. d. ges. Psychol.,* 41, 1921, 172.

[77] H. R. CROSSLAND. A Qualitative Analysis of Forgetting, *Psychol. Monogr.,* 29, 1 (Whole No. 130), 1921, 89.

[78] R. KATZ. Zur Psychologie der Ernährung des Kindes, *Arch. f. d. ges. Psychol.,* 65, 1928, 292-320.

[79] *Ibid.*, 313.

[80] W. JAMES. The Varieties of Religious Experience, N. Y., 1902, 41.

[81] Cf. J. B. PRATT. The Religious Consciousness, N. Y., 1924, Chs. XVII-XX.

[82] SAINTE THERESA. *Oeuvres,* Vol. I, translated into French by Marcel Bouix, S. J., Paris, 1923, 5.

[83] *Ibid.*, 68-69.

[84] *Ibid.*, 168.

[85] *Ibid.*, 170-171.

[86] E. JONES. The Pathology of Morbid Anxiety, *J. Abnor. Psychol.,* 6, 1911, 85.

[87] *Ibid.*, 106.

[88] W. McDOUGALL. Outline of Abnormal Psychology, N. Y., 1926, 269.

[89] T. V. MOORE. Dynamic Psychology, Philadelphia, 1924, 207-208.

[90] *Ibid.*, 207-208.

[91] K. LEWIN. Vorsatz, Wille und Bedurfnis, Berlin, 1926.

Chapter VII

Hedonic Tone in Relation to Maturation and Learning

Hedonic Tone in Early Childhood.—As hedonic tone is defined in terms of report alone, its study in early childhood, when reports are out of the question, is bound to be indirect. This fact is a handicap, but not an unsurmountable one. Inference of hedonic tone from non-emotional behaviour is dangerous. Choice of foodstuffs, for instance, is not necessarily a sign of hedonic preference; it may indicate merely hygienic preference. Inference of hedonic tone from emotional behaviour, on the other hand, appears to be very reliable. Unless we be actors, a situation to which we respond with the behavioural symptoms of grief or rage will in practically every case be judged to be unpleasant. Thus if we confine ourselves to observations of emotional behaviour, there is no reason why we should not seek to increase our knowledge of hedonic tone by the study of early childhood.

The best single source concerning hedonic tone in early childhood is W. Stern's "Psychology of Infancy." [1] According to Stern, behavioural signs of both pleasantness and unpleasantness are present from the first day of life: the infant cries when hungry and displays enjoyment when satiated. Unpleasantness, however, is apparently more frequent than pleasantness (a circumstance which follows, it seems to me, from the fact that sleep is the normal behaviour of an infant, and is only broken by strong internal or external stimulation). At first, hedonic tone occurs predominantly in connection with internal stimulation (e.g. hunger), cutaneous stimulation (e.g. warmth) and loud sounds. Later on it extends to visual and kinaesthetic stimulation. Hedonic idiosyncrasies (e.g. fear of wet sand) appear as early as the eighth month. A striking feature of early infancy is what may be called hedonic (and emotional) lability: pleasantness and unpleasantness alternate without appreciable transition. In 15 minutes, Idelberger observed in his 11 month old son joy, sorrow, curiosity, surprise, anger, dislike, desire, rejection.

This emotional lability persists long after the child has learned to talk. Interference with the child's activities readily brings anger or grief, assistance brings smiles and laughter. As Stern puts it, "the energy of the emotion and desire of the moment is often much greater in a child than in an adult." [2] Whereas in the infant, however, behaviour is largely determined by physiological needs such as hunger, in the child of three or four, it is also determined by wishes, usually wishes for trains of activity, such as playing with blocks. The consequence of this change is two-fold. In the first place, hedonic tone becomes a characteristic not only of objects, but of situations and activities. In the second place, the behaviour accompanying pleasantness, at first limited almost wholly to grasping and placing in the mouth, extends to include almost any kind of response. As a child grows up, the role of *activities* as bearers of hedonic tone markedly preponderates over that of objects. A. Jersild, in a recent study of "pleasures and unpleasures of college men and women" found that "social contacts, visits, dates, social correspondence, and the like, provide the outstanding source of pleasure and unpleasure in the lives of the college students tested." [3] H. Cason, in an earlier study of annoyances alone, found that for a large group of observers ranging from grammar school students to adults the percentages of annoyances involving non-human things and activities was 15% while that of annoyances involving human behaviour was 57%. [4]

Changes in Specific Preferences with Change of Age. —A considerable number of studies are available concerning color-preferences at various ages. In the case of infants, the results are fairly well in accord. In 1903, Marsden published a number of experiments on his son during his first year.[5] In one of them, carried out between the 189th and 203rd day, the child was offered in pairs four colored crochet-work balls and its grasping of the one or the other was observed. The number of times a ball could have been grasped, together with the number of times it actually was grasped, are presented below (each possible pair of balls (6) was presented 12 times, making the possible number of choices for any one ball 36).

TABLE XLIII

```
Number possible .............  36
  "     for Red .............  29
  "      "  Yellow  .........  19
  "      "  Blue  ...........  18
  "      "  Green  .........    6
```

Preference for red and yellow during the second half-year was likewise found by Shinn in her well-known study of the development of a child. Shinn believes that in the *first half-year* preference is wholly a matter of illumination. "When I attempted some tests, at the end of the sixth month, by dangling colored ribbons before the child, she grasped regularly at the one that received the strongest light from the windows; and when we made the objective illumination equal, she turned from one ribbon to the other with equal joy." [6] Shinn believes, however, that there is evidence that in the *second half-year* "Red (including pink), yellow, and orange are overwhelmingly indicated as the colors that attract most." [7] (Earlier observations of Baldwin indicating preference for blue are considered by Miss Shinn as inconclusive.[8]) This preference gradually disappears, she believes: "By the third year the warm colors in some cases lose their advantage, and the cold ones may give as much pleasure." [9] Observations of McDougall on preferences during the first half-year accord well with those of Shinn, but supplement them somewhat. During the sixth month, McDougall found that red, green and blue were not markedly preferred to each other (although there was slight evidence that red was preferred during the fifth month), but that all were preferred to white, and even more to grey.[10] A more recent experiment by Valentine confirms the finding of Marsden and Shinn that warm colors are preferred during the second half-year.[11] Valentine presented to his son, aged seven months, all possible pairs (in both spatial orders) of nine Holmgren wools. The child was allowed to grasp one or both of the wools, and such grasping was interpreted as indicating preference. The rank order of the stimuli according to number of preferences, was found to be as follows: yellow (most preferred), red, pink, grey, violet, white, green, black, blue. Valentine believes, however, that some of his data contradict Miss Shinn's contention that preferences prior to six months are based wholly on brightness. When his son was but three months old, Valentine presented to him, for two minutes, each of the 36 possible combinations of nine colors. The time was recorded during which the infant gazed at one or the other color, or at neither. Taking length of gaze as an index of preference, Valentine found the rank order of the colors to be as follows: yellow (most preferred), white, pink, red, brown, black, blue, green, violet. The high value of yellow and pink, Valentine is willing to attribute to greater brightness, but not so the preference of red and brown to blue, green and violet, which were objectively of very similar luminosities. Thus Valentine would have the child show preference for warm colors as early as the fourth month.

A good many investigations have been made of the color preference of school children in the various grades. One of these investigations, that of Dashiell, indicates that infantile preference for warm colors (red, yellow, orange), which is noticeably decreased, according to Shinn, by the third year, has almost wholly disappeared by the fourth or fifth.[12] Using the method of order of merit, Dashiell compared the preferences of kindergarten children for six colors with those of college students. His results, expressed in average rank orders (most pleasant at top), were as follows:

TABLE XLIV

Girls		Boys	
Kinderg.	College	Kinderg.	College
Blue	Red	Blue	Blue
Violet	Blue	Red	Red
Green	Green	Orange	Green
Yellow	Violet	Yellow	Orange
Red	Yellow	Green	Yellow
Orange	Orange	Violet	Violet

According to Dashiell, the chief difference between the preference of kindergarten and college students was one of variability, the variability being much greater in the case of kindergarten students.

Four other investigations, however, all of them very thorough-going, indicate that the disappearance of infantile preference for warm colors is a gradual process, not fully completed until adolescence. The procedure in the first of these experiments, that of W. H. Winch, published in 1909, was peculiar in that the children were made to judge colors by name, rather than by actual presentation.[13] We shall see presently, however, that according to G. M. Michaels, this should not have influenced the results. The method used by Winch was that of order of merit. His "stimuli" were the following names: Blue, Red, White, Green, Yellow, Black. The results show that for eight years, or rather for "Standard I," a grade averaging 8:10 for boys and 8:00 for girls, Red was preferred to Blue, and Yellow ranked second for the boys. In "Standard II," —ages around 9—Blue achieved first place and remained there for all higher ages. In "Standard II," Yellow ranks in general high, but in subsequent Standards it gradually sinks in rank until it reaches 4th or 5th place in Standard VII. Winch adduces evidence that the changes in preferences shown by his study are due partly to environmental conditions (he found Green abnormally high in high-class schools), but very little to color-work.

Similar results were published in 1924 by T. R. Garth and by G. M. Michaels. Garth's investigation covered one thousand children from grades one to eight.[14] Each child was made to arrange in order of preference seven discs of "standard" Milton-Bradley papers (including white). The results for the different grades were as follows (best liked colors at top):

TABLE XLV

First	Second	Third	Fourth	Fifth	Sixth	Seventh	Eighth Ninth & Tenth
Red	Blue	Blue	Blue	Blue	Blue	Blue	Blue
Blue	Red	Green	Green	Green	Green	Green	Green
Orange	Violet	Red	Red	Red	Red	Orange	Violet
Green	Green	Orange	Orange	Violet	Violet	Violet	Orange
Violet	Orange	Yellow	Yellow	Orange	Orange	Red	Red
Yellow	Yellow	Violet	Violet	Yellow	Yellow	Yellow	Yellow
White	White	White	White	White	White	White	White

The investigation of Michaels covered 535 boys ranging from 6 to 15 years of age.[15] His method was likewise that of order of merit, and the stimuli Milton-Bradley papers. The number of stimuli, however, was only six, white not being included. The results were as follows for the various age-groups:

TABLE XLVI

6	7.2	8.1	9.2	10.3	11.2	12.4	13.4	14.3	15.4
Y	B	B	B	B	B	B	B	B	B
R	R	R	R	O	V	V	R	R	G
G	G	Y	V	R	O	O	V	O	R
V	O	V	O	V	R	R	O	Y	Y
B	V	O	Y	Y	Y	Y	G	V	V
O	Y	G	G	G	G	G	Y	G	O

The results of Garth and Michaels are clearly in accord with those of Winch. In Garth's investigation, orange, red and yellow do not reach their collective minimum of preference until the eighth, ninth and tenth grades, and in the research of Michaels this minimum does not occur before the last age-group (15:4). On the other hand, these results also show that by the 7th year a cold color, blue, has taken the place of red as best liked color. It should be added, however, that an earlier investigation of Garth on the preferences of Indian children makes it likely that the statements above hold strictly only for white children. In the case of the Indian children, it was not until the 8th to 10th grades (these three grades were treated collectively) that blue secured first place, and even then blue was but little preferred to red.[16]

Results published by Dorcus in 1926, finally, agree entirely with those of Winch, Garth and Michaels in showing the gradual nature of the disappearance of preference for warm colors.[17] The number and types of observers used by Dorcus is indicated in the table below:

Table XLVII

Group	No. of Males	No. of Females
8 year old	49	62
9 " "	63	55
10 " "	38	30
College Students	430	401
Psychopaths	19	48
Inhabitants of Homes for Aged (over 60 years)	15	25

With the method of paired comparison, he established the preferences of his observers for two series of six Munsell papers. In both series the hues were green, blue, purple, red, orange and yellow. In one series, however, brilliance and saturation were as constant as possible, the common saturation being low, while in the other they varied from one paper to the next, the saturations being on the whole high. Dorcus interprets his results as showing that " . . . There is not a very wide difference in the order of choice for the different groups. On the whole the order determined by the college group is the one that will suffice for all the groups," [18] although orange is an exception to this rule. His term "wide difference," is obviously meant to be taken textually. If one compare his data for college men and women with those for children one finds that for saturated and unsaturated colors the totals of the percentages of times red, yellow and orange were preferred by girls and by boys of each age-group are greater than the totals of the percentages of times that green and blue were preferred, whereas the reverse is true for college students, both men and women. (Cf. table below.)

TABLE XLVIII

Highly Saturated Colors

	8 Yrs.		9 Yrs.		10 Yrs.		College Students	
	Boys	Girls	Boys	Girls	Boys	Girls	Men	Women
Total Preferences for Red, Or. and Yel.	145	142	148	143	154	138	123	131
Total Preferences for Blue and Green ...	101	109	100	111	106	111	124	137

Unsaturated Colors

	8 Yrs.		9 Yrs.		10 Yrs.		College Students	
	Boys	Girls	Boys	Girls	Boys	Girls	Men	Women
Total Preferences for Red, Or. and Yel.	135	131	133	124	131	124	108	110
Total Preferences for Blue and Green ...	108	111	107	116	110	114	130	138

Concerning color-preferences, then, we may conclude as follows: In the first half-year, preference depends only upon saturation and brilliance: chromatic colors are preferred to greys, but between different chromatic colors preference is a matter of brilliance, not of hue (the more brilliant being preferred). In the second half-year, hue becomes a factor in color-preference, the warm colors (red, yellow and orange) being preferred to the cold ones (blue and green). From the third to the fifteenth year, preference for warm colors over cold ones gradually disappears, so that by adolescence either cold colors are actually preferred to warm ones, or the distinction between warm and cold colors ceases to be a factor in preference.

The preferences of children with respect to *intervals* have been investigated very thoroughly by C. W. Valentine.[19] The 12 musical intervals were presented to 195 boys and girls between 6 and 14 years of age, from two elementary schools, and to 76 girls between the same ages in a high class preparatory school. With the children from the elementary school each interval was presented twice to each child with instructions to state whether he (or she) liked the interval or not. Affirmative answers were scored 1, negative ones — 1. The total scores were then added for each interval in the case of children 6 years old, in the case of those 7 years old, and so forth up to 13 years. As the number of children in the various age-groups was not the same, the original totals were changed to proportionate totals for a group of 30 children, thus allowing direct comparison of figures for different age-groups. The results are shown graphically below (abscissae represent ages, ordinates, total scores; 60 is the maximal score, — 60 is the minimal). For the sake of comparison the graph shows likewise similar (though not exactly corresponding) totals secured by Valentine with 146 adults. Three features stand out in these results. In the first place, differentiation between different intervals is slight for the young children, and increases with age. In the second place, differentiation in general takes the form of a gradual decrease in the liking for discords without any change in the liking for concords, and the change for discords continues until they are actually disliked. In the third place, the rank order of the intervals changes very little from age 6 to adulthood. The correlation of the pleasantness of the intervals for children aged

6 and for adults is .53, which is quite high in view of what we know from the preceding section on the variability of hedonic judgments of children.

With the girls from the preparatory school the general procedure was the same, and the results were stated in similar form. In their case, however, judgments "very"

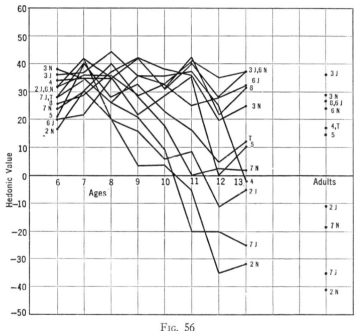

Fig. 56

(*Data from Valentine*)

and "slightly" pleasing (or displeasing) were allowed, and scored $1\frac{1}{2}$ and $\frac{1}{2}$ (or $-1\frac{1}{2}$ and $-\frac{1}{2}$), respectively. Thus when total scores were changed to proportionate totals for 30 children, the maximal possible score was 90, the minimal, -90. Furthermore, the girls of 6 and 7 years were grouped together in calculating results, as were also the girls of 13 and 14. The results are shown on the next page, together with comparable results for adults secured in another experiment.

In contrast with the preceding graph, we find here differentiation of concords and discords even for the youngest children. As to the rank-correlation between the hedonic value of the intervals for the 6 and 7 year group and for

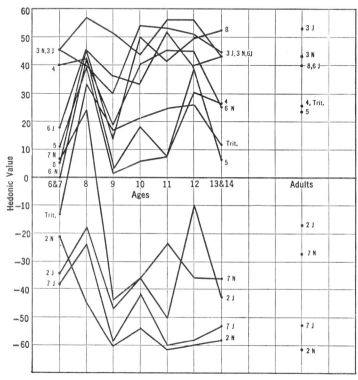

FIG. 57
(*Data from Valentine*)

the adults, we find that it is not only distinctly positive, but very high, namely .76.

Why the difference in the results? One obvious difference between the two groups was that of the first (children from the elementary schools), numbering 195, only 15 had had lessons on the piano, and 2 on the violin, while of the second group (children from a private school), 4 of the 7 children under 8 had studied music, and "practically every" child of 8 or over had done likewise. Valentine himself hesitates to ascribe the difference in results for the two groups to the striking difference in training, for he points out that difference in training might be only a sign of difference in hereditary musical sensitiveness. It seems to me, however, in the absence of any good evidence that musical ability is wholly inherited, that difference in training must be considered as at least a partial explanation of the difference between the two groups.

Valentine's findings have received a general confirmation from a later experiment by Dashiell (who was ignorant of Valentine's results).[20]   Dashiell had 198 kindergarten children and 89 college sophomores express like or dislike for five intervals. The results are given in the table below, the scores indicating the number of judgments of liking minus the number of judgments of disliking.

TABLE XLIX

	Kindergarten Children	College Sophomores
Octave	154	81
Major Third	193	79
Major Fifth	170	73
Minor Second	24	— 87
Major Seventh	66	— 89

As with Valentine's children from the elementary schools, so with Dashiell's kindergarten children the discords are on the whole liked instead of disliked. Again, however, as in Valentine's experiment, the order of preference of the intervals for the kindergarten children and for adults is quite similar, the rank correlation being .60. Dashiell leaves it an open question whether the change from liking discords (though less than concords) to disliking discords, is a matter of maturation or of training.

The facts, then, are quite in accord concerning preferences for intervals at different ages. As early as the sixth or seventh year the order of preference of intervals is quite similar to that for adults (raw correlation of about .50), in the case of musically untrained children, and very similar in the case of musically trained children (raw correlation of about .75). For the musically untrained children discords are not as a rule unpleasant until after the tenth year, but for musically trained children they are unpleasant as early as the seventh year. The interpretation of these facts, however, is not too easy, for, as Valentine has pointed out, training may be a mere cloak for maturation. It seems safe to conclude from the similarity of orders of preference for untrained young children and for adults that preference for intervals is in part independent of learning—in part due to the general characteristics of the organism. All further conclusions must be very tentative. It seems likely that training is indeed effective in influencing the hedonic value of intervals. H. T. Moore has presented good evidence that with frequent repetition an interval changes its consonance relative to other intervals.[21] Again, according to Valentine, "there seems to be a general agreement that to the modern ear the third is the most pleasing interval, whilst during the middle ages the fifth was probably the most popular, and with the Greeks, the octave." [22] Taken together, these circumstances favor the view that the relative hedonic value of intervals is influenced by learning. As to the fact that untrained children find discords absolutely pleasant, while trained children (and adults, of course,) find them absolutely unpleasant, it can readily be understood as a manifestation of hedonic contrast: the untrained children are presumably judging the discords relative to all the sounds in their recent past experience, including the most unpleasant noises, and consequently the discords, being more pleasant than many of these sounds, are judged absolutely pleasant; the trained children are presumably judging the discords relative to musical intervals alone, and consequently, as the discords are the least pleasant of the musical intervals, the discords are judged absolutely unpleasant.

Although preferences for foodstuffs are a matter of daily observation, I know of no reliable data on the constancy or variation of such preferences with increasing age. C. M. Davis, in the investigation mentioned in the preceding chapter, secured very interesting data on the tastes for foodstuffs of a group of children between six months and four years of age.[23] From the time when they were weaned, the children were allowed to select all their food from a very complete list of edible products, eight to eleven different items being presented to them at every meal. This procedure was continued with thirteen children for periods of time ranging from six months to three and one-half years. Although there were marked individual differences, it was found that the foodstuffs fell into three well-defined classes, the one involving foodstuffs "that almost all infants have liked continuously," the second involving foodstuffs "eaten in small amounts or not at all by most of the infants," and the third class, an intermediary one, involving foodstuffs "liked by most of the infants, but not by all, or that have not been eaten by some of the infants for months at a time, and those that have been eaten in much greater quantity at one age than at another." These classes were made up as follows:

TABLE L

Most Popular	Intermediate	Generally Unpopular
Meats	Pineapple	Spinach
Potatoes	Peaches	Lettuce
Carrots	Cabbage	Turnips
Beets	Cauliflower	Barley
Peas	Oatmeal	
Apples	Wheat	
Bananas	Milk (sweet or	
Oranges	lactic or both)	
Egg	Ry-Krisp	
	Cornmeal	
	Bone marrow	
	Glandular organs	
	Sea fish	

Unfortunately no complete data are available for later ages. Until this lack has been overcome, it will be impossible to use these excellent data to secure light on changes of children's tastes for foodstuffs with increasing age.

Maturation vs. Learning.—It is clear from the results presented above that tastes undergo marked changes with development from infancy to adulthood. The interpretation of these changes in terms of maturation and of learning, however, is by no means an easy matter. Consider, for instance, the work of Valentine on preferences for musical intervals. As he himself points out, one cannot be sure that the differences between the students from elementary schools and those from a private school are due to learning, because one cannot be sure that the two groups were equal with respect to musical ability. On the other hand, one cannot be sure that the differences are due to different degrees of maturation, for the training of the two groups was different. So it is with almost all the data above on changes of taste with increase in age. They do indeed suggest the occurrence of maturation or of learning to a greater or lesser degree, but they fail definitely to prove this occurrence. Far more experimentation will have to be done before it will be possible to state with reasonable certainty just what changes in taste may result from maturation and what changes can be achieved by training.

In the meantime, however, we can safely accept as fact that both maturation and learning are capable of changing taste. That maturation may be effective in this respect is not only made likely by several of the investigations reviewed above, but is strongly supported by certain other considerations. It has already been pointed out that whereas in the infant hedonic tone is mainly a characteristic of objects and passive internal states, in the child of three or four it characterizes situations and activities. So marked is the connection of hedonic tone with activity when the child begins to play that Bühler defines play in terms of what he calls "function-pleasure," the pleasure accompanying the effortless functioning of the body irrespective of any end.[24] It seems impossible to interpret the development of this relation between hedonic tone and activity

as anything but maturation, for the development is a feature
not only of the whole human species, but of many animal
species as well.

Again, H. E. and M. C. Jones studied the reactions of
51 children and of about 90 adults to a large, though harm-
less, snake.[25] "Children up to the age of two years showed
no fear of a snake; by three or three and one-half, caution
reactions were common. . . . Definite fear behaviour occurred more often after the age of four years, and was more
pronounced in adults than in children." [26] As the children
were being brought up in an institution, where "the snake
was as novel to them as the unicorn," the authors believe
that the difference in response with increasing age must be
due to maturation—in all likelihood, to perceptual discrimination. If this be so, we have here another instance of the
dependence of hedonic tone upon maturation, for it can
hardly be doubted that fear is as a rule unpleasant.

As to the effectiveness of learning in changing tastes,
this has been demonstrated very convincingly by the work
of J. B. Watson, H. E. Jones and others.[27] In an experiment by Watson and R. Rayner, the experimenters first
made sure that the subject, a child of 11 months, was un-
disturbed by a white rat (the child was accustomed to play
with it), but markedly disturbed by a loud noise.[28] The
experimenters then repeatedly caused the loud noise to occur
just as the child was about to touch the rat. In each case
this combined stimulation resulted in disturbed behaviour.
After seven combined stimulations the rat *presented alone*
called forth the following response: ". . . the baby began
to cry. Almost instantly he turned sharply to the left, fell
over on left side, raised himself on all fours and began to
crawl away so rapidly that he was caught with difficulty
before reaching the edge of the table." [29] This response
to the rat was certainly indicative of unpleasantness and it
certainly was learned. Similar results were secured by H. E.
Jones on a child of 15 months.[30] Before conditioning, the
child's reaction to an electric bell could be described as "mild
interest," shortly becoming "indifference." The bell was

then sounded a number of times while the child was subjected to a light inductive shock, provocative of a "slight, but unmistakable startle reaction" frequently accompanied by murmurs or whimpers. Seventy-two hours later the conditioned reflex was tested by sounding the bell alone. "The first application of the bell resulted in momentary crying; on the second, he cried and withdrew his hand slowly; on the third, he showed a generalized bodily startle reaction." [31] Here, again, then, is a response which indicates unpleasantness and which has definitely been learned. Furthermore, if one accept a wide definition of learning, the evidence from direct conditioning may be supplemented by a host of other data. We have seen that contrast may operate over a considerable period of time (Ch. V). The ensuing shifts can be interpreted as being a matter of learning. We have seen that hedonic tone can be shifted by suggestion (Ch. VI). Such shifts can likewise be interpreted as cases of learning. In the latter connection it is interesting to note that L. J. Roberts, in an investigation of the tastes of children for foodstuffs, finds evidence of the marked effect of "prestige," of the opinions of the parents, or of other adults who occupy an important position in the mind of the child.[32] We have seen, finally, that hedonic tone can be influenced by motor habituation (Ch. V). An experiment by M. C. Jones indicates that this influence is frequently offset by positive conditioning, so that repetition is of little value in controlling tastes.[33] The fact remains, however, that in those cases where motor habituation does operate, it constitutes a form of learning in the wide sense of the term.

Conclusion.—We know, then, that definite changes in taste take place as the individual develops from infancy to adulthood. Furthermore, although we do not know the part played by maturation and learning in most of these changes, we do know that both maturation and learning are capable in certain cases of bringing about changes in taste. This knowledge is both great enough to ensure that further investigation will be profitable and slight enough to make such investigation imperative. The relation of hedonic tone to maturation and learning is of interest both to the psychologist and to the practical educator. R. K. White and C. Landis,[34] for instance, have shown that in the case of silhouettes of faces those silhouettes are disliked which deviate from a standard silhouette. The psychologist interested in aesthetics obviously is very anxious to know whether this correlation between deviation from the standard and dislike is a matter of learning or of maturation. Again, consider the data of C. M. Davis on the likes and dislikes of children with respect to food.[35] The educator concerned with the problem of prescribing a diet, wishes to know whether these likes or dislikes are wholly due to the nature of the organism, or whether they are learned and consequently are subject to control. It is to be hoped that the strict methods of Watson, H. E. Jones and M. C. Jones will soon be used in the investigation of the marked changes of taste described in the early part of this chapter.

FOOTNOTES AND REFERENCES

1 W. STERN. Psychologie der frühen Kindheit, Leipzig, 1914.

2 Ibid., 282.

3 A. JERSILD. A Note on the Pleasures and Unpleasures of College Men and Women, J. Abn. & Soc. Psychol., 26, 1931, 92.

4 H. CASON. Common Annoyances, Psychol. Monogr., 40, 1930, No. 2, 25.

5 R. E. MARSDEN. A Study of the Early Color Sense, Psychol. Rev., 10, 1903, 37-47.

6 M. W. SHINN. Notes on the Development of a Child, II. The Development of the Senses in the First Three Years of Childhood, University of California Publications, Education, Vol. 4, 1907, 150.

7 Ibid., 159.

8 Cf. J. M. BALDWIN. Mental Development in the Child and in the Race, 1906, ch. 3.

9 M. W. SHINN. Op. cit., 172.

10 W. McDOUGALL. An Investigation of the Colour Sense of Two Infants, Brit. J. Psychol., 2, 1908, 338-352.

11 C. W. VALENTINE. The Color Perception and Color Preferences of an Infant During Its Fourth and Eighth Months, Brit. J. Psychol., 6, 1914, 363.

12 J. F. DASHIELL. Children's Sense of Harmonies in Colors and Tones, J. Exper. Psychol., 2, 1917, 466.

13 W. H. WINCH. Colour Preferences of School Children, Brit. J. Psychol., 3, 1909, 42-65.

[14] T. R. GARTH. A Color Preference Scale for One Thousand White Children, *J. Exper. Psychol.*, 7, 1924, 233.

[15] G. M. MICHAELS. Color Preference According to Age, *Amer. J. Psychol.*, 35, 1924, 79-87.

[16] T. R. GARTH. The Color Preferences of Five Hundred and Fifty-nine Full-blood Indians, *J. Exper. Psychol.*, 5, 1922, 392-417.

[17] R. M. DORCUS. Color Preferences and Color Associations, *Pedag. Sem.*, 33, 1926, 399-434.

[18] *Ibid.*, 431.

[19] C. W. VALENTINE. The Aesthetic Appreciation of Musical Intervals Among School Children and Adults, *Brit. J. Psychol.*, 6, 1913, 190-216.

[20] J. F. DASHIELL. Children's Sense of Harmonies in Colors and Tones, *J. Exper. Psychol.*, 2, 1917, 466.

[21] H. T. MOORE. The Genetic Aspects of Consonance and Dissonance, *Psychol. Monogr.*, 17, 1914, No. 73, Ch. V.

[22] C. W. VALENTINE. *Brit. J. Psychol.*, 6, 1913, 191. *Cf.* H. T. MOORE, *Psychol. Monogr.*, 17, 1914, No. 73, Ch. IV.

[23] C. M. DAVIS. What Infants on Self Selected Diet Experiment Eat, *Transactions of the Section on Diseases of Children of the American Medical Association*, Chicago, 1930, 137-146.

[24] K. BÜHLER. Die Geistige Entwickelung des Kindes, 4th Edit., *Jena*, 1924, 457.

[25] H. E. and M. C. JONES. A Study of Fear, *Childhood Educ.*, 5, 1928, 136-143.

[26] M. C. JONES The Conditioning of Children's Emotions, in A Handbook of Child Psychology, C. Murchison, editor, Worcester, Mass., 1931, 74.

[27] An excellent summary of this work is to be found in M. C. JONES, *op. cit.*

[28] J. B. WATSON and R. RAYNER. Conditioned Emotional Reactions, *J. Exper. Psychol.*, 3, 1920, 1-14.

[29] *Ibid.*, 5. *Cf.* also J. B. WATSON, Behaviourism, revised edit., N. Y., 1930, 160-1; J. B. WATSON, Psychology from the Standpoint of a Behaviourist, Phila., 1919, 212.

[30] H. E. JONES. The Conditioning of Overt Emotional Responses, *J. Educ. Psychol.*, 22, 1931, 127-130.

[31] *Ibid.*, 129. Jones has also established in infants conditioned galvanic skin reflexes (so-called psycho-galvanic reflexes). *Cf.* H. E. JONES, The Retention of Conditioned Emotional Responses in Infancy, *J. Genet. Psychol.*, 37, 1930, 485-498.

[32] L. J. ROBERTS. Teaching Children to Like Wholesome Foods, *Hygeia*, 2, 1924, 135-140.

[33] M. C. JONES. Elimination of Children's Fears, *J. Exper. Psychol.*, 7, 1924, 386.

[34] R. K. WHITE and C. LANDIS. Perception of Silhouettes, *Amer. J. Psychol.*, 42, 1930, 431. *Cf.* also WHITE and LANDIS, A Reply to Dr. Murray's Concept of Aesthetics, *Ibid.*, 43, 1931, 289.

[35] C. M. DAVIS. .Trans. Sect. on Diseases of Children of the Amer. Med. Assoc., Chicago, 1930, 137-146.

Chapter VIII

Hedonic Tone in Relation to Muscular and Glandular Responses

The various muscular and glandular responses of interest in connection with hedonic tone may profitably be divided into two groups, the first consisting of what we shall call *vegetative* responses, such as the beat of the heart or breathing, the second of what we shall call *locomotor* responses, such as reaching for an object or adopting a posture. I shall discuss in turn the relation of hedonic tone to the responses in each group, beginning with the vegetative responses.

HEDONIC TONE IN RELATION TO VEGETATIVE RESPONSES

The close relation between feelings and emotions on the one hand, and vegetative responses on the other, has been known for more than two thousand years. It is said of Erisistratus, who practised medicine around 300 B.C., that when asked to diagnose the disease of the son of King Antiochus, he noticed an increase of heart rate in the patient upon the entrance into the room of a certain beautiful maiden, and promptly diagnosed the complaint of the patient as love. Not until the close of the nineteenth century, however, with the experiments of Mosso (1881) and the theories of James and Lange (1884 and 1885, respectively) did this relationship become subject to experimental investigation. Indeed, it was not until 1899, with Wundt's appeal to physiological concomitants in support of his tridimensional theory, that the particular phase of the relationship of interest to us, namely the correlation between hedonic tone and vegetative responses, became an independent subject of laboratory investigation.

It is impossible in the space at our disposal to deal with

each of the dozens of investigations concerned with the relation between hedonic tone and vegetative responses. We shall consequently confine ourselves to the more outstanding of these investigations.

Vasomotor and Respiratory Responses. — Wundt, in his 1899 article, using as a basis results secured in a somewhat different connection by Mentz and Lehmann, advanced the view that the relation between feelings and vasomotor responses was as indicated in the schema below: (P = pleasantness, U = unpleasantness, E = excitement, D = depression, T = tension, R = relaxation.)

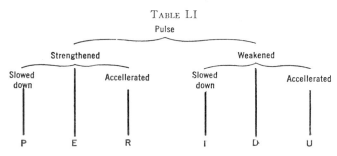

TABLE LI

Pulse

In 1901, Max Brahn[1] published experimental results which supported Wundt's contention that there were definite relationships between his feeling-dimensions and the various characteristics of the pulse. The details of Wundt's schema were altered, however, in accordance with the following table: (alterations in circles).

TABLE LII

Feeling Dimensions	Pulse Strength Increase	Decrease	Pulse Speed Increase	Decrease
P.	+			+
U.		+		(+)
E.	+			
D.		+		
T.			(+)	
R.				(+)

In 1902, in the 5th edition of the "Physiologische Psychologie," Wundt gave a schema indicating the relations of his six qualities not only to pulse-characteristics but also to those of breathing.[3]   This new schema insofar as the pulse is concerned, is identical with Wundt's 1899 schema, in spite of the results of Brahn indicating the necessity of certain changes.   As to that part of the new schema which refers to breathing-characteristics, Wundt states that it is based primarily upon experimental results secured by Gent[4] and by Meumann and Zoneff.[5]

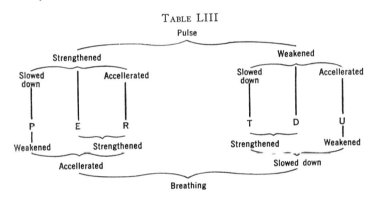

TABLE LIII

Five years later, there appeared Alechsieff's work on both the pulse and breathing correlates of the six Wundtian feelings.   He summarized his results in the following table.[6]

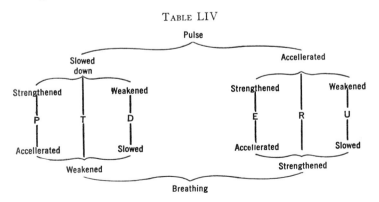

TABLE LIV

Despite the fact that this schema differs markedly from that published in 1902 by Wundt, the latter is to be found in the 1920 edition of the "Gründriss," unchanged except for the breathing-correlates of tension, depression and unpleasantness. In the event of these Wundt made the changes indicated below:

TABLE LV

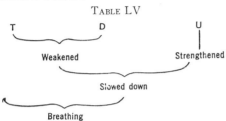

The correlations established by the Wundtian school did not remain unquestioned. In 1906, for instance, J. F. Shephard published an experiment upon the relationship between the six Wundtian feeling-qualities and changes in volume of the hand and brain, changes in heart rate, changes in the extent, depth and rate of breathing, and changes in the form and size of the plethysmographic pulse in brain and hand. His results led him to conclude as follows: "I find that feelings cannot be classified on the basis of vasomotor and heart rate changes. There is no reverse relation even between the accompaniments of agreeableness and disagreeableness; much less are there three such pairs of reactions." [7] Furthermore, a number of the vegetative responses which were at first considered to be the physiological correlates of feelings were shown to be equally much the correlates of other mental processes. Thus Zoneff and Meumann found that slowing of the pulse was not only a concomitant of pleasantness, but of attention in general.[8]

By 1914, the number of experiments upon the physiological concomitants of various forms of experience had so increased as to warrant some tabular representation of their results. Such a tabular representation was provided by E. Leschke.[9] It is reproduced below. Authors are indicated in this table by letters in accordance with the following list.

A	Alechsieff	G	Gent	Me	Mentz
B	Berger	Ki	Kiesow	Mo	Mosso
Br	Brahn	Kü	Küppers	S	Shephard
Bz	v. Bezold	L	Lehmann	W	Weber
Ci	Citron	Lo	Lombardi	Wu	Wundt
D	Dumas	Lv	Loven	Z	Zoneff and
Di	Dittmar	Ma	Martius		Meumann

The findings of these authors are indicated by symbols in accordance with the following key:

+ Increase (for arteries, expansion)

— Decrease (for arteries, contraction)

+ — First increase (expansion), then decrease (contraction)

(+) — First increase, but as essential characteristic a subsequent decrease

± Now increase, now decrease (when in parenthesis means of slight degree)

(+) In a few cases increase, in most decrease

O No change

Examination of the table shows marked agreement of the results of different observers. Thus eight observers investigated changes in pulse rate correlated with "sensory" pleasantness and unpleasantness. All eight found an increase of rate for pleasantness and seven of the eight found a decrease for unpleasantness. On the other hand, the table shows just as strikingly the absence of any definite correlation between hedonic tone in general and vegetative responses, and the relative equivocality of such correlations if they could be established. Pleasantness is accompanied by decrease in pulse rate in the case of "sensory" pleasantness but by increase in the case of the "active" and "passive" pleasantness distinguished by Dumas; it is accompanied by no change in blood pressure "sensory" pleasantness, by increase in the case of "active" pleasantness, by decrease in the case of "passive" pleasantness; it is accompanied by increase in arm volume in the case of "sensory" pleasantness, by no change in the case of "intellectual" pleasantness, and by decrease in the case of "active" pleasantness. The volume of the radial artery, which increases

TABLE LVI (From Leschke)

	Attention		Mental Work		Fear	Strain	Relax.	Excitem.	Depress.	Pleasantness				Unpleasantness								Intention of Movement	
	To Visual and Audit. Stim.	To Tactual Stim.	Normal	During Fatigue						Sensory	Intell.	Active	Passive	Sensory	Pain	Intell.	Fear	Active	Passive	Discouragement	Suffering	Normal	During Fatigue
Frequency of Pulse	(+)−(+)L −N −Me	(+)−−L −S	+L +S +Me ±G (+)Z		(+)−−L −S	O L −W −A −Br −+G	+Wu +A +G	+Wu +A +G	−Wu −A −G −I	Wu −A −I −N +−S	−Wu −A −I −G	+D	+D	Wu −A −S −L −N −G −W	+L +Z +−−I	−L +++S	+L	+D +G	−D −G	−D	+D	+S	
Amplitude of Pulse in Periph. Arteries	(+)−(+)L		−B −G		−L	−Wu −L −L −W +G	+Wu +L +G +Br	+Wu +G +Br	−Wu −G −Br	−L −G +B +W	O G			−G −I −Br −W	−L	−L	−L	−G	−G				
Dicrotic						−Br	−Br			+L +I +W	O Ki	−S	−D	O Ki									
Blood Pressure	(+)−(+)L −G −S (+)Kü	+S −L +We Kü +Lu	+Ki ±W	+We	+Ki −L −W (+)Kü	−Wu −G −L −W −B −S	O D +G +L +S	+Wu +G −S	−Wu −G	(−)+L −+S (+)G (O)Kü	O G	−S	−D	Ki −W	+W +D	−L	(+)Ki −L	−G	−L −G	+D	+D	+W +Ci	−Ci
Volume of the Arm														−Kü	−Kü							+W +Ci	+W +Ci
Volume of the Head			−W −Ci +W	+W +Ci	−W	−W				−W	+W	+W		−W								−W −Ci	+W +Ci
Volume of the Viscera	+B +S		+B +W	+W	+W					−W	−W			+W								−W	+W
Volume of the Brain	+B		+B +Lo	−W	+B	O B		+G +A		−B +S	−B +S			−B +W				+B +Mo				+W	
Amplit. of Pulsation in Brain			+B +Lo		+B	O B				+B	+B	+B		−B				+B +Mo					
Carotid Artery	+L +W		+L +W	−W		O L	O L	+Wu +G +A		+B +W +S	+B +W +S			−L −B −I −I				+B +Mo	−L		+D	+W	
Radial Artery	−L −W	+L +S	−L −W	+W		−L	+L	O G O A	−Wu −G −I	−L +I	−L +L	+L		−L				−D	−L −D −I	−D	+D	+W	
Tibial Artery	−L −W		−L −W							−L	−L	−L		+L					+L				
Frequency of Respiration	(±)L +Z O G		+L (+)Z ±G +Ma		O L +W	O L (−)G O A	O G O A	+G +A	−Wu −I −A	Z +G +A	N +Z +G			(±)L −Z −A	±Ma	−Z		+D +G	−D −G	−D	+D		
Depth of Respiration	−Z −G		−Z −I −Ma			−Wu −G −I −A	+Wu +G +A	O Wu −G −I +A	−Wu −I −A	(±)Z (−)G −I	(±)Z −G			(+)G +Z +A	±Z			+G	−G				

for all forms of pleasantness and decreases for all forms of unpleasantness except moral suffering, increases for attention to touch stimuli and for mental work during fatigue —neither of which need to be pleasant, surely—and decreases for attention to visual and acoustic stimuli and for normal intellectual work—neither of which seem necessarily connected with unpleasantness. Thus it would seem that with respect to the vegetative responses considered so far we must conclude that although there is a definite correlation between certain types of pleasant and unpleasant experiences and certain vegetative responses, there is no exclusive correlation between the latter and pleasantness in general or unpleasantness in general such that we can infer the hedonic tone from response or response from hedonic tone. At best there is but a statistical tendency for pleasantness and unpleasantness to be accompanied by vaso-motor and breathing changes in accordance with the table below.

TABLE LVII

	P	U
Pulse frequency	—	+
Pulse height (strength)	+	
Blood pressure	O	+
Arm volume	+ ?	—
Breathing frequency	+	— ?
Breathing depth (strength)	— ?	+ ?

In view of the conclusion that there is no general correlation between hedonic tone and changes in pulse and breathing, there is no point in asking whether the former precedes the latter or vice-versa. Some readers, however, either because they cannot accept the conclusion above, or because of historical interest, may desire mention of the problem of temporal priority. For such readers I point out that Lehmann,[10] basing himself on his own work and that by Zoneff and Meumann, Brahn, Gent, Berger and Kelchner, argues that feelings *precede* the changes in pulse and breathing correlated with them; that Cannon[11] draws a somewhat similar conclusion from a comparison of the latent times of hedonic judgments and of contractions of smooth muscles; but that Newman, Perkins and Wheeler[12] in a recent discussion of Cannon's evidence, do not consider this evidence to be conclusive.

The Psychogalvanic Reflex.—Much work has recently been done upon another supposed accompaniment of hedonic experience, namely the psychogalvanic reflex.[13] A clear and concise characterization of the psychogalvanic reflex is to be found in Wechsler's excellent monograph, "The Measurement of Emotional Reactions." [14] Wechsler writes: "If two points on the human skin are connected with unpolarizable electrodes to a sufficiently sensitive galvanometer, the points of the galvanometer will be seen to deviate, indicating the passage of a current due to the difference of potential between the two connected points. . . . If now, while a person is so connected with the galvanometer and, provided that at least one of the points is a part of the skin that contains sweat glands, he be subjected to a mental stimulus, e.g., a simple multiplication, the initial galvanometric deflection will be seen to increase after a short latent time of two or three seconds, indicating an apparent augmentation in the difference of potential. This electrical variation of the human skin following mental excitation without any exterior electromotive force passing through it, was first observed by Tarchanoff in 1888. . . . If, maintaining the above conditions of the experiment, we introduce in series with the subject and galvanometer a small source of current, e.g., two volts, then when the circuit is closed the galvanometer will register a deflection due to the passage of the current across the body as a resistance. If now the subject is again caused to experience a psychic excitation, the initial galvanometric deflection will, as before, be seen to increase (after a similar latent time) indicating an augmentation of the current passing through the circuit. . . . The electrical variation of the human body in response to a mental stimulus during the passage of an exsomatic current was first reported by Charles Féré in 1887 . . . but it was not until 1906 that Otto Veraguth made a systematic study of the phenomenon to which he gave the name of 'psychogalvanic reflex.' The term 'psychogalvanic reflex' is now used to include the electrical variations of the skin to psychic stimuli obtained both with and without the use of an external current in the circuit." [15]

Wechsler inquires at length into the nature of the psychological correlates of the psychogalvanic reflex. Beginning with the question of the nature of the stimuli capable of provoking it, he points out that such stimuli may be arranged into the five following classes: "1. Outright emotion-provoking stimuli, as when a person is frightened or angered; 2. Affectively toned ideational processes centrally aroused: (a) conscious, as when a subject recalls a pleasant experience; (b) unconscious, as in the case of an evoked complex response to association stimulus; 3. Strong sensations, as sound of a gun or prick of a pin; 4. Mental effort, as exemplified by the mental process employed in the solution of arithmetical problems; 5. Changes in state of attention." [16] According to Wechsler, stimuli belonging to the first two classes obviously involve "affective tone," and those belonging to the third class may be shown to be effective only in proportion as they likewise involve "affective tone." Stimuli in class 4 are effective only at the beginning and end of the mental task involved, when it is reasonable to assume that the experience is "affectively toned." As to stimuli in class 5, Wechsler contends that the close connection between emotions and instinct on the one hand and between instinctive adaptation and attention on the other suggests a close connection between attention and emotion. This latter connection leads him to believe that "psychologically the important differentiating aspect of the mental state known as attention is as in the case of the emotion, that which has been termed affective tone." [17] Thus stimuli belonging to the 5th class may also be considered to determine "affective tone." Wechsler concludes that examination of the nature of the stimuli provoking the psychogalvanic reflex supports the general proposition that " . . . at least as far as humans are concerned, the psychogalvanic reflex is primarily, if not exclusively, an index of affective tone." [18]

This view is further supported, he believes, by the results of studies upon variations in magnitude of psychogalvanic reflexes. According to both his experiments and those of the majority of other investigators who have studied the problem, the magnitude of the galvanic reaction is in no way dependent upon the intensity of the physical stimulus involved, but varies roughly as the intensity of the "affective tone" accompanying such stimulation. Thus Wechsler had ten observers give associations to 25 words and determined in each case the galvanometric deviations involved. He then had his observers classify the words in five groups, according to the emotional value of the response elicited by them during the actual experiment. He found considerable correlation between the average of the galvanometric deflections recorded for a given word from the ten observers and the average of the emotional values assigned by the ten observers to the responses elicited by that word. Individual records did show discrepancies with the general relationship—occasionally large galvanic deflections occurred when the observer failed to report any concomitant emotion, and vice versa—but Wechsler believes at least many of these discrepancies to be only apparent, as subsequent free association experiments showed that in many such cases the electrical changes were probably accompanied by affective reactions which were not conscious at the moment of their occurrence.

In connection with this latter point, Wechsler describes an experiment in which he sought to determine whether the psychogalvanic reflex could be elicited in a sleeping observer by stimuli adequate to do so in observers who are in a waking state. He found that the psychogalvanic reflex could indeed be elicited during sound sleep, and concluded that although the psychogalvanic response is to be taken as an index of the occurrence of an affective reaction in response to an exciting stimulus, ". . . Neither the affective response nor the exciting stimulus need be consciously perceived by the subject experiencing them." [19]

Wechsler's evidence must, I think, be considered as

definitely supporting his general conclusion that the psychogalvanic reflex is an index of "affective tone" in his sense of
the term. It must also, however, be considered definitely
to support the conclusion that the psychogalvanic reflex is
not an index of hedonic tone in our sense of the term.
Wechsler's concept "affective tone" is obviously broader
than our concept hedonic tone. It includes the latter and
much more besides. Hedonic tone for us is pleasantness
or unpleasantness. Affective tone for Wechsler is a much
broader term akin to "emotionality," as shown by his contention that affective tone is psychologically the important
differentiating characteristic of attention. Consequently
Wechsler's conclusions insofar as they state positive relationships, do not imply like conclusions involving hedonic
tone as defined by us. On the other hand, Wechsler's negative conclusion that the "affective tone" correlated with the
psychogalvanic reflex need not be conscious implies a very
definite conclusion in connection with hedonic tone. In
connection with the problem of a special hedonic attitude
we found good reason to deny that inferred phenomenal
entities—including, naturally, unconscious ones—can be
characterized as having hedonic tone. If this be so, the
fact that the "affective tone" correlated with the psychogalvanic reflex need not be conscious clearly implies that
hedonic tone may be absent when the reflex is present. From
this in turn follows that although there are doubtless relationships between special types of hedonic events, e.g., emotions, and the psychogalvanic reflex, there is no relationship
between hedonic tone in general and the psychogalvanic reflex such that hedonic tone can be predicted from the reflex.
Whether there is a converse relationship between hedonic
tone in general and the psychogalvanic reflex, i.e. whether
the reflex can be predicted from the hedonic tone, is a question which can be answered neither affirmatively nor nega-
tively from Wechsler's data. This question is answered,
however, by another experiment, that of H. C. Syz.[20] A
large number of observers were given supposedly emotional
verbal stimuli while they were connected with a galvan-

ometer. All galvanometric reactions were recorded photographically, and at the close of the experiment the observers were asked to give an account of their emotional experiences. Syz found that: "None of the subjects reported more than 37 per cent. of his galvanic reactions; most of them gave account of only 10 to 25 per cent. On the other hand, there were reports of emotional responses with many words where the galvanic curve did not indicate any deflection." [21] As emotions are very frequently characterized by marked hedonic tone, it is reasonable to infer that it is no more possible to predict the psychogalvanic reflex from hedonic tone than it is to predict hedonic tone from the reflex.[22] The results of Wechsler and of other investigators show, however, that *there is some tendency for hedonic tone to be accompanied by a psychogalvanic reflex,* i.e. that there is some connection, though not an invariable one, between the two processes. This positive conclusion must not be lost sight of just because of the negative conclusions arrived at above. Just what the reason is for this connection cannot at present be stated with certainty. Recent work on the reflex, indicating that it is essentially a manifestation of the activity of the sympathetic nervous system,[23] suggests that the connection is mediated by emotion. According to such a view hedonic tone would of itself have no relation to the galvanic reflex, but would appear to have one in the case of hedonically toned emotional experiences because of the sympathetic activity involved in the emotion. This view is strongly supported by the striking fact that when hedonic tone is accompanied by a galvanic reflex, the reflex is the same for a given degree of either pleasantness or unpleasantness. A. Gregor, in an experiment published in 1913, found that "the direction of the excursion in the psychogalvanic reaction is determined by the position of the limbs relative to the poles of the galvanometer. The form of the psychogalvanic reaction, however, is independent of the quality of the feeling aroused by the stimulus." [24] In the case of one observer, for instance, the photographic records of the galvanic responses to introspectively pleasant Eau de

Cologne and to introspectively unpleasant asafoetida were practically identical. This is exactly what would be expected if the connection between hedonic tone and the reflex is mediated by emotion, for Cannon has demonstrated clearly that the sympathetic responses to all intense emotions, whether pleasant or unpleasant, are of a single type.[25]

HEDONIC TONE IN RELATION TO LOCOMOTOR RESPONSES

The close connection between hedonic tone and locomotor responses is attested by the prevalence throughout the ages of psychological hedonism among both laymen and scientists. Nor is there any lack of experimental proof of this connection. Sherrington, for instance, in his "Integrative Action of the Nervous System," writes: "It would seem a general rule that reflexes arising in species of receptors which considered as sense organs provoke strongly affective sensations caeteris paribus prevail over reflexes of other species when in competition with them for the use of the 'final common path.' "[26] This connection has been studied from two different points of view, namely with reference to changes in the energy involved in the responses, and with reference to their type. We shall deal with these two points of view successively.

Energy Involved in Responses. —O. Külpe, in his "Outlines," wrote: "Pleasurable states are regularly accompanied by increase of the force of voluntary muscular action, and unpleasurable states as regularly by its diminution."[27] In his "Experimental Psychology," Titchener described two methods of demonstrating this relationship to laboratory classes, and gave for both methods what he called typical results. In the case of the first method, in which the apparatus used is a finger dynamometer, the typical results are indicated by Titchener in two curves, reproduced on page 331. The ordinates are force exerted, the abscissae, time elapsed since the exertion began. The stars indicate the application of a stimulus. It will be noticed that these curves are absolutely univocal and in complete agreement with the statement of Külpe mentioned above.[28]

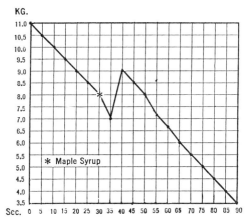

FIG. 58.—Typical curve for high degree of pleasantness.

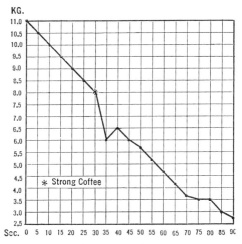

FIG. 59.—Typical curve of unpleasantness.

Neither Külpe nor Titchener refer the reader to specific experiments proving the propositions which they assert. It may be that such exist, but if so, I have been unable to find them. Féré, it is true, published in 1885 a series of papers upon the dynamometric effects of "agreeable and disagreeable sensations" in which he concluded that the former increase motor energy, while the latter decrease it.[29] A. Ernst has recently pointed out, however, that these papers describe not only experiments in which "agreeable sensations" increased motor energy as measured by a dynamometer and "disagreeable sensations" decreased such work, but also experiments in which obviously disagreeable experiences brought about increases of motor energy.[30] In support of this statement, Ernst cites the following passage from one of the papers by Féré: "The study of a great number of induced hallucinations has shown us that when it is a question of a disagreeable sensation, like the sight of a viscous toad, the smell of rotten eggs, a bitter taste, etc., there was a sufficiently notable decrease. We were tempted to conclude from this that sensations are agreeable or disagreeable according to whether they determine an increase or a decrease of energy; but this conclusion is at least premature, for on the same observer and on ourselves the painting of the back of the throat with sulphate of quinine, the breathing of ammonia, which do not constitute agreeable sensations, constantly determine an increase of dynamometric force." [31] After citing a number of other experiments by Féré in which habitually unpleasant stimuli such as quinine produced increase in motor energy and not decrease, Ernst concludes—with right, it would seem—that Féré's conclusions do not follow from his own results. It would seem wise, therefore, before accepting the law stated by Külpe, to make a careful examination of available facts. These facts may conveniently be divided into two groups, according to whether the hedonic tone involved occurs in connection with a "major emotion" or not. We shall first consider the relation of hedonic tone to energy of voluntary muscular contraction during major emotional states.

In his monograph on joy and sorrow—a much too little known work, incidentally—G. Dumas reports observations upon the strength of hand-contraction of psychiatric patients under ordinary conditions and when in a state of marked *joy.* For two patients he found the following values (in kilograms).[32]

TABLE LVIII

Patient	Normal	During Joy
Eugénie	20	27
	18	24
Antoinette	24	36
	20	30

In the case of the latter patient, the measurements representing force during joy were made on the day of her departure from the hospital. Dumas points out that these observations agree with the view expressed by Lange: "The functional excitation of the voluntary muscles and nerves make the joyful man feel enervated like all those whose muscles are powerful. He feels the need of moving, he bestirs himself with promptness and vivacity, he gesticulates with force." [33]

The observations of Dumas are confirmed by the results of what might be called an accidental experiment performed upon himself by U. Mosso.[34] In 1889, Mosso, then at the University of Turin, was training himself in the use of the ergograph. In the previous year he had been given a scholarship which had enabled him to work with Schmiedeberg at the University of Strassburg, but at the close of the year he had been obliged to return to Turin, and although he was very anxious to get back to Strassburg, could not see his way clear to do so. One morning, after completing around 9 a. m. a session at the ergograph in which, lifting a 5 kg. weight with his finger until he could no longer move the weight, he had made 14 lifting movements and produced work to the extent of 1.500 kilogrammeters—the usual amount for him,—he was suddenly informed at 10 a. m. by his brother, a professor at the University of Turin, that he could return to Strassburg and Schmiedeberg. This news created in him a strong emotion. At 10.50, he carried out the second session of the day at the ergograph under the same conditions as earlier. This time he was able to make

21 lifting movements and to produce 2.555 kilogrammeters of work. He then went home to tell the good news to his parents and found there a letter informing him officially that he was to be sent to Strassburg. He writes feelingly: "It was a great joy that I experienced that day." [35] At 12.50, having returned to the laboratory, he carried out a third session at the ergograph. This time he was able to make 30 finger movements and to produce 4.320 kilogrammeters of work. Mosso concluded as follows: "It follows from this experience, that a strong and agreeable emotion influences the activity of the muscles and makes them develop twice and three times the normal energy. I did not continue the experiment because the state of mind in which I found myself did not allow me to busy myself longer with ergographic curves." [36] Clearly the work of Mosso agrees with that of Dumas in showing that joy is correlated with an increase in the energy of voluntary muscular contraction.

With respect to *sorrow,* the case seems to be equally clear, and equally in accord with Külpe's law. Dumas found in psychiatric patients who were in a state of great sadness a marked decrease of the strength of contraction of the hand. In the case of three men patients, he measured this strength with a dynamometer and compared the results with those secured from average men. The figures which he gives are as follows (force in kilograms).[37]

TABLE LIX

| | Depressed Men | | Normal for Men | |
	right hand	left hand	right hand	left hand
Edouard	18	16 (4 trials)	45	40
T	14	22 (6 trials)		
F	30	28 (3 trials)		

In the case of a woman patient, Dumas determined the strength of contraction of the hand during 8 days of sadness and during 8 days of joy. The results are given on next page.[38]

When we consider, however, the relation between *anger* and energy of voluntary muscular contraction, we find data

TABLE LX

Sadness		Joy		Normal for Women	
r.h.	l.h.	r.h.	l.h.	r.h.	l.h.
13	14	28	20	30	25
15	12	28	25		
17	13	26	26		
14	14	30	28		
18	15	28	27		
17	16	30	28		
15	15	31	26		
18	16	28	25		

distinctly contrary to Külpe's law.   In 1894, while professor of experimental pharmacology at the University of Genoa, Mosso undertook an investigation of the effects of sugar upon muscular contraction.[39]   In order to note these effects, he carried out successive trials at the ergograph every five minutes, in each case working until complete exhaustion.   On the 5th of January, the first trial of the day, made at 9 a. m., gave a total output of energy of 2.910 kgm. with 26 lifts.   The second trial, at 9.05, gave 2.090 kgm. with 20 lifts, and the third, at 9.10, 1.490 kgm. with 17 lifts. In these three trials there is a continuous decrease of energy output, and with a continuation of the trials this decrease should likewise have continued.   At the close of the third trial, however, a colleague of Mosso came into the room to solicit his vote in a matter involving the faculty with respect to which Mosso was well known to hold views divergent from those of his colleague.   There followed an animated discussion.   In the meantime Mosso continued his experiment, but his mind was troubled.   The fourth trial, at 9.15, gave 2.305 kgm. with 21 lifts; the fifth, at 9.20, gave 2.395 kgm. with 22 lifts; the sixth, at 9.25, 2.380 kgm. with 24 lifts.   Thus instead of a decrease in output of energy, there occurred a marked increase in this output. The discussion continued very animated, Mosso being dominated by a feeling of rebellion.   The eighth trial, at 9.25 gave 1.800 kgm. with 21 lifts.   Following this trial the discussion became so acrimonious that Mosso was obliged to ask his colleague to leave the room. The ninth trial, at 9.40, gave 1.545 kgm. with 26 lifts, and the eleventh, 1.855 kgm. with 21 lifts. The succeeding trials continued to give results greater than those of the third trial until 11.10. Mosso concluded that this is striking evidence that an emotion may increase muscular energy very markedly, even though unpleasant. In connection with this experiment by Mosso, it is interesting to note that unpleasantness may correlate with striking increases of metabolic rate. I quote Miss Washburn: "Fourteen neurotic war veterans were asked by Ziegler and Levine[40] to recall unpleasant war experiences, and their basal metabolism during recall was compared with the normal rate. Ten of them showed a rise, two a fall. Some showed an increased rate when they were unaware of any emotion. This is like what happens with the galvanic reflex." [41]

It seems obvious from the foregoing data that major emotional states have a marked relation to the strength of voluntary muscular contractions, but that this relationship is not properly described by Külpe's law. Pleasant emotions may indeed be accompanied by increase of the voluntary strength of the individual, but unpleasant ones likewise. It appears that in the case of emotions, energy of the voluntary musculature is univocally related not to hedonic tone, but to presence or absence of excitement. This conclusion is quite obviously in accord with Cannon's findings that all intense emotions, whether pleasant or unpleasant, involve a similar set of sympathetic responses, many of which are antagonistic to fatigue.[42]

Is it not possible that the relationship just mentioned— that between energy and excitement—obscures the relation between energy and hedonic tone in the case of the emotions? In order to answer this further question, let us turn to the data on the relation of hedonic tone to energy under conditions not involving any major emotions.

We have already seen that Féré's own results do not support Külpe's law.[43] Féré did indeed find that pleasant stimuli were generally followed by increased energy of voluntary contraction, but so were in some cases unpleasant stimuli. In 1906, G. Störring published some observations on the effect upon strength of voluntary muscular contraction, as measured by the dynamometer, of unpleasant sensory experiences (Empfindungsunlust) occasioned by such stimuli as vinegar, salt solution, and tintura gentianae.[44] The results showed a distinct increase in the force registered by the dynamometer. Rose confirmed Störring's results, concluding that "Sensory unpleasantness (Empfindungsunlust) of both weak and strong degree determines an increase of the motor effect, irrespective of the reaction-set and of the mode of reception of the stimulus." [45] Störring's results were again confirmed by Ernst, who found that unpleasant sensory experiences (Empfindungsunlust) markedly increased muscular power as registered with a dynamometer. Ernst writes: "Thus in our results unpleasantness invariably brings about an average increase of the motor impulse and of the effect of the force developed." [46]

It is patent from the foregoing that Külpe's law, according to which pleasantness is accompanied by an increase of voluntary muscular power and unpleasantness by a decrease, finds experimental support neither in the case of hedonic tone during major emotions nor in the case of hedonic tone in the absence of emotional stress. Can we not conclude from the latter data, however,—from the work of Störring, Rose and Ernst—that a law holds which is exactly the converse of Külpe's? The results in question do indeed agree in showing that unpleasant stimuli are accompanied on an average by increased energy. There is no proof, however, that the change in energy is due to the unpleasantness rather than to some co-variant of unpleasantness such as stimulus-intensity. This question is at present being investigated by W. A. Bousfield in the Harvard Laboratory. Until it has received at least a partial answer it will be wisest to refrain from any positive conclusion concerning the relation of hedonic tone to the energy of locomotor responses.

Types of Response. —The problem whether pleasantness and unpleasantness are correlated with specific types of responses is one of great importance to the theory of motivation. In his "Fundamentals of Human Motivation," L. T. Troland distinguishes very aptly between three forms of hedonism: hedonism of the future, which holds that conduct is determined by future hedonic tone; hedonism of the present, which holds that conduct is determined by present hedonic tone; and hedonism of the past, according to which conduct is determined by past hedonic tone.[47] Hedonism of the future is nowadays usually assimilated to hedonism of the present, the hedonic tone of a "future" phenomenon being considered as the hedonic tone of a present phenomenon referred to the future. Hedonism of the past will be dealt with in the next chapter in connection with the relation of memory to hedonic tone. As to hedonism of the present, its validity clearly depends on the accompaniment of pleasantness by movements towards the object of attention and of unpleasantness by movements away from it, i.e. on a specific correlation between hedonic tone and types of movements. Consider, for instance, the quasi-hedonism which K. Lewin believes to obtain in children.[48] The essence of this doctrine is that the condition of the child with respect to needs determines certain objects in its psychological environment ("phenomenal" objects, not physical ones) to be endowed with psychological "valences" (Aufforderungscharaktere). "These imperative psychological facts (the valences) . . . determine the *direction* of the behaviour. . . . One may distinguish two large groups of valences according to the sort of initial behaviour they elicit; the positive valences (+), those affecting approach; and the negative (—), or those producing withdrawal or retreat."[49] But to say that an object has a positive or negative valence is apparently equivalent to stating that it is pleasant or unpleasant. Lewin does not make this point explicitly, but it is an implication of many passages in his articles. In discussing the forcing of children to complete tasks by making threats, for instance, he writes: "In this case one uses . . . a second negative valence, a further unpleasantness." [50] Thus Lewin's doctrine of motivation in children presupposes that in children pleasantness is accompanied by initial movements *towards* the object of attention, unpleasantness by initial movements *away* from it.

What are the facts concerning the relation of hedonic tone to types of movements? In a paper read before the 2nd International Congress of Psychology in London in 1892, Münsterberg described an experiment on the relation of hedonic tone to the contraction and extension of voluntary muscles. The observer shut his eyes and then sought to move an indicator sometimes 10 centimeters, sometimes 20 centimeters, both towards himself and away from himself. The error made by the observer was recorded and also his feelings during the trial. The averages of the errors (in millimeters) made in the case of the various feelings recorded are given in the table below, copied from Münsterberg:

TABLE LXI

	Centrifugal		Centripetal	
	10 cm.	20 cm.	10 cm.	20 cm.
Fatigue	— 12 mm.	— 17 mm.	— 15 mm.	— 21 mm.
Excitement ...	16	22	19	26
Sorrow	— 7	— 11	— 12	— 16
Joy	17	16	12	14
Unpleasantness	— 10	— 13	12	19
Pleasantness ..	10	16	— 20	— 24

Insofar as pleasantness and unpleasantness are concerned, there is a marked opposition between centrifugal and centripetal accompaniments. "For unpleasantness, movements of extension are too small, those of flexion, too large; for pleasantness, the movements of flexion are too small, those of extension, too large." [51]

Münsterberg's results have been confirmed to greater or lesser degree by three subsequent investigations. The first of these confirmations is the more striking because it occurred without the knowledge of its author. In his remarkable work on joy and sorrow, Dumas cites a description of Münsterberg's experiments from Ribot's "Psychologie des Sentiments." [52] This description mentions only the results secured by Münsterberg with respect to pleasantness and unpleasantness. Dumas goes on to say that he has sought confirmation upon his patients, but only with indifferent success. Three of his "mélancholiques déprimés" were tested according to Münsterberg's technique, one of them quite thoroughly. Results showed for all a negative error—indicating decreased mobility—in the case of *both* flexion and extension. Three of his manic patients, in a joyfully excited condition, were likewise tested. These showed positive errors in the case of both flexion and extension. Dumas, apparently judging solely from the description by Ribot, considers these results to be contrary to Münsterberg's findings. If we consult, however, the table on the preceding page we note that in the case of depression Münsterberg found a negative error for both extension and contraction and in excitement and joy a positive error for both types of movements—exactly the results of Dumas. The second confirmation of Münsterberg comes from an experiment by H. H. Remmers and L. A. Thompson, Jr., in which 84 observers were made to draw forty lines, half while thinking of very pleasant past experiences, the other half while thinking of very unpleasant ones. [53] The observers were instructed to draw the lines free-hand, and to make them 2 to 5 inches long. Computation of the average lengths of line under the two conditions showed that the two average lengths were significantly different (from the statistical point of view) and that the average length for pleasant experiences was greater than the average length for unpleasant ones (avg. for pleasant, 83.481 mm.; avg. for unpleasant, 80.904 mm.). The investigators consider these results to substantiate the view that there is a positive relationship between pleasantness and motor activity. And in a sense, they do so. It seems to me, however, that they may be considered more appropriately to substantiate Münsterberg's contention that pleasantness increases muscular extension, while unpleasantness decreases

it. Free-hand drawing of a line involves for the great majority of observers a movement of extension, and consequently the results above may be interpreted as indicating
differences in the relations of pleasantness and unpleasantness to extension of voluntary muscles. As there is some
doubt, in view of Münsterberg's own results, whether pleasantness would increase motor activity more than unpleasantness when this activity is contraction, it seems to me that
the conclusions of Remmers and Thompson involve excessive generalization and that it is wiser to interpret the results in a more modest fashion as a partial confirmation of
Münsterberg's findings. A third experiment supporting
Münsterberg, finally, is that of H. E. Burtt and W. W.
Tuttle on the relation of hedonic tone to the patellar reflex. These investigators measured the knee jerks of subjects during word reaction experiments in which 120 stimulus-words were grouped in such a fashion that five supposedly indifferent stimulus-words were followed by five
supposedly unpleasant stimulus-words, these in turn by five
supposedly pleasant stimulus-words, and these in turn by
five supposedly indifferent stimulus-words, etc.[54] From their
results, the investigators conclude as follows: "There is a
depression of the reflex on the average for unpleasant stimulus-words amounting to 16%. There are slight and less consistent indications of a similar depression for pleasant stimulus-words."[55] The slight indication of depression for pleasant stimulus-words obviously takes much force from these
results. The depression with unpleasant stimulus-words,
however, is entirely what one would expect if Münsterberg's
results could be extended to involuntary movements, for the
patellar reflex is evidently a movement of extension. As
far as available data are concerned, then, we must conclude
that there is indeed for voluntary movements, and probably
also for involuntary ones, a relation between hedonic tone
and type of response such that pleasantness is accompanied
by excess of extension, unpleasantness by excess of flexion.
Very different from Münsterberg's work in method, but
closely related in purpose, is an experiment by Young pub-

lished in 1921.[56] Instead of using the method of expression, Young studied the relation of hedonic tone to types of movement by having his observers report motor experiences accompanying pleasant and unpleasant stimuli. Each observer—there were seven in all, five men and two women —was seated in a morris chair, with eyes closed. His instructions were as follows: "In this experiment, be passive and receptive. Let the experimental situation have its full normal effect upon you. Report all muscular tendencies and organic sensations in any way related to the affective reaction. Report whether the experience was pleasant, unpleasant, or indifferent; and indicate the intensity of the feeling (using, for example, such terms as 'very weak,' 'weak,' 'moderate,' 'strong,' 'very strong.')." [57] As stimuli, Young used a large variety of smells, tastes, touches and sounds, each presented singly. The results showed in the first place that pleasantness and unpleasantness were frequently reported without organic or kinaesthetic accompaniments, although there was a marked correlation between unpleasantness and muscular strain (tension) and between pleasantness and relaxation. In 28 reports, strain was associated with unpleasantness; in only three was it associated with pleasantness. In 31 reports, muscular relaxation was associated with pleasantness; in none with unpleasantness. The results showed further that the average number of organic-kinaesthetic processes mentioned in a report was greater for unpleasantness than for pleasantness of the same intensity; and that this number was less for indifference than for any intensity of either pleasantness or unpleasantness. With respect to this last fact it was further found that if strain and relaxation were omitted from the count the average number of organic-kinaesthetic processes mentioned in a report was the same for pleasantness as for indifference, while for unpleasantness it remained distinctly greater. Young further studied his reports with a view to determining the relation between hedonic tone and seeking and avoiding movements. He found that unpleasantness was indeed associated in a large number of cases—though not by any means always—with tendencies "to react away," "to put the stimulus object away from oneself or to prevent its action," "to inhibit or resist the normal response (tension)," and to experience "bodily twitches, shocks, waves of sensation, and other reverberative reflexes." [58] Pleasantness, however, was found to be associated but very seldom with seeking movements, and then only with deliberate ones, not reflex-like ones such as those accompanying unpleasantness. From these results, Young draws the following conclusions: " . . . There is no organic-kinaesthetic *sine qua non* of affection. . . . However a number of tendencies toward correlation can be made out, and of these the most probable is that between muscular strain and U and muscular relaxation and P. U is associated with a positive bodily response which becomes more intense and widespread as the feeling becomes stronger, while with P the bodily response is relatively slight. When one reacts away from the stimulus-object, or puts it away from oneself, or resists it (strain), or when bodily reverberations are present, U is apt to be felt. P, on the other hand, so far as our data go, is organically-kinaesthetically negative. P is felt when one relaxes, or simply 'does nothing'; there are no reflex responses to the stimulus-object and no bodily 'reverberations.' " [59]

One of these conclusions, that stating that the typical involuntary reaction to pleasantness is a relaxation and not a seeking movement, is strikingly at variance with psychological tradition. This fact, together with the mention by Young himself that his results might be peculiar to the special conditions of his experiment, led G. H. Corwin to carry out a further experiment upon the involuntary responses associated with pleasantness.[60] Instead of placing his observers in a morris chair and instructing them to be passive, Corwin sought to create a situation in which they would have to seek if they desired to retain a pleasant experience, and gave them instructions under which they might move without disobeying the instructions. Corwin used olfactory, cutaneous and auditory stimuli. In the case of the olfactory stimuli, the observer was made to sit in an ordinary chair and the stimulus, first placed directly under the observer's nose, was made to recede from him at the rate of 1.7 mm. per second; with the cutaneous stimuli, the various stimulus-objects were moved slowly across the observer's forehead or nose; in the case of auditory stimuli, finally, the free end of a tube conducting the sound to the observer from another room was gradually moved away from the observer. The instructions made no mention of passivity but required merely a report on the quality and intensity of the feeling experienced and on all muscular tendencies and organic sensations in any way related to the affective reaction. The results of this experiment were very different from those of Young's. Definitely seeking or maintaining reactions to pleasant stimulation were found in 89.3% of the total number of pleasant cases. In 55.7% of the total number of pleasant cases the observers reported definite movement or tendencies to move, while in 66.6% of the cases they reported secondary reactions—e.g. changes in breathing and expansion—characteristic of pursuit or desire to maintain the experience. Furthermore, these results were verified by graphic records of movements of the head made in the experiments involving olfactory stimuli. Corwin concluded that Young's results were determined by the particular situation in which he placed his observers. He wrote: "There is no doubt that the most natural response to U is a movement of withdrawal. The direct response of the organism to P is . . . either relaxation *with a certain degree of expansion,* if the stimulus is weak or stationary; or, if the stimulus is intense, and the source of the P is withdrawn, a definite activity of pursuit or of tendencies to pursuit." [61]

Corwin's article failed to convince Young that his results were entirely dependent upon his experimental setting. He felt in particular that the pursuit-movements found by Corwin might not be genuine expressions of pleasant feelings. He consequently undertook a further investigation of the problem with a view to answering the question: "Is pursuit, as a matter of fact, correlated with pleasant feeling and avoidance with unpleasant feeling?" [62] Young's procedure involved throughout both an introspective and an objective check upon the movements correlated with the hedonic experience. With respect to the objective check, Young attached one end of a tape to the observer's head and the other to a Porter lever equipped with a straw pointer which indicated movements by its position with reference to a radial scale. With respect to the introspective check, the observers—two in number—were given instructions practically identical with those used by Corwin, making no mention of passivity and requiring a report on the quality and intensity of the feeling experienced and on all muscular tendencies and organic sensations related to the hedonic reaction. The stimuli were olfactory substances contained in bottles. Each bottle was placed 1 cm. below the observer's nose, and the observer was allowed to take two and, rarely, three full inhalations. The bottle was not withdrawn, in order not to suggest movement to the observer. On the other hand, the bottle being 1 cm. below the O's nose, there was opportunity for both seeking and avoiding movements. The results showed a marked correlation between pleasantness and forward movements of the head and between unpleasantness and backward movements. Out of 52 cases of pleasantness, 35 involved forward movement of the head; out of 49 cases of unpleasantness, 34 involved backward movement of the head; out of 20 cases of indifference, 10 involved no appreciable head movement. From these results, Young draws the preliminary conclusions that "There is probably a tendency for forward movements to occur when S reports pleasantness, and also a tendency for backward movements to be associated with unpleasantness." [63] Examination of the introspective reports, however, showed a number of cases in which forward movements of the head were seemingly associated not with pleasantness, but with olfactory attention to weak stimuli. Young consequently carried out another experiment to determine objectively the relation between attention and seeking movements. In this second experiment, hedonic tone was eliminated by the use of a normally indifferent stimulus, the ticking of a watch. Young recorded the lateral head movements of the two observers previously instructed to attend to the sound as the watch was gradually moved away from them. He found in every case definite movements towards the stimulus, and these movements were of the same order of magnitude as those found in the olfactory experiment involving hedonic tone. These results led him to doubt whether the forward movements which occurred in the first experiment, when the observer reported pleasantness, were to be considered as expressions of pleasantness. He wrote: "Now if pleasant feeling is normally associated with attentive response and unpleasant feeling is accompanied by inhibition of the normal reaction, or by avoidance, or by some other response which may be called inattentive, then attentional pursuit should correlate in the long run, with P, and its absence or opposite with U. It is extremely doubtful whether the pursuit movements observed in the present experiment express anything more than sensory attention. The actual extent of the movement of S's head is very slight—usually less than .5 cm., and never more than 2 cm. at the very most. Certainly such movements cannot be interpreted directly and unequivocally as expressions of pleasant feeling." [64] Young concludes his article with a general discussion of the relation between hedonic tone and seeking and avoiding movements. Corwin's experiment, he agrees, shows that pleasantness may be correlated with what may be interpreted as seeking movements. His own experiments, however, indicate that this correlation occurs only under special conditions, when there is an incentive to such movement due to withdrawal or weakness of the stimulus and when the stimulus is normally pleasant. Furthermore, every-day experience furnishes innumerable cases in which this correlation does not hold. Thus when seated in a chair facing a source of music determining a pleasant experience, one usually settles back in the chair—a withdrawal move-

ment. Again, a drowning rat "seeks" air—but the experience correlated with these seeking movements is surely
not pleasant. With respect to unpleasantness, Young considers his own earlier experiment (1921) as evidence that
unpleasantness frequently correlates with what may be interpreted as avoidance movements. Here again, however,
the correlation is by no means invariable. Consider the
play of courtship, which may be assumed to be pleasant.
It is generally considered to involve pursuit by the male
but avoidance by the female. Again, when one puppy runs
away from another in play, this avoidance is surely not
unpleasant. *What may be considered as avoidance movements, then, although frequently correlated with unpleasantness, are by no means always so correlated.* Young goes a
step further—and a long one—by adding that "seeking"
and "avoiding" are teleological terms which refer not so
much to different forms of behaviour as to different inter-
pretations of behaviour. "One can easily read into the same
response either the purpose of 'seeking' or the purpose of
'avoiding.' "[65] This circumstance makes the use of these
terms equivocal, and consequently—for the present at least
—undesirable.

So far I have dealt only with experiments carried out
with the express intention of studying the relation of hedonic
tone to locomotor responses. I now turn to a series of
experiments whose purpose was somewhat different, but
whose results are very rich in suggestions concerning this
relation. As was pointed out in Chapter 3, Nafe in 1924
published an experiment in which the observers identified
pleasantness with bright pressure and unpleasantness with
dull pressure.[66] Young repeated the experiment, but secured identification only in the case of one of three observers, and that one a previous observer of Nafe.[67] He concluded that Nafe's results were due to a particular "set"
of the observers. As Nafe had maintained that reports of
bright and dull pressure could only be secured with a specific
attentive set, the issue seemed to have reached an impasse.
W. A. Hunt, however, by comparing hedonic judgments

elicited by a set of stimuli on one occasion with judgments
of the brightness or dullness of the pressure experiences
occasioned by these stimuli on another occasion, was able
to confirm in the main the results of Nafe without opening
himself to the criticisms of Young.[68] He found that although no hint had been given the observers about the relation of hedonic tone to pressures, the correlation between
the pleasantness-unpleasantness ascribed to the stimuli on
one occasion and the brightness-dullness of the pressures
elicited by the stimuli on another occasion was extremely
high. Although these results do not prove conclusively a
relation between hedonic tone and muscular responses, they
very strongly suggest such a relationship. It is hard to
understand how pressures could originate without some
form of muscular response, and differences in pressures presumably indicate differences in muscular responses.

But are these differences in muscular responses differences of degree or differences of type? It is too early to
answer this question with confidence, but the results of a further experiment of Hunt point definitely to the latter alternative. The work of Nafe,[69] and later that of Horiguchi,[70]
showed that bright pressures were frequently localized in
the neck and chest, while dull pressures were frequently
localized in the abdomen. Hunt had a group of observers
judge on one occasion the hedonic tone of a set of Milton-
Bradley colors, and on another occasion the position of the
bright or dull pressures elicited by these stimuli on a scale
representing the vertical axis of the body.[71] He then compared the position of pressures elicited by stimuli judged
pleasant with that of pressures elicited by stimuli judged
unpleasant. For six out of seven observers (and for the
seventh, after a certain amount of training in introspection)
the average position of the pressures elicited by the pleasant
stimuli was definitely above that of the pressures elicited
by the unpleasant stimuli. Clearly, these results make it
very likely that the responses corresponding to pleasantness
are different in localization—and thus in type—from those
corresponding to unpleasantness, and not merely different

in degree. It is to be hoped that this promising line of research will be continued, and that the responses involved will thus be defined with greater specificity. An obvious step in this direction would be to localize the bright and dull pressures in a transverse plane. In the meantime, however, we may conclude tentatively from the work of Nafe and Hunt that pleasantness and unpleasantness are accompanied by different types of responses within the trunk—presumably of the postural muscles—the responses corresponding to pleasantness being more in the chest, those corresponding to unpleasantness more in the abdomen.

The data on the relation of hedonic tone to type of locomotor response have been sufficiently numerous to require some form of summary. First, we have the results of Münsterberg and of three subsequent investigators indicating that pleasantness is accompanied by excess of extension, unpleasantness by excess of flexion—at least in the case of voluntary movements. Second, we have the results of Young and Corwin indicating that pleasantness and unpleasantness very frequently, though not invariably, have organic or kinaesthetic accompaniments; that under instructions to remain passive pleasantness usually correlates with relaxation, unpleasantness with tension; and that in a situation allowing movements of seeking and avoidance pleasantness very generally correlates with seeking, unpleasantness with avoidance. Third, we have the results of Nafe and Hunt, indicating that pleasantness and unpleasantness are accompanied by different types of muscular responses within the trunk, those accompanying pleasantness being more in the chest, those accompanying unpleasantness more in the abdomen.

What is the bearing of these facts upon the specific problem of hedonism of the present? Clearly a narrow interpretation of the doctrine is wholly out of the question, for such an interpretation would require complete concomitance of pleasantness with avoiding. Is this also true, however, of a broader interpretation, according to which hedonic tone would indeed be a determinant of conduct, but not the sole determinant? In the latter case we should certainly not expect the complete concomitance mentioned above, because of the intervention of other contrary determinants. We should expect merely that for any constant set of conditions there would be more seeking, or less avoidance, with pleasant stimuli than with unpleasant ones. Whether or not this be so is hard to judge from the experiments described above, for all were carried out with reference only to hedonism in the narrow sense. The results of Young, involving a correlation between relaxation and pleasantness under instructions to remain passive, do indeed suggest that even when interpreted broadly hedonism of the present is not a valid doctrine. They suggest rather that the co-variation which is observed under other conditions between hedonic tone and direction of movement is the manifestation merely of an indirect relationship such as that which appears to obtain between needs and hedonic tone. They constitute no more than suggestions, however, and it is to be hoped that they will soon be supplemented by further data.

What, now, is the bearing of the facts summarized above on the general problem of the relation of hedonic tone to type of response? The facts are so heterogeneous that before drawing a general conclusion from them we should obviously like to know their interconnections. Thus we should like to know whether pleasantness and unpleasantness are accompanied respectively by excess extension of the torso (by the so-called anti-gravity musculature) and by excess flexion of the torso and, if so, whether these accompaniments are judged introspectively to involve bright and dull pressures, respectively. We should also like to know whether relaxation and seeking, on the one hand, and tension and avoidance, on the other, are accompanied respectively by flexion and extension of the torso and whether they are judged introspectively to involve respectively bright and dull pressures. It is to be hoped that both of these questions will soon be subjected to experimental investigation. In the meantime, two alternatives present themselves. We may be positivistic and simply suspend judgment. On the other hand, we may be speculative and conclude—very tentatively, naturally—that pleasantness correlates with exaggeration of the contraction of the skeletal muscles involved in holding the body upright, unpleasantness with exaggeration of the contraction of the abdominal muscles involved in flexing the torso. I myself prefer the latter alternative because I believe that the questions stated above are more likely to be investigated experimentally if they constitute tests of a particular view, and because suspension of judgment is apt to cause disregard of the excellent data already available concerning the relation of hedonic tone to type of locomotor response.

FOOTNOTES AND REFERENCES

[1] W. WUNDT. Bemerkungen zur Theorie der Gefühle, *Philos. Stud.,* 15, 1899, 163.

[2] MAX BRAHN. Experimentelle Beiträge zur Gefühlslehre, I. Theil. Die Richtungen des Gefühls, *Philos. Stud.,* 18, 1901, 127.

[3] W. WUNDT. Grundzüge der physiologischen Psychologie, 5th Edit., Vol. II, 1902, 298.

[4] *Cf.* W. GENT. Volumpulscurven bei Gefühlen und Affekten,*Philos. Stud.,* 18, 1903, 715.

[5] *Cf.* E. MEUMANN and P. ZONEFF. Ueber Begleiterscheinungen Psychischer Vorgänge in Atem und Puls, *Philos. Stud.,* 18, 1903, 1.

[6] N. ALECHSIEFF. Die Grundformen der Gefühle, *Psychol. Stud.,* 3, 1907, 156.

[7] J. F. SHEPHARD. Organic Changes and Feeling, *Amer. J. Psychol.,* 17, 1906, 557-558.

[8] P. ZONEFF and E. MEUMANN. Ueber die Begleiterscheinungen Psychischer Vorgänge in Atem und Puls, *Philos. Stud.,* 18, 1901.

[9] E. LESCHKE. Die Ergebnisse und die Fehlerquellen der bisherigen Untersuchungen über die Körperlichen Begleiterscheinungen Seelischer Vorgänge, *Arch. f. d. ges. Psychol.,* 31, 1914, 30-31.

[10] A. LEHMANN. Hauptgesetze des Menschlichen Gefühlslebens, Leipzig, 1914, 59-73. *Cf.* for criticism of Lehmann's earlier utterances on the subject R. LAGERBORG, Das Gefühlsproblem, Leipzig, 1905, 56-68.

[11] W. B. CANNON. The James-Lange Theory of Emotion: a Critical Examination and an Alternative Theory, *Amer. J. Psychol.,* 39, 1927, 112.

[12] E. B. NEWMAN, F. T. PERKINS and R. H. WHEELER. Cannon's Theory of Emotion: a Critique, *Pschol. Rev.,* 37, 1930, 311.

[13] *Cf.* for an excellent review of the literature concerning the psychogalvanic reflex: C. LANDIS and H. N. DeWICK, The Electrical Phenomena of the Skin (Psycho-galvanic Reflex), *Psychol. Bullet.,* 26, 1929, 64-119.

[14] D. WECHSLER. The Measurement of Emotional Reactions, *Arch of Psychol.*, 12, 1925 (No. 76).

[15] *Ibid.*, 20-21.

[16] *Ibid.*, 112.

[17] *Ibid.*, 115.

[18] *Ibid.*, 116-117.

[19] *Ibid.*, 166.

[20] H. C. SYZ. Observations on the Unreliability of Subjective Reports of Emotional Reactions, *Brit. J. Psychol.*, 17,, 1926, 119-125.

[21] *Ibid.*, 121.

[22] *Cf.* F. AVELING. *Proc. of the VIII Internat. Congress of Psychol.*, Groningen, 1927, 232; R. J. Bartlett, *Brit. J. Psychol.*, 18, 1927-28, 30.

[23] *Cf.* C. LANDIS. The Expression of Emotion, in The Foundations of Experimental Psychology (C. Murchison, editor), Worcester, 1929, 515.

[24] A. GREGOR. Die Hautelektrischen Erscheinungen in Ihren Beziehungen zu Bewusstseinsprozessen, *Arch. f. d. ges. Psychol.*, 27, 1913, 247.

[25] W. B. CANNON. Bodily Changes in Pain, Hunger, Fear and Rage, 2nd Edit., N. Y., 1929, 341-345.

[26] C. SHERRINGTON. Integrative Action of the Nervous System, N. Y., 1906, 231.

[27] O. KÜLPE. Outline of Psychology, transl. by E. B. Titchener, New York, 1895, 245.

[28] E. B. TITCHENER. Experimental Psychology, Vol. I, Part II, New York, 1901, 164-165.

[29] CH. FÉRÉ. Contribution à la physiologie de l' esthétique, *C. R.* de la *Soc. de Biol.*, 37, 1885, 348-351. *Cf.* also *ibid.*, pp. 270-273, 629-632.

[30] A. ERNST. Dynamographisch-plethysmographische Untersuchungen, über die Einwirkungen von Unlustgefühlen auf äussere Willenshandlungen, *Arch. f. d. ges. Psychol.*, 57, 1926, 445.

[31] CH. FÉRÉ. Sensation et Mouvement, *C. R. de la Soc. de Biol.*, 37, 1885, 271.

[32] G. DUMAS. La Tristesse et la Joie, Paris, 1900, 343.

[33] LANGE. Les Emotions, Paris, 1895, 46-47. Quoted from Dumas, *Op cit.*, 343.

[34] U. MOSSO. Influence des Emotions sur la Force des Muscles, *Arch. Ital. de Biol.*, 50, 1908, 292.

[35] *Ibid.*, 294.

[36] *Ibid.*, 5.

[37] G. DUMAS. *Op. cit.*, 332.

[38] *Ibid.*, 332.

[39] U. MOSSO. *Loc. cit.*, 5 ff.

[40] L. H. ZIEGLER and B. S. LEVINE. The Influence of Emotional Reactions on Basal Metabolism, *Am. J. Med. Sci.*, 169, 1925, 68-76.

[41] M. F. WASHBURN. Feeling and Emotion, *Psychol. Bullet.*, 24 1927, 579.

[42] *Cf.* W. B. CANNON. Bodily Changes in Pain, Hunger, Fear and Rage, 2nd Edit., N. Y., 1929, 193-219. *Cf.* also J. F. FULTON, Muscular Contraction and the Reflex Control of Movement, Baltimore, 1926, 409.

[43] CH. FÉRÉ. *C. R. de la Soc. de Biol*, 37, 1885, 271.

[44] G. STORRING. Experimentelle Beiträge zur Lehre vom Gefühl, *Arch. f. d. ges. Psychol.*, 6, 1906, 316 ff.

[45] H. ROSE. Der Einfluss der Unlustgefühle auf den Motorischen Effekt der Willenshandlungen, *Arch. f. d. ges. Psychol.*, 28, 1913, 179.

[46] A. ERNST. *Arch. f. d. ges. Psychol.*, 57, 1926, 480.

[47] L. T. TROLAND. The Fundamentals of Human Motivation, New York, 1928, 276 ff.

[48] K. LEWIN. Environmental Forces in Child Behaviour and Development, in Handbook of Child Psychology, C. Murchison, editor, Worcester, Mass., 1931, 94-127.

[49] *Ibid.*, 101-102.

[50] K. LEWIN. Die Psychologische Situation bei Lohn und Strafe, Leipzig, 1931, 9. Two passages with a like implication will be found on page 112 of the chapter by Lewin in C. Murchison's Hand-book of Child Psychology, Worcester, Mass., 1931.

[51] H. MÜNSTERBERG. Die Psychophysische Grundlage der Gefühle, *International Congress of Experimental Psychology*, 2nd Session, London, 1892, 132. We are not concerned here with the theory of hedonic tone, but I cannot refrain from stating that Münsterberg concludes from these observations to the theory that "die psychophysische Wirkung der reflektorisch ausgelösten Streckungen oder Beugungen ist eben das, was wir Lust oder Unlust nennen." (133.)

[52] G. DUMAS. La Tristesse et la Joie, Paris, 1900, 334-335 and 344.

[53] H. H. REMMERS and L. A. THOMPSON, JR., *J. of Applied Psychol.*, 9, 1925, 417. The authors point out that this is essentially the experiment described on pp. 146 ff. of "An Elementary Course in Laboratory Psychology" by H. S. LANGFELD and F. H. ALLPORT.

[54] H. E. BURTT and W. W. TUTTLE. The Patellar Tendon Reflex and Affective Tone, *Amer. J. Psychol.*, 36, 1925, 553-561.

[55] *Ibid.*, 561.

[56] P. T. YOUNG. Pleasantness and Unpleasantness in Relation to Organic Response, *Amer. J. Psychol.*, 32, 1921, 38-53.

[57] *Ibid.*, 39.

[58] *Ibid.*, 51.

[59] *Ibid.*, 52-53.

[60] C. H. CORWIN. The Involuntary Response to Pleasantness, *Amer. J. Psychol.*, 32, 1921, 563-570.

[61] *Ibid.*, 570.

[62] P. T. YOUNG. Movements of Pursuit and Avoidance as Expressions of Simple Feelings, *Amer. J. Psychol.*, 33, 1922, 512.

[63] *Ibid.*, 516.

[64] *Ibid.*, 519.

[65] *Ibid.*, 523.

[66] J. P. NAFE. *Amer. J. Psychol.*, 35, 1924, 507.

[67] P. T. YOUNG. *Amer. J. Psychol.*, 38, 1927, 175.

[68] W. A. HUNT. *Amer. J. Psychol.*, 43, 1931, 87.

[69] J. P. NAFE. The Sense of Feeling, in The Foundations of Experimental Psychology (edited by C. Murchison), Worcester, Mass., 1929, 411.

[70] *Cf.* L. B. HOISINGTON. Pleasantness and Unpleasantness as Modes of Bodily Experience, Wittenberg Symposium on the Feelings and Emotions, Worcester, 1928, 237-240.

[71] W. A. HUNT. The Pressure Correlates of Hedonic Tone, Thesis, Harvard University, 1931, 29-42.

Chapter IX

Memory in Relation to Hedonic Tone

When one first considers the relation of memory to hedonic tone, one cannot but feel that a valid formulation of the relation is beyond the ability of modern psychology. Certain psychologists accept in its *strictest sense* the doctrine which L. T. Troland calls *hedonism of the past*,[1] according to which pleasantness enhances learning while unpleasantness diminishes it. McDougall, for instance, writes: ". . . On recurrence of a situation of the kind in which we have striven successfully before, our tendency to strive again in the same way is stronger, the tendency seems to be confirmed by the previous experience of success, and this confirmation of the tendency may fairly be regarded as a consequence or result of the pleasure experienced on the former occasion. Conversely, pain, arising during striving, tends to divert the striving to other directions, and on renewal of the situation in which we have striven unsuccessfully and (in consequence) painfully, our tendency to strive again in the same way is weakened or abolished or diverted to some new direction; these weakenings and diversions of the impulse seem to be the effects or consequences of the pain experienced on the foregoing occasion." [2] Other psychologists, like Troland and Hunter, accept a modified form of hedonism of the past according to which learning is influenced, not by hedonic tone itself, but by its neutral correlate. Hunter writes: "In our own mind there is every reason to believe that frequency, recency and the *neural processes underlying pleasure* are the important factors (in learning). . . . A child is given disagreeable medicine and thereafter refuses it. I make a mistake in my English-French vocabulary. Since it is unpleasant I do not make it *again,* thereby eliminating that random movement; and if

354

the elimination is thoroughgoing, I do not even have an image of the mistake made. But how can pleasantness and unpleasantness, which are conscious processes, influence chemical or electrical processes in the synapses? This has been the universal objection which is well founded. There can, however, be little doubt that something connected with these conscious states affects learning, that in some way the neural processes underlying pleasure facilitate those other neural processes contiguous to them. We would, therefore, agree with Thorndike, but speak more objectively, and not imply that consciousness affects the body. On the other hand, we would explicitly recognize the effect of pleasure's neural basis rather than . . . deny any effect." [3] Yet others, finally, like Carr, Cason and Watson, deny completely the validity of hedonism of the past. Witness Watson's scornful statement that most psychologists "believe habit formation is implanted by kind fairies. For example, Thorndike speaks of pleasure stamping out the unsuccessful movement." [4] With such marked differences of opinion, is it not a foregone conclusion that the experimental data concerning the relation of hedonic tone to memory are hopelessly equivocal?

The more one thinks the problem over, the more one wonders whether such pessimism is warranted. What is really the difference between the hedonisms of the past of McDougall and Hunter? Acceptance or rejection of interactionism, a metaphysical doctrine. Disregarding this difference, both forms of hedonism may be formulated in the following single proposition: Given two cases of learning differing only in involving different degrees of hedonic tone, the effectiveness of the learning will be greater in the case involving the greater pleasantness. Again, what is Watson's position? Not so much that hedonism of the past is false as that it involves one of the "subjective" concepts which he considers to be unserviceable in psychology. True, Watson would never agree to McDougall's interactionism. When one reads his admission, however, that Behaviourism is essentially a methodological approach—the best,

naturally, but, by implication, not the only one possible—
one cannot help feeling that he might well agree with the
foregoing formulation of the common, non-metaphysical
residuum of the hedonisms of McDougall and Hunter, provided only that he were not obliged to include it in his own
system of psychology.[5] To one who disregards metaphysical
issues,[6] then, the modern divergence of opinion concerning
hedonism of the past is no proof whatever that the data
relating memory to hedonic tone are incapable of satisfactory interpretation.

A word, now, concerning form of presentation. There
is no question but that results in psychology are very much
a function of method. Elimination of methodological factors in the interpretation of results is bound to be hazard-
ous when dealing with a relationship so little known as that
between memory and hedonic tone. Rather than jeopardize
the validity of my exposition, I shall consequently forego a
systematic classification of the data, which would involve
at least some degree of interpretation, and shall present
them under purely methodological headings. In particular,
I shall deal quite separately with the experiments involving
the relation of memory to hedonic tone occurring *during*
the learning of a task and with those involving the relation
of memory to hedonic tone occurring *after* the learning
task (sometimes called experiments on retroactive affective
inhibition).[7]

Memory in Relation to Hedonic Tone During Learning

**Proportion of Pleasant and Unpleasant Events in
Free Recall.**—A first group of facts relates to the proportion, among memories recalled by observers under hedonically unselective instructions, of events believed to have been
pleasant to events believed to have been unpleasant. The
world at large unquestionably believes that pleasant events
are remembered better than unpleasant ones. Colgrove,[8] in
a questionnaire sent to a large group of adults, included the

question: "Which do you remember better, pleasant or unpleasant experiences?" The replies indicated that more pleasant impressions were remembered than unpleasant ones. A similar question, put by Kowalewski to 270 boys and girls, gave the same results.[9]

Such opinions are interesting, but hardly convincing. Appreciating this, Kowalewski early sought to supplement his first inquiry by an experimental investigation.[10] On the day following a public holiday, he had a group of school children write down during ten minutes their pleasant experiences on the preceding day, and then during a similar time-interval their unpleasant experiences. The same procedure was repeated ten days later. The results showed a marked preponderance of what Kowalewski called "memory-optimists," i. e., individuals in whose records pleasant experiences were numerically predominant over unpleasant ones. Similar results were secured by a somewhat different procedure in an experiment published in 1914 by Peters and Nemecek.[11] In this experiment the observers were required to react to a stimulus word with the memory of some previous personal experience. After each successful recall the observers were asked a number of questions, including questions upon the original hedonic tone of the recalled experience. The results of this experiment, confirming those of a previous similar experiment published by Peters alone,[12] showed that of the hedonically toned experiences which were recalled, more were pleasant than unpleasant.

At first sight these experiments appear to prove that memory for pleasant events is better than that for unpleasant ones. As far back as 1911, however, E. N. Henderson pointed out that such need not be the case.[13] In the preceding year, Hollingworth had written an essay upon "The oblivescence of the disagreeable," in which he had contended that "The disagreeable, once lived through, oblivesces; the agreeable becomes enriched, magnified and embellished with tone and color that it did not originally possess." [14] Henderson, doubtful of the validity of this proposition, determined to put the matter to an experimental test.

His procedure was much the same as had been that of Kowalewski, although he seems to have been unfamiliar with the latter's work. Ten observers were asked to recall incidents from their life, and 100 such incidents were recorded in the case of each observer. The observers were then asked to grade each of their memories according to whether they represented incidents which, when they happened, were very agreeable, indifferent, moderately disagreeable, or very disagreeable. "The thousand incidents recalled were divided as follows: Very agreeable, 28.3 per cent; agreeable, 26.8 per cent; indifferent, 11.8 per cent; disagreeable, 12.6 per cent; very disagreeable, 20.5 per cent. Classifying the experiences into the three cases of agreeable, indifferent and disagreeable, we get:

"Agreeable, 55.1 per cent. Average deviation, 6.7 per cent.
Indifferent, 11.8 per cent. Average deviation, 4.6 per cent.
Disagreeable, 33.1 per cent. Average deviation, 4.7 per cent." [15]

Henderson does not think, however, that these results indicate a greater oblivescence of the disagreeable, for he feels "It is quite likely that in the lives of most of us the agreeable incidents far outnumber the disagreeable ones." [16]

Henderson's position has since turned out to be well founded. In repeating Kowalewski's experiments on a larger scale with a somewhat different point of view, Wohlgemuth completely verified the former's results. [17] He found that in the case of a very large number of children who, after a half-term holiday, were made to write down separately as many as possible of their pleasant and unpleasant experiences during the holiday, the total number of pleasant experiences recorded was 6735, while the total number of unpleasant ones was only 3491. [18] In commenting upon these results, Wohlgemuth points out, as had Henderson, that the mere preponderance of pleasant memories over unpleasant ones does not prove that pleasant experiences are better remembered than unpleasant ones, unless it be certain that the frequency of occurrence of both types of events was the same. Instead, however, of confining himself, as had Henderson, to a statement that such probably is not the case, Wohlgemuth definitely proves that such is not the case by invoking the experimental work of J. C. Flügel. In an attempt to determine experimentally the relative proportion of pleasantness and unpleasantness encountered in human life, Flügel[19] had nine observers record in notebooks their hedonic experiences during the waking hours of each of thirty days. The observers were instructed to record their feelings as frequently as possible in order to avoid memory distortion, and to state in each case the duration of the feelings and their quality and intensity. Quality and intensity were to be stated in terms of a scale of seven steps, running from 3 (maximal pleasantness ever experienced by the observer) through O (indifference) to — 3 (maximal unpleasantness ever experienced by the observer). From the data thus secured, there were computed in the case of each observer the percentages of waking time during which there were experienced feelings of the seven types indicated by the scale. The results of this computation showed in the case of each observer that the sum of the percentages for pleasant feelings was greater than that for unpleasant ones. The averages of these percentages for all observers are given in the table below:

TABLE LXII

	Pleasantness			Indiff.	Unpleasantness		
Degrees of Hedonic Tone ...	+ 3	+ 2	+ 1	0	— 1	— 2	— 3
Duration in per cent	1.1	10.4	38.6	27.8	17.5	4.2	0.4
		50.1				22.2	

These results, if generalized, indicate, according to Flügel, that ". . . Pleasure occupies a very considerably larger proportion of human life than does unpleasure." [20] But clearly, if this be so, it is to be expected that human experience will involve a greater number of pleasant experiences than unpleasant ones, and consequently that more pleasant experiences will be recalled than unpleasant ones, even though the "memory value" of these two classes of experiences be the same. From this in turn it follows that the general excess of pleasant memories over unpleasant ones—a fact which is proved conclusively by the results of Kowalewski and Wohlgemuth—in nowise implies that an event is more readily recalled if it be pleasant than if it be unpleasant.

Another set of data which show that the general predominance of pleasant memories cannot be interpreted as support for the doctrine of hedonism of the past are those derived from studies of temperamental influences. D. A. Laird[21] had sixty-two students in psychology write down the names of the first ten people they thought of, and then write down the names of ten people in order of likeableness. Averaging results for all observers, it was found that the most likeable persons were thought of spontaneously more than five times as often as the least likeable ones. When, however, the observers were fractionated into three groups, optimists, mixed and pessimists, according to ratings by themselves and by others, it was found that, although the optimists had thought spontaneously of the best-liked persons in 72% of the cases, and of the least-liked ones in only 15% of the cases, the pessimists had thought of the best-liked persons in only 27% of the cases, and of the least-liked in 45%. It would then seem that "memory optimism" holds only in the case of temperamental optimism, while in the case of pessimists, unpleasant memories preponderate. This fact, taken with Flügel's findings that pleasant experiences are in general more frequent than unpleasant ones, makes it impossible to draw from the unquestionable general preponderance of pleasant memories over unpleasant ones any conclusions whatever concerning "hedonism of the past."

Frequency of Recall of Pleasant and Unpleasant Events.—In the course of an extensive (but by no means intensive) investigation of the relation between memory and attitudes. W. D. Tait[22] sought to determine the relative proportion of pleasant and unpleasant words which could be recalled by observers after having heard them once. Tait used three types of lists consisting of twenty words each, one type involving supposedly pleasant words, another supposedly unpleasant words, a third supposedly indifferent words. After each list had been read to the observers once, the observers (eleven in number) were asked to report the words which they could remember.[23] Tait found that the average proportion of words remembered was for supposedly pleasant lists 10.5%, for supposedly unpleasant lists, 8.2%, and for supposedly indifferent lists, 6.2%. More recently, the problem has been investigated in a similar but far more thorough way by R. H. Thomson, with results wholly in accord with those of Tait.[24] In one experiment, Thomson had observers record in a diary for five days all pleasant and unpleasant experiences. Two weeks later, and again a month later, the observers were asked to recall those experiences. In another experiment, each observer was asked to make up two lists of twenty words each, the words in one list having very pleasant connotations; those in the other, very unpleasant ones. At the end of a month, the observers were asked to recall the lists. In a third experiment, observers were made to rate as pleasant or unpleasant each of 47 narrative poems read in connection with work in English. A month later, after reviewing the poems for a test, the observers were asked to write the titles of all the poems they could remember. A fourth and a fifth experiment consisted of repetitions of the first and second experiments described above with another and larger group of observers, except that the diary was kept for but a single day. In a sixth experiment, finally, the large group of observers was made to tabulate pleasant and unpleasant items from a current events magazine, and a month later required to recall the tabulated material. The results of all of these experiments are given in the table below, which summarizes a more complete table presented by

Thomson. N indicates number of observers, and $D/\sigma D$ indicates the ratio of the difference between the names given in the second and third columns of the table and the standard error of this difference.[25]

TABLE LXIII

Tests (Small group of Os)	N	Mean number of *pleasant* items recalled	Mean number of *unpleasant* items recalled	$D/\sigma D$
1. Diary records				
First recall	29	33.20	31.13	.48
Second recall	28	25.39	18.78	1.76
2. Word lists	27	37.92	23.55	4.10
3. Titles of poems ..	27	56.44	31.62	6.02
(Large group of Os)				
4. Diary records	101	32.05	16.21	7.04
5. Word lists	101	37.69	15.47	10.95
6. Current events ...	104	20.86	13.50	4.43

These results obviously confirm those of Tait. As Thomson writes: "Although not all of the tests showed significant differences between the recall of the pleasant and the unpleasant, all of the results point in the same direction —namely, to the more ready recall of the pleasant." [26] Furthermore, in six out of eight cases the differences are more than three times the standard error.

Strikingly out of harmony with the results of both Tait and Thomson are those secured by K. Gordon in an inquiry concerning the recollection of pleasant and unpleasant odors.[27] Gordon made her observers smell once of each of twenty bottles, ten of which contained olfactory substances, while ten were empty. As each bottle was smelled, Gordon announced a name. These names were for the ten odorous bottles the names of the corresponding odors. In the case of the ten empty bottles, each was given one of the ten names used for the odorous bottles. Thus the name "lemon" was pronounced both in conjunction with the smelling of the bottle containing oil of lemon and also in conjunction with the smelling of one of the empty bottles. The bottles were presented in two spatial series of ten bottles each. In the case of each series, the observers were instructed to smell the bottles one after the other, beginning at one end. They were further instructed to remember as many names as possible and the position of the corresponding bottles. At the close of each series, each observer was asked to "Give all the names you can and point to the bottles where they belong." In scoring, a credit was given for each name correctly located. No partial credits were given. After an observer had completed this first part of the experiment, the ten odorous bottles were placed before him and he was asked to arrange them in an hedonic series and to indicate in this series the rank where unpleasantness and pleasantness began.

From the data secured in the first part of the experiment there were calculated for each name the number of times that it had been correctly recalled in connection with an odorous bottle, and the number of times it had been recalled in connection with the empty bottle. The difference between the first and the second of these numbers was considered to be an index of the average memorial clue of the odor in question. From the data secured in the second part of the experiment there were computed the average hedonic ranks of the ten odors. The odors were then arranged in two series, in the one according to average memorial value, in the other according to average hedonic rank, and these series were compared. The correlation between the two series was found to be very slight. Lemon, for instance, first in the hedonic rank order, had a lower average memorial value than asafoetida, last in the hedonic series. The Spearman coefficient of correlation between the two series was indeed actually negative: — .07. Gordon concluded that ". . . Pleasant odors are not more likely to be recalled than the unpleasant. If any difference has been shown, it is in favor of the unpleasant, but we are inclined to doubt the validity of this difference. We must search for other factors than affective tone if we would understand why some impressions are recalled and others are not." [28]

At first sight it would seem that we have here three experiments upon the frequency of recall of pleasant and unpleasant events whose results are incompatible. But is this really the case? The title under which Miss Gordon published her experiment is indeed "The recollection of pleasant and unpleasant odors," but her results concern the recollection of the *names* of pleasant and unpleasant odors and of the *positions* of their containers. Furthermore, the psychological event in which was combined the name of an odor, the odor itself, and the position of the odor was of appreciable duration and not particularly unitary. Each such event was approximately as follows: The observer picked up a bottle from a series of bottles before him and unscrewed a metal cap which covered it. He then took "one good smell," during which the experimenter spoke the name of the odor. The observer finally screwed the top on and put the bottle back on the table. It seems much indeed to expect of hedonic tone that it should correlate not merely with ability to recall the odors themselves, but with the ability to recall names pronounced simultaneously with their presentation and positions which may have been perceived an appreciable time before their presentation. Consequently I feel that Gordon's results do not have any bearing upon the frequency of recall of pleasant and unpleasant events. The only experiments which do have such a bearing are those of Tait and Thomson, and both indicate that pleasant events are recalled more frequently than are unpleasant ones. This, then, must be our conclusion pending further experimental investigation.

Adequacy of Recall of Pleasant and Unpleasant Events.—In an experiment published in 1905, K. Gordon sought to determine whether "the pleasantness or unpleasantness of certain visual experiences has any influence on the exactitude of memory for those experiences." [29] Seven observers were shown a variety of colored and black and white figures from one to three seconds. Immediately after the presentation the observers were asked to give a detailed description of the figures and to state whether they were pleasant, indifferent or unpleasant. It was found that the number of items in the description did not vary significantly as between pleasant and unpleasant figures. Miss Gordon concluded that pleasantness and unpleasantness have no direct differential effect upon memory, i.e., that they do not have a differential effect upon associative and reproductive tendencies.

The same problem was dealt with incidentally by Crossland in an experiment directed towards a qualitative analysis of forgetting.[30] Various materials, mostly visual, were presented to observers for 30 seconds with instructions to learn them with a view to subsequent recall. The materials in each case bore a distinguishing caption. After intervals of time varying from 30 minutes to 300 days, the observers were asked to recall the material corresponding to a certain caption, and to express this recall orally, or orally and by drawing, or by drawing alone, depending upon the nature of the material. Crossland does not give any quantitative data with respect to the relation between hedonic tone and adequacy of recall, but he states that "There was no discoverable correlation between presence of affection in learning and accuracy and correctness of recall." [31] As these are to the best of my knowledge the only two experiments bearing upon the relation between the hedonic tone of an event and the adequacy of its subsequent recall, I conclude that there is no evidence of the dependence of the latter upon the former.

Frequency of Recognition of Pleasant and Unpleasant Events.—In the inquiry mentioned in the last but one section, Tait[32] also experimented upon the relation between hedonic tone and recognition. His observers were first shown a series of fifteen colors and asked to judge their hedonic value on a scale of seven degrees. Two or three alterations were then made in the series, and it was shown again in a different order to the observers, with the same instructions as previously. In this second case, however, the observers were asked after the exposure of each color if that color had been in the preceding series. Tait found that the average number of colors recognized was, in the case of pleasant colors, 63.4% ; in the case of unpleasant colors, 47.2%, and in the case of indifferent colors, 27.3%. In complete harmony with these results are those secured by A. Peters[33] upon the recognition of pictures. Peters presented to his observers portraits taken from illustrated periodicals. After intervals varying from a few minutes to 15 days, the same portraits were again shown to the observers. This time, however, they were mixed in with portraits not previously shown. At the second presentation the observers were instructed to state in the case of each picture whether it had been shown previously, and also to judge its affective value. Peters found that the percentages of portraits recognized were, in the case of the originally pleasant portraits, 75.6% ; in the case of the originally unpleasant portraits, 65.7%, and in the case of the originally indifferent ones, 64.4%.

Rate of Forgetting of Pleasant and Unpleasant Events.—In dealing above with Wohlgemuth's results, I mentioned that they were incidental to the main purpose of his investigation. This main purpose was to test the statement so often made by psychoanalysts that *unpleasant experiences are more easily forgotten than pleasant ones*— that they are "suppressed" or what not. Ten to fourteen days after the experiment mentioned above, Wohlgemuth gave the same children the same task over again. He found that of the 6735 pleasant experiences reported in the first experiment, 2700, or 40.1%, were omitted in the second experiment, and that of the 3491 unpleasant experiences reported on the first occasion, 1406, or 39.8%, were omitted on the second occasion. In view of the practical identity of these two percentages Wohlgemuth concludes: "There is no difference whatever between the two feeling tones, pleasure and unpleasure, in their influence upon memory." [34]

Diametrically opposed to these findings are those in a very similar experiment by H. Meltzer. On the day following a Christmas vacation, 132 students were asked to list all their experiences during the vacation, and to mark pleasant ones with a P, unpleasant ones with an U. Six weeks later the same procedure was repeated. "Of the 2231 experiences given on the first recall, 1092, or 48.97%, were forgotten at the end of six weeks. Of the total pleasant experiences given the first time, 593, or 42.06%, were forgotten, and of the total unpleasant, 499 experiences, or 59.53%, were forgotten." [35]

It is obviously difficult to reconcile the results of Wohlgemuth and Meltzer. The former used children, whereas the latter used adults, and it may consequently be that the relation between hedonic tone and rate of forgetting varies with age. For the time being, however, the only safe conclusion is that more evidence is needed before we are justified in making any formulation of the relationship.

Associative Learning in Relation to Hedonic Tone.—Little information is to be found dealing with the relation between hedonic tone and experimentally controlled associative learning, but this little fortunately is univocal in its implications. Some attention was given to this relationship by J. W. Harris[36] in a study of the associative power of odors. The experimental procedure in this study was to have observers form associations between odors and two-digit numbers. Among other results Harris found that "The affective qualities of the odors seem to have played a certain subordinate role in the fixing of the associations, some distinctly pleasant (and in a few instances some distinctly unpleasant) having formed especially prompt and lasting associations with their numbers, but our evidence on this matter is meagre." [37]

Further light on the relationship under discussion was secured by C. Fox[38] in an attempt to determine experimentally the relative values of two learning methods. Fox had twenty-four observers learn two sonnets, the one by a "mixed" method, the other by the "entire" method. In the case both of immediate recall and of delayed recall (seven days), the adequacy of the two methods measured in terms of number of promptings proved to be practically identical. When the subjects were asked, however, to state which of the two sonnets they preferred, it was found that, irrespective of method, the number of promptings necessary for the preferred sonnet was markedly less than for the less liked one. Fox concludes that ". . . Memory, as evinced both by immediate and delayed recall, is more efficient in those cases where there is a distinct subjective preference for what is learnt." [39]

Entirely in accord with these results are those of a study by E. B. Sullivan[40] of the effect of knowledge of previous success or failure upon memorizing series of non-sense syllables. The general procedure involved two steps. All observers were first made to learn series of non-sense syllables under uniform instructions. One or more days later they were made to learn similar series of non-sense syllables, having been told at the beginning of the experimental period either that they had made the best score of the group on the preceding occasion, or the worst. The results showed in general that "the time taken to learn a memory series is increased by the knowledge of failure in a previous performance" and that "the value for recall, measured by abbreviation of time taken to learn, is less in the case of the failure report and greater in the case of the success report." [41] Sullivan does not deal with the bearing of her experiment upon hedonism. This bearing, however, is easy to infer. After completing the second step of the experiment each observer was asked for an introspective report. Of these Sullivan writes: "A great variety of terms was used to characterize the experimental task and period. These, in most cases, are not descriptive introspective terms, but do give an indication of the subject's attitude for the period in question. They, therefore, are indications of the conscious accompaniments of the variations in responses noted. A list of some of the phrases and terms used shows the emotive nature of this process:

"Expected to do poorly, dislike of task, don't care about doing well, critical of self, confusion, all at sea, discouraged, disappointed, unpleasant, despair, annoyance, insecurity, odious, difficult, emotionally disturbed, anxious, dislike, impatient, hopeless, depressed, confused, irritation, limp, hot cheeks, tightness in throat, tendency to squirm, suspicious, angry, disgusted.

"Relief, interested, curiosity, happy, feeling of well being, contented, desire to do well, confidence, pleasurable, easy, satisfied, calm, excited, liked the exercise, sure of myself, full of zest, cheerful, attempt to get quickly, intention to do well, encouraged, collected, etc." [42]

Although Sullivan does not state so explicitly, the words in the first group above may, I think, be taken safely as descriptive of attitudes correlated with knowledge of previous failure, and those in the second group as referring to attitudes accompanying knowledge of previous success. But clearly the first group refers to predominantly unpleasant experiences, while the second refers to predominantly pleasant experiences. We may consequently infer that the learning tasks carried out with knowledge of previous failure were predominantly unpleasant, while those carried out with knowledge of success were predominantly pleasant. From this in turn we may infer that in this experiment, as in the preceding ones, associative learning accompanied by unpleasantness is less efficient than that accompanied by pleasantness.

Association-times in Relation to Hedonic Tone.— A further group of facts which is sometimes invoked as having a bearing upon our present problem deals with the relation between hedonic tone and association-times. Mayer and Orth[43] found that in the case of association-times for mediate associations, i. e., for associations where "one or more conscious processes are interposed between the stimulus and the word-reaction . . . the feeling-tone of the interposed conscious processes slows down the associative process, negative feeling-tone doing so more than positive feeling-tone." [44] Much the same results were secured by Wreschner.[45] He found that when associations were accompanied by hedonic tone (most frequently though not always referred to the stimulus word), the association-times were longer than for non-hedonic associations, and that the association-times for associations accompanied by unpleasantness were longer than those accompanied by pleasantness. In 1912, Birnbaum[46] determined for five observers the association-times of twenty supposedly pleasant words, twenty supposedly indifferent words and twenty supposedly unpleasant words. Comparison of the median times for the words of each of the three types showed these times to be practically identical for all five observers. A very similar experiment by Tolman and Johnson,[47] however, yielded very different results. In this experiment the investigators likewise determined the association-times of three groups of words supposed by them to involve respectively pleasant words, indifferent words and unpleasant words. The results showed that "The pleasant words as stimuli were not noticeably different from the indifferent words, but the unpleasant words showed a decided tendency to cause longer association-times." [48] In order to make sure that the lengthening of reaction-times in the case of supposedly unpleasant stimulus words was not due to the tendency of some of these words to arouse complexes, the writers repeated the experiment, including this time in the case of each of the three groups of ten words one which referred to simple sense qualities. The results of the second experiment were the same as those of the first, and the lengthening of reaction times was found to occur as much for words describing simple sense qualities as for other words. The writers concluded that "Simple unpleasantness as such lengthens association-times." [49] Except for the experiment by Birnbaum, then, the evidence agrees in indicating that reaction-times accompanied by pleasantness are quicker than those accompanied by unpleasantness.

Conclusion.—So many different types of experiments— and so many experiments of each type—have been dealt with in the present section that it will be well to bring the results together in brief form before attempting to interpret them. In the table below will be found, for each heading, a statement of the conclusion which appears to follow from

the experiments discussed under the heading, together with
an indication of the degree to which the experiments agree
in supporting the conclusion:

TABLE LXIV

Heading	Conclusion	Agreement
Proportion of pleasant and unpleasant events in free recall.	Greater for pleasant.	Evidence agrees completely.
Frequency of recall of pleasant and unpleasant events.	Greater for pleasant.	Two experiments in favor, one against.
Adequacy of recall of pleasant and unpleasant events.	Equal.	Evidence agrees completely.
Frequency of recognition of pleasant and unpleasant events.	Greater for pleasant.	Evidence agrees completely.
Rate of forgetting of pleasant and unpleasant events.	?	Evidence disagrees badly.
Associative learning in relation to hedonic tone.	Greater with pleasantness.	Evidence agrees completely.
Association-times in relation to hedonic tone.	Shorter with pleasantness.	Evidence agrees fairly well.

It will be noticed that in the table above there is no
mention of hedonic indifference. The reason for this is two-
fold. In the first place, we have found good reason to believe (Chapter I) that indifference does not represent a definite concept distinct from pleasantness and unpleasantness,
but only an ideal boundary between the two. In the second
place—and this ground is the more telling—although indifference is involved in the results of some of the experiments described above, it is not even mentioned in the results of others. Thus any conclusion involving the concept
of indifference would of necessity be based upon only a part
of the data presented. The fact, however, that in several
experiments—more especially in those upon the relation of
association-times to hedonic tone—the memorial value of indifference seems to be not intermediate between the me-

morial values of pleasantness and unpleasantness, but smaller than the latter, raises a problem in great need of further investigation.

How, now, shall we interpret the contents of the table above? Clearly, available evidence supports on the whole the proposition that *learning accompanied by pleasantness is more effective than learning accompanied by unpleasantness*. It is just as clear, however, that the evidence is far from constituting satisfactory proof of this proposition. In the first place, there is need that contrary results such as those of Gordon be accounted for not merely in terms of a likely hypothesis, but in terms of an actual experiment. In the second place, there is need that the proposition be verified by experimentation in which hedonic tone is varied without simultaneous variation of the stimulus or of the instructions. It might well be that in the confirmatory experiments the correlation between learning and pleasantness of stimulation or of general bodily state is really indicative of a functional relation between learning and stimulation or general bodily condition rather than between learning and hedonic tone. A technique adequate to such a verification has already been used in studying the relation of memory to hedonic tone occurring after learning, and will be discussed in the next section. Although we are justified, then, in accepting for the time being the proposition formulated above, we should consider this proposition more as an hypothesis suggestive of verificatory experimentation than as an answer to the problem of the relation of memory to hedonic tone occurring at the time of learning.

Memory in Relation to Hedonic Tone Following Learning

The problem of the relation of memory to hedonic tone following learning has sometimes been referred to as the problem of *affective retroaction* or of *retroactive affective facilitation and inhibition*. Use of these expressions, however, has not been sufficiently frequent to give them a position in psychology independent of appropriateness, and their appropriateness seems excessively slight. It would appear that in these expressions reference to retroaction is due wholly to equivocation between learning in the usual sense of *entire learning-process,* including acquisition, retention and reproduction, and learning in the pedagogical sense of *acquisition alone.* We shall consequently refrain from using these expressions.

It is obvious that the data from experiments on the relation of performance to reward and punishment in animal-training constitute indirect evidence concerning the relation of memory to hedonic tone subsequent to learning. This evidence is on the whole favorable to the view that memory is better when learning is followed by pleasantness than when it is followed by unpleasantness. J. B. Watson, it is true, found that a delay of thirty seconds in giving rats their reward had no appreciable influence upon the rate of acquisition,[50] and C. J. Warden and E. L. Haas partially confirmed this result, using delays of one minute and five minutes.[51] More recent work by one of the latter experimenters, however, indicates that, under carefully controlled conditions, delays in feeding do indeed appreciably decrease the rate of acquisition.[52] Furthermore, there is a very large number of experiments whose results are wholly in accord with some form of the law of effect. In a review of experimental work upon habit-formation in animals from 1921 to 1925, Tolman, after citing seven experiments upon the effect of rewards or punishments, concludes: "Thus the law of effect in some sense certainly holds, and cannot be dispensed with in the simple fashion originally proposed by Watson."[53] The same conclusion could be drawn equally well from subsequent experiments at the University of California by M. H. Elliott,[54] K. A. Adams,[55] H. C. Blodgett[56] and Tolman and C. H. Houzik.[57]

The evidence from experimentation on animals, however, cannot possibly be considered as proof of a specific relationship between memory and hedonic tone after learning. In the first place, many psychologists would refuse to make the necessary assumption that reward is pleasant to animals and punishment unpleasant. In the second place—and this I consider much more important—even if one makes the assumption just mentioned one cannot even be reasonably sure that the data show a relationship between memory and hedonic tone. Reward and punishment have many characteristics besides hedonic tone which may well be related to memory. They often involve important reflex responses and effects upon the general metabolism of the animal. How, in our present relative ignorance, is one to judge whether in these experiments hedonic tone is a mere apparent co-variant of memory or a real one?

When we turn to the evidence from experimentation upon human beings we find three relevant experiments. The first is that of W. D. Tait, unfortunately very sketchy.[58] Neutral lists of words were read to the observers, and immediately thereafter "something pleasant, optimistic and cheerful" or "something unpleasant and depressing" was read to them. The observers were then tested for recall of the lists of words. Tait summarizes his results in the following table:

TABLE LXV

	Average % of words remembered
When list was followed by pleasant ideas	21
When list was followed by unpleasant ideas	15

So far as this evidence goes—unfortunately not very far—it clearly supports the proposition that memory is better when learning is followed by pleasantness than when it is followed by unpleasantness.

The second relevant experiment upon human beings is that performed by E. J. Ludvigh and J. D. Frank in the Harvard Laboratory.[59] Each of twelve observers was first made to associate each pair of a list of ten pairs of nonsense syllables. Each pair was shown singly for two seconds, and the list was repeated ten times. Thirty seconds after the close of this period of learning the observer was subjected to a period of stimulation with a group of six normally indifferent odors. The odors were presented in pairs, according to the method of paired comparison, and the observer was asked to state for each of the fifteen pairs which odor was the more pleasant, and also whether each was very pleasant, pleasant, indifferent, unpleasant or very unpleasant. Following this stimulation with odors the observer was given a ten-minute rest period, during which he was supplied with back copies of the "Nation" for reading matter. Then his recall was tested by presenting the first member of each of the ten pairs of non-sense syllables, with instructions to give the *second member*.

After a period of five minutes, during which the observer was told "to forget all about the list you have just had," the same procedure was repeated, except that a new list of syllables was used, and the odors, instead of being normally indifferent ones, were normally pleasant ones. The procedure was again repeated with a new list and normally unpleasant odors, and finally again with a new list and the normally indifferent odors used at the beginning. For half of the observers, unpleasant odors were used in the second part of the experiment and pleasant ones in the third. The four lists were used in random order for the various observers in order to nullify the effect which a particularly easy or difficult list might have on the results. At the end of the entire experiment, finally, each observer was asked to arrange all eighteen odors in order from most pleasant to least, and to divide the odors into three groups, pleasant, unpleasant and indifferent.

Comparison of the recall-scores of the observers when learning had been followed by the normally pleasant, normally indifferent and normally unpleasant odors yielded the following results. (Figures for "indifferent" represent averages of the scores for indifferent stimulation at the beginning and at the end of the experiment.)

TABLE LXVI

Average Scores

	Learning followed by pleasant stimulation	Learning followed by indifferent stimulation	Learning followed by unpleasant stimulation
Six observers with whom pleasant odors were used before unpleasant ones	100	106	85
Six observers with whom unpleasant odors were used before pleasant ones	111	79	69
All observers	211	185	154
Per cent of scores for learning followed by indifferent stimulation.	114	100	83

These results are wholly in accord with those secured by correlating the rank of individual trials with respect to hedonic value, as determined by averaging the actual judgments of the observer, and with respect to learning value, as defined by the ratio of the recall-score of the trial to the sum of the scores of the particular observer in all four parts of the experiment. The coefficient of correlation thus secured was .52, P. E. 7.32.

From these results and other similar ones secured by slightly different treatments of the data, the experimenters feel warranted in drawing the following conclusions: "(1) Pleasant odors have a retroactive facilitative effect on learning; unpleasant odors have a retroactive inhibitory effect on learning. (2) The degree of retroactive facilitative and inhibitory effect is proportional to the degree of pleasantness and unpleasantness of the odors as judged by S." [60] They point out, however, that this conclusion does not necessarily mean that "pleasantness and unpleasantness *per se,* as opposed to pleasant and unpleasant stimuli, have this retroactive effect," and consequently are unwilling, pending further experimentation, to generalize their conclusion into a proposition relating memory and hedonic tone.

The fundamental issue thus raised by Ludvigh and Frank led to a subsequent experiment by Frank alone.[61]

Commenting upon the results which he had secured with Ludvigh, he points out that they can be interpreted in terms of either of two hypotheses. These are: "(1) that the affective value of odors is the primary determinant of the degree of reproduction, or (2) that the odors themselves determine both the affectivity and the degree of reproduction, there being no direct causal relation between the reproduction and the affectivity. These hypotheses may be expressed diagramatically (the observed variables are in italics) :

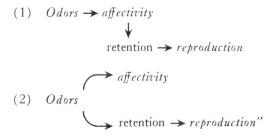

(1)   *Odors* → *affectivity*
                          ↓
           retention → *reproduction*

            ⌒→ *affectivity*
(2)   *Odors*
            ⌎→ retention → *reproduction*"

In order to decide between these two hypotheses, Frank determined to repeat the experiment which he had carried out with Ludvigh, with a slight but very important variation. This consisted of inducing experiences of different hedonic tone, not by the use of different sets of stimuli, but by the use of the same set of stimuli after their hedonic tone had been shifted in different directions by different contrast stimuli. The procedure with two of the four observers was as follows: First, a set of six normally indifferent odors was combined with a set of six normally unpleasant odors, and the twelve odors were presented to the observer in fifty pairs over a period of one hour. As in the previous experiment, the observer was required to give both relative and absolute judgments. From the results obtained, the experimenter determined for each observer six "test" odors, namely, the six odors which had been judged on the average to be the most pleasant, and it was these "test" odors which were used for that particular observer in the subsequent trials involving learning. Two days later, the observers were given ten repetitions of a list of ten pairs of non-sense syllables, as in the previous experiment with Ludvigh. They were then stimulated with the six "test" odors and their judgments of the odors were recorded. Thereupon their recall was tested by asking them to give for each first member of a pair of non-sense syllables the second member previously presented with it. After a week, the whole procedure, including the preliminary presentation of twelve odors, was repeated. At least two weeks were then allowed to elapse. After this the six "test" odors were again presented for hedonic judgment, but this time they were combined with six normally pleasant odors. Both relative and absolute judgments were required as before. This combined presentation was continued at intervals of from two days to a week until through contrast the hedonic tone of the test odors, as indicated by the absolute judgments, had been markedly shifted towards unpleasantness. Two days after the last combined presentation, the observers were given the learning test, just as before. After a week's interval, the "test" odors were again presented with the normally pleasant ones, and two days later the learning test was repeated. With two other observers, the procedure was the same, except that the "test" odors were originally the six most unpleasant of a combination of six normally indifferent and six normally pleasant odors, and that their hedonic tone was subsequently shifted towards pleasantness by repeated presentation with six normally unpleasant odors.

Comparison of the recall-scores of the observers when learning had been followed by different degrees of hedonic tone (evoked by the same set of stimuli) is afforded by the table below, reproduced from the article by Frank:

TABLE LXVII

Showing for Every S the Affective and Recall Scores at
Every One of the Test Periods

	1		2		3		4	
S	Aff. score	Recall score	Aff. score	Recall score	Aff. score	Recall score	Aff. score	Recall score
We ...	− 10	9	− 24	3	+ 6	6	+ 10	4
Tw ...	− 9	16	− 17	30	− 2	52	− 4	28
Lo	+ 29	15	+ 25	15	+ 17	26	+ 19	18
Cu ...	+ 5	13	+ 1	24	− 18	24	− 15	29

This table can be summarized in two ways. First, one
may compare for each observer the difference between the
average hedonic value of the odors in the first two periods
and the difference between the corresponding average recall-
scores. If pleasantness *per se* is accompanied by better
memory than unpleasantness, a positive difference in hedonic
scores should correspond to a positive difference in recall-
scores and a negative difference in the former to a negative difference in the latter. Obviously, such is not the case.

TABLE LXVIII

Observer	Difference in hed. value	Difference in recall scores
We	+ 25	− 1
Tw	+ 10	+ 7
Lo	− 9	+ 7
Cu	− 19.5	+ 13

Another way of summarizing the table next above is
to determine the coefficient of correlation between shift in
hedonic score and shift in recall-score from one trial of an
observer to another. If hedonic tone *per se* and memorial
efficiency co-vary in the manner described above, this coefficient should be positive. Actually the coefficient turns out
to be − .16, P. E. .21. The conclusion which Frank draws
from these results is best stated in his own terms. "Due
to the slender proportions of this experiment," he writes,

"its chief value lies rather in its suggestion of a method of attacking the problem than in the conclusions to be drawn from the results. Since the data all seem to point in one direction, however, we may conclude tentatively that, when the odors remain constant, a shift in their affective value, as determined by absolute judgments, has no corresponding effect on the reproduction of the syllables. It follows that of the two hypotheses presented at the beginning of this paper, the second is presumably the correct one. It would seem that the odors themselves determine the degree of reproduction, and that there is no direct causal relation between the reproduction and the affectivity." [62]

The evidence presented above concerning the relation of memory to hedonic tone subsequent to learning is so clear and so self-consistent that it is hardly necessary to formulate any general interpretation. Experiments on animals, we saw, are on the whole consistent with the proposition that learning followed by pleasantness is more effective than learning followed by unpleasantness. The experiments of Tait and of Frank and Ludvigh provide positive support for this proposition, but fail to be in any way conclusive, because their procedure does not allow variation of hedonic tone independently of stimulus. The experiment of Frank, finally, devised to obviate this shortcoming, provides a limited amount of evidence flatly contradicting the proposition above. Clearly, we are justified in holding that learning followed by pleasantness is *as a rule* more effective than learning followed by unpleasantness, but we are by no means justified in omitting the qualification "as a rule" and transforming this proposition into a statement of strict functional relationship. Indeed, if Frank's results are confirmed, we shall be obliged definitely to deny the existence of such a relation.

General Conclusion

As to the general conclusion to be drawn concerning the relation of memory to hedonic tone, it again is obvious. In the case both of hedonic tone during learning and of hedonic tone immediately following learning there is little doubt but that *learning accompanied by pleasantness is as a rule more effective than learning accompanied by unpleasantness.* This proposition, however, is a mere statement of tendency. For it to become a truly predictive law, a strict functional relationship, it would be necessary to eliminate the qualifying expression "as a rule." This step is certainly not warranted so long as the only available evidence involves co-variation of memory not with hedonic tone alone, but with both hedonic tone and such important determinants of consciousness and behavior as either the stimulus or the instructions to the observer. With respect to hedonic tone *during* learning, no data are available on the co-variation of memory and hedonic tone when the stimulus and the instructions are held constant. With respect to hedonic tone *after* learning, however, such "pure" data are available, although they come from an experiment which is more an illustration of technique than an attempt to establish facts. These data, as we have just seen, are contrary to the existence of a functional relation between memory and hedonic tone of the type suggested by the qualified proposition above. Although it is obvious that these data sorely need confirmation, we cannot but entertain the possibility that the qualified proposition above is indicative of no functional relation between memory and hedonic tone, but of a functional relation between memory and a close correlate of hedonic tone, namely, the nature of the stimulus-situation. We cannot but refrain, in consequence, from accepting any form whatever of hedonism of the past.

FOOTNOTES AND REFERENCES

[1] As I have pointed out in the preceding chapter, L. T. Troland aptly distinguishes between three forms of psychological hedonism in which responses are considered to depend respectively upon future hedonic tone, present hedonic tone and past hedonic tone. The latter form he terms hedonism of the past. *Cf.* L. T. TROLAND. The Fundamentals of Human Motivation, N. Y., 1928, 276-280.

[2] W. McDOUGALL. Outline of Psychology, N. Y., 1923, 270.

[3] W. S. Hunter. General Psychology, revised edition, Chicago, 1923, 331-332.

[4] J. B. Watson. Behaviourism, N. Y. 1924, 166. *Cf.* also H. A. Carr, Principles of Selection in Animal Learning, *Psychol. Rev.*, 21, 1914, 157; H. Cason, Criticism of the Laws of Exercise and Effect, *Psychol. Rev.*, 31, 1924, 397 ff.

[5] *Cf.* J. B. Watson. Behaviourism, N. Y., 1924, 17-19; revised edition, N. Y., 1930, 18-19. In the latter edition Watson, though admitting that Behaviourism is essentially a methodology, contends that as a successful methodology it is a science, presumably Psychology. From this point of view no statement of hedonism would be a true *psychological* proposition, but this would not mean that it could not be a *true* proposition.

[6] For an illustration of the difficulties involved in settling differences of opinion concerning metaphysical aspects of hedonism, *cf.* W. McDougall, Dr. Lloyd Morgan on Consonance of Welfare and Pleasure, *Mind*, N. S., 38, 1929, 77.

[7] For an excellent summary of the experimental work on the relation of memory to hedonic tone, *cf* H. Meltzer, The Present Status of Experimental Studies on the Relationship of Feeling to Memory, *Psychol. Rev.*, 37, 1930, 124-139.

[8] F. W. Colgrove. Memory, N. Y., 1900; Individual Memories, *Amer. J. Psychol.*, 10, 1898-99.

[9] A. Kowalewski. Studien zur Psychologie des Pessimismus, *Grenzfragen des Nerven und Seelenlebens*, IV, No. 24 (quoted from H. R. Crossland).

[10] A. Kowalewski Arthur Schopenhauer und Seine Weltanschauung, Halle a/S., 1908.

[11] W. Peters and O. Nemecek. Massenversuche über Errinerungsassoziationen, *Fortschritte der Psychol. und Ihrer Anwendungen*, 2, 1914, 226-245.

[12] W. Peters. Gefühl und Errinerung, Beiträge zur Errinerungsanalyse, *Psychol. Arbeiten*, 1911, VI, 197-260.

[13] E. N. Henderson. Do We Forget the Disagreeable? *J. Philos., Psychol. and Sc. Meth.*, 8, 1911, 432-437.

[14] H. L. Hollingworth. The Oblivescence of the Disagreeable, *J. Philos., Psychol., and Sc. Meth.*, 7, 1910, 710.

[15] E. N. Henderson. *Op. cit.*, 434.

[16] *Ibid.*, 435.

[17] A. Wohlgemuth. The Influence of Feeling on Memory, *Brit. J. Psychol.*, 13, 1922, 405-416.

[18] This preponderance of pleasant memories has since been verified again with a very similar procedure by Metzger. *Cf.* H. Metzger, *J. Educ. Psychol.*, 21, 1930, 399.

[19] J. C. Flügel. A Quantitative Study of Feeling and Emotion in Everyday Life, *Brit. J. Psychol.*, 15, 1925, 318-355.

[20] *Ibid.*, 328.

[21] D. A. Laird. The Influence of Likes and Dislikes on Memory as Related to Personality, *J. of Exper. Psychol.*, 6, 1923, 249-303.

[22] W. D. Tait. The Effect of Psycho-physical Attitude on Memory, *J. Abn. Psychol.*, 8, 1913, 10-37.

[23] Tait's description of his procedure is very meagre. I cannot consequently be sure that my exposition of his work is wholly correct.

[24] R. H. THOMSON. An Experimental Study of Memory as Influenced by Feeling Tone, *J. Exper. Psychol.*, 13, 1930, 462.

[25] Thomson fails fully to define the symbols in her table, but I feel reasonably sure that my interpretation of the table is correct.

[26] R. H. THOMSON. *Op. cit.*, 467.

[27] K. GORDON. The Recollection of Pleasant and Unpleasant Odors, *J. Exper. Psychol.*, 8, 1925, 225.

[28] *Ibid.*, 239.

[29] K. GORDON. Ueber das Gedächtnis fur Affecktiv Bestimmte Eindrücke, *Archiv. f. d. ges. Psychol.*, 4, 1905, 437-458.

[30] H. R. CROSSLAND. A Qualitative Analysis of the Process of Forgetting, *Psychol. Monogr.*, 29, 1921, No. 1 (whole No. 130).

[31] *Ibid.*, 88.

[32] W. D. TAIT. The Effect of Psycho-physical Attitude on Memory, *J. Abnor. Psychol.*, 8, 1913, 10-37.

[33] A. PETERS. Gefühl und Wiedererkennen, *Fortschritte der Psychologie und Ihrer Anwendungen* (edited by Marbe), 4, 1917, 120-133.

[34] A. WOHLGEMUTH. The Influence of Feeling on Memory, *Brit. J. Psychol.*, 13, 1923, 416.

[35] H. MELTZER. Individual Differences in Forgetting Pleasant and Unpleasant Experiences, *J. Educ. Psychol.*, 21, 1930, 402.

[36] J. W. HARRIS. On the Association Power of Odors, *Amer. J. Psychol.*, 19, 1908, 557-561.

[37] *Ibid.*, 561.

[38] C. FOX. The Influence of Subjective Preference on Memory, *Brit. J. Psychol.*, 13, 1923, 398-404.

[39] *Ibid.*, 404.

[40] E. B. SULLIVAN. Attitude in Relation to Learning, *Psychol. Monogr.*, Vol. 36, No. 3 (whole No. 169), 1927, 149.

[41] *Ibid*, 141-142.

[42] *Ibid.*, 117.

[43] A. MAYER and J. ORTH. Zur Qualitativen Untersuchung der Assoziation, *Zeitschr. f. Psychologie und Physiologie der Sinnesorgane*, 26, 1901, 1-13.

[44] *Ibid.*, 12-13.

[45] A. WRESCHNER. Die Reproduktion und Assoziation von Vorstellungen, *Zeitschr. f. Psychol.*, Erg.-Band 3, 1. Teil, 1907, 172-179, 190-194; 3. Teil, 1909, 566.

[46] K. BIRNBAUM. *Monatschr. f. Psychiat. u. Neurol.*, 32, 1912, 95-123, 194-220.

[47] E. C. TOLMAN and I. JOHNSON. A Note on Association-time and Feeling, *Amer. J. Psychol.*, 24, 1918, 187-195.

[48] *Ibid.*, 189.

[49] *Ibid.*, 193.

[50] J. B. WATSON. The Effect of Delayed Feeding Upon Learning, *Psychology*, I, 1917, 51-59.

[51] C. J. WARDEN and E. L. HAAS. The Effect of Short Intervals of Delay in Feeding Upon Speed of Maze-learning, *J. Comp. Psychol.*, 7, 1927, 107-161.

[52] E. L. Hamilton. The Effect of Delayed Incentive on the Hunger Drive in the White Rat, *Genet. Psychol. Monogr.,* V, 1929, 137.

[53] E. C. Tolman. Habit Formation and Higher Mental Processes in Animals, *Psychol. Bullet.,* 24, 1927, 10.

[54] M. H. Elliott. The Effect of Change of Reward on the Maze Performance of Rats, *Univ. of Calif. Public. in Psychol.,* 4 (No. 2, 1928), 19; The Effect of Appropriateness of Reward and of Complex Incentives on Maze Performance, *Univ. of Calif. Public. in Psychol.,* 4 (No. 6, 1929), 91; The Effect of Change in "Drive" on Maze Performance, *Univ. of Calif. Public. in Psychol.,* 4 (No. 11, 1929), 91.

[55] K. A. Adams. The Reward Value of a Conditioned Stimulus, *Univ. of Calif. Public. in Psychol.,* 4 (No. 3, 1929), 31.

[56] H. C. Blodgett. The Effect of the Introduction of Reward Upon the Maze Performance of Rats, *Univ. of Calif. Public. in Psychol.,* 4 (No. 8, 1929), 113.

[57] E. C. Tolman and C. H. Houzik. Degrees of Hunger, Reward and Non-reward, and Maze Learning in Rats, *Univ. of Calif. Public. in Psychol.,* 4 (No. 16, 1930), 241.

[58] W. D. Tait. The Effect of Psycho-physical Attitudes on Memory, *J. Abn. & Soc. Psychol.,* 8, 1913, 10-17.

[59] E. J. Ludvigh and J. D. Frank. The Retroactive Effect of Pleasant and Unpleasant Odors on Learning, *Amer. J. Psychol.,* 43, 1931, 102-108.

[60] *Ibid.,* 107-108.

[61] J. D. Frank. Affective Value v.s. Nature of Odors in Relation to Reproduction, *Amer. J. Psychol.,* 43, 1931, 479-483.

[62] *Ibid ,* 483.

Chapter X

Hedonic Tone in Relation to Nervous Processes

Indirect Evidence.—Very interesting indirect evidence of the relation of hedonic tone to nervous processes is to be found in the literature of physiology. Bechterew, in 1887, reported observations of the emotional expressive movements of animals some of which had been deprived of the cerebral hemispheres, while others had suffered lesions of the thalamus.[1] In the case of dogs deprived of the cerebral hemispheres, Bechterew was able to observe expressive movements normally indicative of both pleasant and unpleasant states. "Painful stimulation of the face elicited baring of the teeth, retraction of the mouth-corner, wrinkling of the nose and continuous whining. . . . When I subsequently began to stroke the animal's back, its face at once assumed the usual peaceful aspect, and in the case of some dogs it was even possible to observe weak waggling of the tail."[2] As to the cases where the thalamus had been transsected or destroyed by rotating a blade in its approximate location, they were most strikingly characterized by disappearance of almost all emotional expressive movements. Painful stimuli still caused marked activity, frequently including whining (although the whining never was as varied nor as protracted as in normal animals). These stimuli, however, never caused expressive movements of the face. "Even with the strongest stimuli (pinching, pricking, compressing) in the region of the nose and lips it was not possible to elicit even the slightest grimace, although simple reflex responses (e.g., the closing of one eyelid, the slight retraction of the mouth corners) were still retained."[3] Nor could expressive movements be elicited by habitually pleasant

385

stimuli: ". . . Neither stroking nor patting of the back would elicit the supple movements of the back and tail expressive of joy, which, as I have often observed, can easily be called forth in dogs even after serious operations on the cerebral hemispheres." [4] In a further series of experiments, Bechterew confirmed the importance of the thalamus by demonstrating that mechanical and electrical stimulation of this region results in vocal and bodily movements (e. g., in dogs: crying, barking, movements of the back, baring of the teeth, wagging of the tail) reminiscent of various expressive movements. He concluded that "the thalamus plays an outstanding role with respect to the expression of various conscious states. It is a motor centre, through which are carried out in the main the innate expressive movements elicited either under the influence of involuntary psychical impulses, as in the case of emotions, or in reflex fashion by tactual stimuli and stimulation of other sense-organs. In view of the fact, however, that strong cutaneous stimuli still produce in the operated animals general unrest with escape-efforts and monotonous crying, it is evident that the reflex elicitation of a few expressive movements, namely, of those which according to their character are closer to simple reflexes, takes place through the agency of lower centres (independent of the thalamus). These centres lie . . . according to my investigations in the upper part of the medulla oblongata." [5]

Bechterew's findings and conclusions have been confirmed to a large extent by subsequent experimentation. In 1892, Goltz published his famous account of a dog who lived eighteen months after complete removal of both hemispheres.[6] As in the corresponding cases observed by Bechterew, movements expressive of unpleasantness were remarkably retained: "If one grasps the dog at any point (while he is asleep) . . . he not only awakens, but answers immediately with a definite growl. If one then goes further and attempts to lift the awakened animal out of the cage, he develops a thoroughgoing fit of rage, stamps in the most violent manner with all members, barks very loudly and bites in all directions." [7] Movements expressive of pleasantness were also retained, but to a lesser degree. "Everyone who saw the animal eat and drink derived the impression that the animal was striving to consume the nourishment and swallowed it with satisfaction." [8] On the other hand, the pleasant emotion of joy seemed to have been eradicated: "Our dog without a cerebrum lacks all expressions of joy; gentle stroking of the skin appears to leave him wholly unaffected. Occasionally he does move his tail, but it was never possible to observe in his case a sweeping wagging of the tail which could have been interpreted as the expression of a pleasant mood." [9] In addition, Goltz noted that his dog was much more subject to explosions of rage than normal dogs. Sufficient stimulation for such explosions was provided by merely bumping a table or by being handled relatively gently by the experimenter. Further confirmation of Bechterew's findings and of the additional observation of Goltz is to be found in an experiment by Cannon and Britton.[10] These investigators used as subjects cats decorticated in such a way as to leave the basal ganglia of the brain intact. In summarizing the results in his paper at the Wittenberg Symposium, Cannon wrote: "As soon as recovery from anesthesia was complete, a remarkable group of activities appeared, such as are usually seen in an infuriated animal—a sort of sham rage. A complete list of these quasi-emotional phenomena which we observed is as follows: Vigorous lashing of the tail; arching of the trunk, and thrusting and jerking of the limbs in the thongs which fasten them to the animal board, combined with a display of claws in the forefeet and clawing motions, often persistent; snarling; rapid head movements from side to side with attempts to bite, and extremely rapid, panting respiration. These activities occur, without special stimulation (apart from the operative trauma and confinement to the holder), in 'fits' or periods, lasting from a few seconds to several minutes. During the intermediate quiet stages a 'fit' could be evoked by slight handling of the animal, touching the paws or jarring the table." [11]

With respect to the specific localization of the neural centres, it seems likely that Bechterew was slightly in error. This is not surprising, when one considers that his work was that of a pioneer. Working in Cannon's laboratory, P. Bard[12] recently carried out an extensive investigation of the neural centres controlling the " 'sham rage' regularly developed after removal of all parts of the brain cranial to the middle of the diencephalon and after removal of the dorsal part of the thalamus. It invariably failed to appear after sections which separated the ventral and most caudal fractions of the lower half of the diencephalon from the midbrain." [13] He concluded that "sham rage" was probably conditioned by neural mechanisms in the hypothalamus.[14] Evidence comparable to that of Bard is still lacking with respect to emotional expressions other than those of rage. When one considers, however, the great similarity demonstrated by Cannon between the internal bodily changes for all emotions,[15] it seems reasonable to infer that it is not the thalamus which is the primary centre for all emotional expressive movements, as Bechterew believed, but a lower and more ventral portion of the diencephalon, probably the hypothalamus.

Two conclusions concerning the relation of hedonic tone to nervous processes may readily be drawn from the experiments described above. In the first place, the observations of Bechterew, Goltz, and Cannon and Britton indicate that the movements expressive of hedonic states are in all likelihood dependent upon centres either identical with or in close juxtaposition to the centres responsible for movements expressive of major emotions. Deprived of their cerebral hemispheres, the animals still show manifold expressive movements, including those expressive of pleasantness and unpleasantness. Deprived of the thalamus and of neighboring centres, the animals show practically no expressive movements at all. In the second place, the work of Bard, when viewed in the light of the close relationship between movements expressive of hedonic tone and of emotions, indicates that the central mechanisms controlling movements expressive of hedonic tone are in the hypothalamus or in its immediate neighborhood.

Direct Evidence.—The evidence above bears only on the relation of movements expressive of hedonic tone to nervous processes, not on the relation between such processes and hedonic tone itself. The only evidence available, as far as I know, concerning this latter relationship is that published by Head and Holmes.[16] These investigators made a very complete study of the sensory and affective experiences of two groups of patients suffering from cerebral lesions. One group involved patients with lesions of the optic thalamus. The other involved patients with lesions of the cerebral cortex. Observations upon the latter group of patients showed marked blunting and sometimes complete abolition of recognition of posture and of passive movement, of two point discrimination, of localization and of thermal discrimination. On the other hand, it was found that cortical lesions never abolish sensibility to contact. It was also found—and this is the most interesting point to us—that ". . . Stationary cortical lesions, however extensive, which cause no convulsions or other signs of irritation and shock, produce no effect on sensibility to pain. Destruction of the cortex alone does not disturb the threshold for the painful or uncomfortable aspects of sensations." [17]

In striking contrast with these observations were those upon the patients suffering from thalamic lesions. Head and Holmes wrote: "The most remarkable feature in that group of thalamic cases with which we have dealt in this work is not loss of sensation, but an excessive response to affective stimuli. This positive effect, an actual overloading of sensation with feeling-tone, was present in all our twenty-four cases of this class. . . . This excessive response may be accompanied by much or by little loss of sensation, but the extent of this loss bears no relation to the amount of the over-reaction to painful stimuli. It is only necessary that sufficient sensory impulses capable of exciting discomfort should still be able to reach consciousness. If this is possible, the affected half of the body will respond more

profoundly than normal parts to all painful stimuli, in spite
of the gross loss of sensation. . . . But the characteristic
thalamic response does not consist in an excessive reaction
to painful stimuli only.   In suitable cases we have shown
that the response to pleasurable stimuli, such as warmth,
is also greater on the affected side.   Moreover, the manifestations of general mental states of pleasure and discomfort may be more pronounced on the abnormal half of the
body." [18]

Illustrations of excessive reactions to unpleasant stimuli
are afforded by observations such as the following: When
a pin was lightly dragged from right to left across the face
or trunk of one of the patients suffering from a lesion
affecting the left side, she exhibited intense discomfort as
soon as it had passed the middle line.   Not only did she call
out that it hurt more, but her face became contorted with
pain.   Yet careful examination with algesimeters showed
that on the affected side her sensitivity to such stimulation
was, if anything, slightly lowered.   This striking over-
response to prick without raising of sensitivity was present
in twenty out of twenty-two patients examined in this respect.   "Many of these patients complained that they could
not be shaved on the affected cheek because it seemed as if
the razor was 'passing over a raw surface.'   Some objected
to have the hair cut on the affected half of the head, because
of the discomfort, and others complained of the pain caused
by the attempt to cut their nails." [19]   Not only were there
excessive reactions to unpleasant external stimuli applied to
the affected side, but there were furthermore excessive
emotional responses on the affected side which were experienced as particularly unpleasant.   Thus the authors wrote:
"One of our patients was unable to go to his place of wor-
ship because he 'could not stand the hymns on his affected
side,' and his son noticed that during the singing his father
constantly rubbed the affected hand.   Another patient . . .
went to a memorial service on the death of King Edward
VII.   As soon as the choir began to sing, a 'horrid feeling

came on in the affected side, and the leg was screwed up and started to shake' ...." [20]

As to excessive hedonic reactions to pleasant stimuli, the following cases will serve as illustrations: "In one case we were able to show that the patient could not recognize any thermal stimulus as such, and yet over the affected half of the chest large tubes containing water at from 38° C. to 48° C. evoked intense pleasure. This was shown not only by the expression of her face, but by her exclamations, 'Oh! that's lovely, it's so soothing, so very pleasant.' . . . Several of our patients were able to appreciate heat as low as 34° C. on the affected half of the body. Here, whenever the sensation evoked was one of pleasant warmth, the pleasure was obviously greater on the affected side. In one case, a tube containing water at 38° C. applied to the normal palm was said to be warm, but the patient cried out with pleasure when it was placed in the affected hand. His face broke into smiles and he said, 'Oh! that's exquisite,' or 'That's real pleasant.' " [21]

From the fact that cortical lesions alone do not "disturb the threshold for the painful or uncomfortable aspects of sensations," whereas thalamic lesions are associated with excessive hedonic reactions to stimuli applied to the affected side, even though the sensory threshold for these stimuli remains unchanged or is even increased, Head and Holmes concluded: (1) That lesions determining enhanced hedonic tone do so by impeding the inhibitory effect of the cortex upon thalamic activity, and (2) that the thalamus is the seat of the neural processes underlying hedonic consciousness. Concerning the neural paths which are known to run from the cortex to the thalamus, they wrote: "The only function which can be ascribed to these cortico-thalamic paths is that through them the cortex controls, in some way, the activity of the thalamus. If this view is correct, lesions which interrupt these paths, but leave intact the main substance of the optic thalamus, must lead to a permanent over-activity of functions exercised by that organ. Any afferent impulses which are capable of exciting this part of the brain will act on an uncontrolled centre and must, consequently, evoke an excessive effect." [22] Concerning the role of the optic thalamus, they wrote: ". . . We believe that the essential organ of the optic thalamus is the centre of consciousness for certain elements of sensation. It responds to all stimuli capable of evoking either pleasure or discomfort, or consciousness of a change in state. The feeling-tone of somatic or visceral sensation is the product of thalamic activity, and the fact that a sensation is devoid of feeling-tone shows that the impulses which underlie its production make no thalamic appeal." [23]

General Conclusion.—The conclusion of Head and Holmes is startling, although as far back as 1892, Goltz, in his article on the dog without an end-brain, insisted that consciousness is not a direct function of the cortex alone, but to some extent also of infra-cortical centres. [24] Startling or not, however, it appears to be incontrovertible in the present state of our knowledge. In the first place, there is no direct evidence whatever which contradicts it. In the second place, the experiments described in the first section of this chapter, indicating the dependence of movements expressive of hedonic tone on the hypothalamus, obviously suggest a very close relationship between hedonic tone and the diencephalon. Furthermore, the well-known experiment of Lashley, [25] indicating the lack of any cortical mechanism essential to brilliance-discrimination, constitutes strong evidence against the traditional view that the cortex is the sole immediate determinant of consciousness. As far as available evidence is concerned, therefore, the only possible conclusion concerning the relation of hedonic tone to the nervous system is that hedonic tone depends directly upon neural processes in the thalamus.

FOOTNOTES AND REFERENCES

[1] W. BECHTEREW. Zur Bedeutung der Sehhügel auf Grund von Experimentellen und Pathologischen Daten, *Archiv. f. Pathol. Anat. u. Physiol.*, 110, 1887, 102-154, 322-365.

[2] *Ibid.,* 120.

[3] *Ibid.,* 330.

[4] *Ibid.,* 330.

[5] *Ibid.,* 335-336.

[6] FR. GOLTZ. Der Hund ohne Grosshirn, *Archiv. f. d. ges. Physiol.,* 51, 1892, 570-614.

[7] *Ibid.,* 572.

[8] *Ibid.,* 580.

[9] *Ibid.,* 577. It is this passage, presumably, which led Sherrington to write that Goltz's experiment confirmed Bechterew's "except for the striking absence of 'signs of pleasure' " and to conclude that "pain centres seem to lie lower than pleasure centres." (C. S. SHERRINGTON, The Integrative Action of the Nervous System, New Haven, 1906, 255-266). I feel that my previous quotation from Goltz, together with passages on pages 600, 608, 609 indicate that Sherrington's interpretation is erroneous.

[10] W. B. CANNON and S. W. BRITTON. Pseudaffective Medulliadrenal Secretion, *Amer. J. Physiol.,* 72, 1925, 283.

[11] W. B. CANNON. Neural Organization for Emotional Expression, Feelings and Emotions, The Wittenberg Symposium, Worcester, Mass., 1928, 259.

[12] P. BARD. A Diencephalic Mechanism for the Expression of Rage with Special Reference to the Sympathetic Nervous System, *Amer. J. Physiol.,* 84, 1928, 490-515.

[15] W. B. CANNON. Bodily Changes in Pain, Hunger, Fear and Rage, N. Y., 1929, 345.

[16] H. HEAD and G. HOLMES. Sensory Disturbances from Cerebral Lesions, Brain, 34, 1911, 102-254.

[17] *Ibid.,* 181.

[18] *Ibid.,* 177-178.

[19] *Ibid.,* 133.

[20] *Ibid.,* 135-136.

[21] *Ibid.,* 134.

[22] *Ibid.,* 180.

[23] *Ibid.,* 181.

[24] FR. GOLTZ. *Arch. f. d. ges. Physiol.,* 51, 1892, 570.

[25] K. S. LASHLEY. Brain Mechanisms and Intelligence, Chicago, 1929, 45.

Chapter XI

The Theory of Hedonic Tone

Modern Theories

Theoretical discussions of hedonic tone during the last thirty years have dealt with two very different problems, that of the nature of the *conscious carrier* of hedonic tone, and that of the *immediate conditions* or causes of hedonic tone. Most theories have dealt with both problems, but some have greatly emphasized the one, some the other. It will be advisable, therefore, to arrange these theories in two groups according to their emphasis, and to deal with these groups successively. We shall first consider theories concerned solely or primarily with the nature of the conscious carrier.

Theories Emphasizing the Nature of the Conscious Carrier.—We have seen in Chapter III that psychology at the close of the nineteenth century was imbued with the doctrine of mental elements. To such a psychology the chief problem concerning hedonic tone was to determine its relation to mental elements. Was it an attribute of sensations or of special affective elements? If the former, was it an attribute of all sensations, or only of some? All three possible answers to these questions were maintained by eminent psychologists, and continue to have proponents to this very day.

The view that hedonic tone is an attribute of sensations in general is well illustrated by the theory held by Wundt until 1893[1] and by the theories of H. R. Marshall[2] and T. Ziehen.[3] The best known of these theories is that of Ziehen. For him, "insofar as the nature of hedonic tone is concerned, it is obviously an attribute (Eigenschaft) of sensation." Sensations may, however, be devoid of hedonic tone. Thus it is not a *necessary* attribute of sensation. Hedonic tone never occurs independently, but it may occur in conjunction not only with sensations, but with images. The hedonic tone of an image, however, can always be reduced to sensory hedonic tone. Hedonic tone occurring in conjunction with an image is very easily transferred to other conscious contents: "When I have suffered an accident at a certain place, a hurt, for instance, at future times not only will the recollection of this accident be accompanied by unpleasantness, but frequently the recollection of the place itself will be spoiled, i. e., also accompanied by unpleasantness." [5] The basis of such a transfer is the law of association. Its operation is illustrated diagramatically by Ziehen as follows: Let S' be a visual sensation evoked by the locality, and S'' that evoked by the hurt. Let S' be

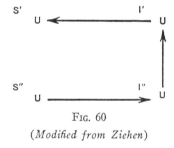

FIG. 60

(*Modified from Ziehen*)

accompanied by no hedonic tone, and S'' by unpleasantness (U). Let I' and I'' be the images determined respectively by S' and S''. I' and I'', having simultaneous origins, are associatively related. At the outset I' is devoid of hedonic tone, but it acquires from I'' part or all of its unpleasantness. (*Cf.* figure above.)

Not only can the hedonic tone occurring with an image be transferred to another image, but it can be transferred to the sensation at the basis of this image—in the figure above, from I' to S'. This is what Ziehen calls a reversion. It explains, in his mind, that in the case cited above as an illustration, the sensation evoked subsequently by the locality where the hurt occurred may be unpleasant, though the image of the hurt never enter consciousness. As to the mechanism underlying the hedonic attribute of sensation, Ziehen has little to say. He assumes that hedonic tone depends upon some cortical physiological process which occurs in the case of certain sensations, in conjunction with the cortical physiological process underlying the sensory attributes of the sensation. He further assumes that the cortical process at the basis of hedonic tone must depend to a large extent upon variable characteristics of the cortex in view of the differences in "taste" of different individuals and of the same individual at different times. As to the nature of this physiological process, Ziehen admits that we know as yet nothing.

The view that hedonic tone is an attribute of certain special sensations is best exemplified by the theory of Stumpf.[6] For Stumpf, pleasantness and unpleasantness are special types of sensations, namely, hedonic sensations (Gefühlsempfindungen). There are two types of hedonic sensations, pleasant and unpleasant ones. The latter are exemplified by pain, though there may be other unpleasant sensations. The former include tickle, itch, lust and certain organic sensations. Hedonic sensations may be aroused by stimulation of peripheral end organs, as is usually the case for tickle and itch, or they may be aroused by central processes, as is the case for pleasant and unpleasant colors. They may give rise to corresponding images. As to a physiological explanation of pleasantness and unpleasantness, it is clear that such an explanation is partially provided by theories of sensation such as that of von Frey concerning pain. No explanation exists in the literature, however, and none is provided by Stumpf for centrally aroused pain, tickle, itch, etc., in so far as these processes differ from imaginal pain, tickle and itch.

The view that hedonic tone is an attribute of special affective elements is admirably set forth in Titchener's theory of affection.[7] According to Titchener, pleasantness and unpleasantness are qualities of a special mental element, affection, of the same general type as sensation, but differing from the latter in involving qualitative opposition and in lacking the attribute of clearness. This special mental element is a more primitive kind of element than sensation, one that might under favorable conditions have developed into sensation. Its peripheral organs are assumed by Titchener to be the free nerve endings distributed to the various tissues of the body, which he considers to represent a lower level of development than specialized end organs. Another well-known theory which makes hedonic tone an attribute of a special type of mental element is that held after 1893 by Wundt.[8] The main difference between this theory and that of Titchener is that for Wundt the qualitative variations of the affective element are not merely unidimensional, but tridimensional. The three dimensions involved are pleasantness-unpleasantness, excitement-depression and strain-relaxation.

Besides the three main views mentioned above, a fourth view has been advanced concerning the relation of hedonic tone to mental elements, namely, that hedonic tone is not an attribute of the elements themselves, but of complexes of elements. This view is well exemplified by the theory of H. C. Warren, according to which pleasantness and unpleasantness are qualities of combinations of systemic (organic) sensations.[9] It is also held by J. P. Nafe, who believes that pleasantness and unpleasantness are characteristics of patterns of specific sensory experiences, namely, bright and dull pressures: "Psychologically, an emotion and an affection must be defined alike, and both are complexes of sensory experiences." [10]

Just as the emphasis on elements by Wundt and his contemporaries brought forth the views above concerning the relation of hedonic tone to mental elements, so the more recent emphasis upon conscious configurations has brought forth the view that it is these which are the carriers of hedonic tone. A good illustration is the theory of F. Krueger.[11] For Krueger, feelings, including pleasantness and unpleasantness, are "complex qualities of the momentary total whole, of the totallity of experience." [12]

Opposed to feelings in their character are the cognitive qualities of the simplest parts into which experience can be analyzed. As for the partial wholes, intermediate between total wholes and simple parts, their qualities are intermediate between feeling and cognition. The more a partial whole includes of the total whole existing at any moment, the less it stands out from the background of this whole, and the less it is structuralized, the more feeling-like will be its quality. As to a physiological basis for this view, Krueger gives none. He considers it necessary "that attempts at explanation be for the time being omitted as premature; not only physical analogies such as those so ingeniously proposed by Köhler, but also Wertheimer's cerebral 'cross-functions.' What one wishes to explain scientifically must first of all be accurately known with respect to its nature. We must undertake seriously the task of providing a pure and thoroughgoing description of phenomena." [13]

What shall be said of these five views? The last view, in its general formulation, appears to be the obvious premise of all research upon hedonic tone. Experiments upon the hedonic tone of colored surfaces, of tones, of forms, of musical pieces clearly imply that hedonic tone is a characteristic of configurations. In the special formulation given to it by Krueger, however, this view appears to be wholly fanciful. Krueger presents no evidence that large configurations are more readily judged to be pleasant or unpleasant, or judged to be more intensely pleasant or unpleasant, than small configurations. He merely asserts it. On the other hand, the extreme unpleasantness of simple and circumscribed pains is definite proof that very small configurations may be characterized by marked hedonic tone.

As to the four other views, those relating hedonic tone to mental elements, it was pointed out in Chapter III that their validity rested not on observed relations of hedonic tone, but upon general systematic premises. Mental elements, it was agreed—whether special affective ones or sensations—are not found, but made. They are scientific constructions. If Titchener constructs a sensation involving only necessary attributes (attributes which can never have zero value), then hedonic tone cannot be an attribute of sensation. If Ziehen and Stumpf construct a sensation, including, besides necessary attributes, attributes which may or may not be present, hedonic tone may be an attribute of sensation. Again, if the systematic point of view of Warren involves mental elements, but only elements related to specific receptors and having attributes related to specific characteristics of the stimulus,[14] then hedonic tone cannot be an attribute of elements themselves, but only of combinations of elements. Thus evaluation of the views relating hedonic tone to mental elements must depend upon evaluation of various forms of elementarism. Divergence of opinion concerning fundamental issues is still too great to allow much assurance in the performance of such a task. The fertility of present psychology, however, largely devoid of elementarism, suggests that the wisest course is to do away entirely with the problem of the relation of hedonic tone to mental elements by refraining from the construction of any such elements.

We have seen that none of the current theories concerning the nature of the conscious carrier of hedonic tone is acceptable. What view should be held in their stead? A wealth of experimental evidence shows that pleasantness or unpleasantness may be ascribed by observers to any conscious configuration whatever. In Chapter IV, we dealt with experiments in which odors, colored patches, tones, forms, melodies and many other "objective" configurations were readily judged with respect to hedonic tone. In Chapter III, we dealt with experiments in which a variety of "subjective" configurations—pressures, pains, organic experiences, total bodily feeling—were judged to be pleasant or unpleasant. Attempts to interpret these findings in highly sophisticated fashion have led to a variety of conflicting theories involving very doubtful systematic assumptions. It seems far wiser to accept the observer's reports at their face value and to conclude that hedonic tone may characterize—may be carried by—any conscious configuration whatever.

Theories Emphasizing the Immediate Conditions of Hedonic Tone.—These theories fall into two groups, according to whether they seek the immediate conditions—the fundamental causes—of hedonic tone in the *psychical realm* or in the *physiological realm*.

The former group includes two very well-known theories, those of Herbart[15] and of McDougall.[16] Herbart's theory, later taken over by Nahlowsky,[17] and for many years accepted by German pedagogical circles together with the rest of Herbartian psychology, maintains that hedonic tone depends upon the harmony or disharmony of the forces involved at any moment in the interplay of ideas. Suppose that an act of perception a arouses the idea α, united with a into a complex a + α. Suppose further that when α comes forward, it meets in consciousness an idea β, opposed to it. "Then α will be, at the same time, driven forward and held back. In this situation, it is the source of an unpleasant feeling which may give rise to desire, viz., for the object represented by α provided the opposition offered by β is weaker than the force which α brings with it." [18] Suppose now that an act of perception a' calls forth an idea α', and that its progress into consciousness is favored by the presence in consciousness of an idea β' consonant with it. "This favoring is part of the process which takes place in consciousness, but in no way is it anything represented or conceived. Hence it can only be called a feeling—without a doubt a feeling of pleasure." [19]

McDougall's theory, which comes from Aristotle and was advocated by von Hartmann,[20] maintains that hedonic tone depends upon the satisfaction or non-satisfaction of conative tendencies. It asserts that: ". . . Conation (action, attention, striving, desire, volition, activity of every kind) is immediately determined by cognition, and that pleasure and pain result from the conation, are determined by the striving; pleasure, when the striving attains its natural goal

or progresses towards it; pain, when striving is thwarted
or obstructed and fails to achieve, or progress toward, its
goal." [21] This theory draws a sharp distinction between
pain in the sense of unpleasantness, in which sense it is used
above, and pain in the sense of pain sensation. The latter
is not dependent upon conation, but rather initiates it, for
it is a specific provocative of fear. The theory furthermore
does not consider pleasantness and unpleasantness as mere
epiphenomena: "Pleasure and pain influence the further
course of mental processes very powerfully; each influences
it in two ways which, although closely allied, may be use-
fully distinguished. First, pleasure, arising in the course
of mental activity, supports that activity, sustains our striving in the direction, or of the kind, which brings pleasure;
it strengthens and prolongs the impulse or conative tendency
at work in us. Secondly, on recurrence of a situation of
the kind in which we have striven successfully, our tendency
to strive again in the same way is stronger; the tendency
seems to be confirmed by the previous experience of success, and this confirmation of the tendency may fairly be
regarded as a consequence or result of the pleasure experienced on the former occasion. Conversely pain, arising
during striving, tends to divert the striving to other directions, and on renewal of the situation in which we have
striven unsuccessfully and (in consequence) painfully, our
tendency to strive again in the same way is weakened or
abolished or diverted to some new direction. These weakenings and diversions of the impulse seem to be the effects
or consequences of the pain experienced on the former
occasion." [22]

One of the most difficult problems for a theory like
McDougall's is that of accounting for the pleasantness and
unpleasantness determined by stimuli which are apparently
neutral so far as the welfare of the organism is concerned—
e. g., color stimuli and tonal stimuli. In a recent article,
McDougall has proposed the following solution: "The psychologists of the Gestalt school have taught us that even
a simple patch of color or a simple tone cannot properly

be treated as an isolated sensation; that, rather, the color or the tone always appears to us as standing out from a background; that is, as a feature of a larger whole; or in other words, that here also we have to do, not with an isolated sensation, but rather with a perceptive activity. And in such cases the pleasantness of the clearly bounded patch of color must, I submit, be regarded as due to the fact that the color facilitates the perceptive activity, enables us to distinguish readily the object from its ground. The truth of this view becomes apparent if we complicate the colored area, making of it a repeating pattern; then, in so far as the pattern does not become too complex for assimilation by our perceptual organization, each increase of complexity adds to the pleasantness of the perceptive activity, because rendering it fuller and richer. Similar considerations hold good for pure tone. The clearcut quality is faintly pleasurable because it promotes ready discrimination of tone from background and, if we add other tones, the total activity of perception becomes more pleasant in so far as the additional tones are in relations that are readily apprehended, relations of quality and rhythm such as lend themselves to complete perception, such as facilitate the perception of the whole complex or series as a distinctive object, a clang or a melody. On the other hand, a surface covered with ill-defined patches of color having no definite or significant relations, qualitative or spatial, is found disagreeable, because our perceptive organization cannot cope with it, and a complex or inharmonious tones or a series of tones in no orderly relations of quality and rhythm is disagreeable because we have no perceptive organization that can cope with, can assimilate, the complex." [23]

Herbart's theory is based upon a "mechanics of ideas" which has long been relegated to historical treatises. It is consequently unacceptable on purely systematic grounds. Such is not the case with McDougall's theory. It is stated in terms of concepts accepted by many—though by no means all—modern psychologists. It has considerable explanatory value, accounting well for the dependence of hedonic tone upon motivating factors, for its frequent association with definite types of overt movements, and for some, at least, of its relations to the stimulus. It has one great fault, however, namely, lack of specificity. This is due in the first place to the necessary indefiniteness of McDougall's conception of instinct, an entity devoid of spatio-temporal localization and consequently defined only in terms of more or less remote antecedents and consequences. It is due in the second place to the fact that McDougall has never developed his theory in relation to the more recent facts concerning hedonic tone. Thus the theory is simply neutral with respect to hedonic contrast, to the correlation between hedonic tone and bright and dull pressure, to the dependence of hedonic tone upon thalamic nervous processes. McDougall's theory is probably true, but it represents an early stage of development of the psychology of hedonic tone, a stage which has now been exceeded.

The second group of theories emphasizing the immediate conditions of hedonic tone is directed not towards mental or psychical conditions, but towards physiological ones. This group involves two main types, that which relates hedonic tone to processes specific in their nature, but not in their localization, and that which relates it to processes in a specific part of the nervous system. The former type is well illustrated by the theories of Lehmann, Marshall, Thorndike, Troland and Herrick.

Starting from the general principle that pleasantness and unpleasantness are closely connected with the weal and harm of the organism, Lehmann suggests that the physiological correlate of hedonic tone is the degree to which assimilation counteracts dissimilation during the activity of any group of central neurones.[24] If assimilation (A) entirely counteracts dissimilation (D), i. e., if $\frac{A}{D} = 1$, then the concomitant experience will be pleasant. If not, i. e., if $\frac{A}{D} < 1$, then the experience will be unpleasant. The degree of pleasantness he further believes to increase with the absolute value of D, while the degree of unpleasantness increases both with the absolute value of D and with the decrease of the value of the proportion $\frac{A}{D}$.

The theories of Marshall and of Thorndike are alike in emphasizing the readiness or lack of readiness of neurones to conduct. Marshall's is the simpler of the two.[25] It holds that when a neural element is stimulated this stimulation will determine unpleasantness if the capacity of the neural element to react is subnormal, that it will determine pleasantness if this capacity to react is hypernormal, and that it will determine indifference if the capacity to react is normal. Thorndike's theory is stated in terms not of pleasantness and unpleasantness, but of *satisfaction* and *annoyance*.[26] In so far as the latter terms are interpreted subjectively, however, they must correspond closely to the former. Thus Thorndike's theory may readily be interpreted as a theory of hedonic tone. It is based upon the view that neurones may constitute unitary systems such that actual conduction over one neuron is accompanied by the readiness of others to conduct. "The sight of the prey," writes Thorndike, "makes the animal run after it, and also puts the conductions and connections involved in jumping upon it when near, into a state of excitability or readiness to be made."[27] Satisfaction and annoyance Thorndike believes to be related to such "readiness to conduct" in accordance with the three following laws: "1. When a conduction unit is ready to conduct, conduction by it is satisfying, nothing being done to alter its action. 2. . . . For a conduction unit ready to conduct not to conduct is annoying, and provokes whatever responses nature provides in connection with that particular annoying lack. 3. . . . When a conduction unit not ready for conduction is forced to conduct, conduction by it is annoying."[28]

Troland's theory, like that of Lehmann, starts from the close connection of pleasantness and unpleasantness with biological advantage and disadvantage.[29] Unlike the former theory, however, it considers the physiological processes underlying hedonic tone to be not mere correlates of biological welfare, but determinants of this welfare through their influence upon learning. According to Troland, "The affective intensity of any individual consciousness is proportional to the average rate of change of conductance in the synapses, the activities of which are responsible for that consciousness."[30] This proposition may be expressed mathematically. If affective intensity be represented by a (plus values being pleasant and minus values unpleasant), and average conductance of the synapses by c, one can write

$$a = k \frac{dc}{dt},$$

k being a constant, $\frac{dc}{dt}$ being the expression for the rate of change of c with respect to t. Change in the conductance of synapses, the activities of which underlie consciousness at any given moment, is determined by two factors: (1) By two opposed types of sensory processes, namely, beniception and noci-ception, the former increasing conductance, the latter decreasing it; (2) by exercise (increasing conductance) and disuse (decreasing conductance). Such change definitely alters the neural responses of the organism to stimulation, increase or decrease in the conductance of synapses evidently making the paths involving these synapses more liable or less liable to subsequent nervous conduction. Thus the neural correlates of pleasantness and unpleasantness may be considered to influence learning by "stamping in" and "stamping out" neural patterns.

Simpler than the preceding theories, finally, and at the same time similar to them, is the theory of C. J. Herrick. According to Herrick, "Normal discharge . . . of definitely elaborated nervous circuits resulting in free, unrestrained activity is pleasurable, in so far as the reaction comes into consciousness at all. . . . Conversely the impediment to such discharge, no matter what the occasion, results in a stasis in the nerve centers, the summation of stimuli and the development of a situation of unrelieved nervous tension which is unpleasant until the tension is relieved by the appropriate adaptive reaction." [31]

As to the theories relating hedonic tone to nervous processes in specific portions of the nervous system, the most prominent are those of F. H. Allport and W. M. Marston. Allport's theory is based upon three main premises.[32] The first is that "Every emotion has an affective element; that is, it may be classed as either pleasant or unpleasant." [33] Thus disgust, fear, rage, grief and intense bodily pain are unpleasant, while elation, mirth and love are pleasant. The second premise is that the cranio-sacral and sympathetic divisions of the autonomic nervous system "are allied with two groups of emotions having opposed qualities of feeling, pleasant and unpleasant, respectively." [34] Thus it is the sympathetic system which functions during anger, fear and bodily pain, and the cranio-sacral during digestion and sex behavior. The third premise is that certain forms of pleasantness, those involved, for instance, in exercise and habit, excitement of games, elation and mirth, occur without any accompanying autonomic activity and appear to depend upon unimpeded cerebrospinal impulses. From these premises, Allport develops the following theory: "The cranio-sacral division of the autonomic, supplemented under certain conditions by the cerebro-spinal system, innervates those responses whose return afferent impulses are associated with the conscious quality of pleasantness. The sympathetic division produces visceral responses which are represented in consciousness as unpleasantness." [35]

Marston's theory, essentially a reinterpretation of Herrick's view in the light of the results secured by Head and Holmes, is based primarily upon the analysis of emotions.[36] Fear, he points out, involves conflict of motor impulse, and the type of fear which is accompanied by the most fundamental type of unpleasantness is that "where the competing impulses are of almost equal strength, producing an alternation in control of their common motor path, resulting in trembling of that part of the body or limbs innervated." [37] From this and similar considerations he proceeds to define unpleasantness as "the conscious correlate of motor antagonism between impulses or groups of impulses seeking outlet over a common efferent path," [38] and he adds that the unpleasantness must be considered to be determined not by a partial blocking of the successful impulse, but by "unrelieved, thalamic summation of sensory impulses, in the sensory circuit of the unsuccessful competing impulses." [39]

As to pleasantness, Marston suggests that "the passing of any subminimal sensory impulse to unimpeded motor discharge over any thalamic nerve path correlated with consciousness is accompanied by the feeling of pleasantness." [40] These subminimal sensory impulses he conceives to gain motor outlet by alliance among themselves or with supraliminal sensory impulses, in accordance with the observations of Sherrington that stimuli which singly are unable to evoke a response may, if applied together, elicit such a response. Marston further suggests that indifference obtains "Whenever the controlling groups of sensory impulses are able to find simultaneous motor outlet without passing over a final common path." [41] Marston summarizes his theory in the following table:

TABLE LXIX

Affective States

	Positive	Negative	Neutral
Name of affect.	Pleasantness.	Unpleasantness.	Indifference.
Sensory content.	Awareness of free, harmonious, sub-sensation.	Awareness of blocked, disruptive, super-sensation.	Qualitatively differentiated sensations only.
Correlated relationship of motor impulses.	Allied in final common path.	Antagonistic in final common path.	Unrelated, with separate final paths.

Of these various theories seeking to relate hedonic tone to physiological processes, one stands out strongly because of its definiteness and its consequent wealth of verifiable implications. This is the theory of Allport. Unfortunately, this virtue leads to its undoing. In the first place, Cannon, upon whose experimental results Allport has largely based his theory, states explicitly that joy may, if strong enough, be accompanied by the functioning of the sympathetic division of the autonomic nervous system. In his opinion, this division is distinguished by response to *any* violent emotion. Of crying, one of the most easily observed manifestations of activity of the sympathetic system, Cannon writes: "We do not 'feel sorry because we cry' as James contended, but we cry because when we are sorry or overjoyed or violently angry or full of tender affection—when any one of these diverse emotional states is present—there are nervous discharges by sympathetic channels to various viscera, including the lachrymal glands." [42] But if joy, which is beyond doubt pleasant,[43] involve activity of the sympathetic division of the autonomic, then Allport's theory, stating definitely that "the sympathetic division produces visceral responses which are represented in consciousness as unpleasantness" cannot be maintained. In the second place, Allport points out that his theory implies that unpleasantness is slower of arousal than pleasantness. After reviewing the conditions of conduction in the sympathetic system, he writes: "These conditions—namely, greater synaptic resistance and slower rate of transmission—both indicate that the effects produced by the sympathetic fibres must be slower to appear than those of the cranio-sacral." [44] Allport appeals to "common experience" for verification of this implication. He writes: "Compare, for example, the latency of unpleasant feelings with the quick thrill of pleasure derived from pleasant tastes or erotic sensations. The case of stumbling on the stairs is a good example. In the writer's experience there is a sudden reflex recovery of balance, and then, when several steps have been descended, there wells up gradually a mass of unpleasant organic sensations." [45] It is undeniable that *some* cases of unpleasantness involve a longer latency than *some* cases of pleasantness, but as we saw in Chapter IV, Miss Washburn has shown that for a single type of stimulus hedonic reaction-times are the same for the same degrees of pleasantness and of unpleasantness (i. e., for 1 and -1, for 2 and -2, etc.). Clearly such results are absolutely incompatible with Allport's theory.

When we turn to the other attempts to relate hedonic tone to physiological processes, we find no such striking incompatibility with facts. We do find a disadvantage, however, which to the experimentalist is even more serious. In every case the fundamental relationship involved—in the case of Troland, for instance, the relationship between hedonic tone and change in rate of conductance of the cortical synapses underlying consciousness—is one which, though potentially observable, is not actually so with our present limitations of technique. It follows that these theories cannot be judged by direct observation of the fundamental relationship which they involve, but only by observation of the subordinate relationships which they imply. But—and here is the difficulty—so little is known concerning the processes involved in the fundamental relationship, concerning changes in cortical conductance, for instance, that these fundamental relationships have but very general implications, much the same for all the theories, and these general implications will admit of almost any variety of facts. Troland's theory illustrates this well, although it is by far the most specific of all the theories under discussion. According to this theory, both learning and pleasantness depend upon increase in the conductance of cortical synapses. Does this not mean that learning must invariably be pleasant? Not at all. Hedonic tone depends upon the *average conductance of the cortical synapses, the activity of which underlies consciousness at any given moment.* If a child learns under the influence of punishment, it may well be that the *average* conductance of synapses is decreasing while the conductance of some (concerned with the learning) is increasing. A similar lack of verifiable implications could be demonstrated even more strikingly in the case of the less well-developed theories—those of Marshall and Herrick, for instance. There is no need to do so, however, for the difficulty of verifying all of these theories is sufficiently proved by the fact that none is ever attacked on experimental grounds.

With respect to modern theories of hedonic tone, then, the situation is about as follows: Of the theories emphasizing the relation of hedonic tone to conscious processes, one, that of Krueger, is contrary to fact, and the others involve the construction of a variety of conscious elements which seem to be entirely superfluous for systematic psychology. Of the two leading theories emphasizing the relation of hedonic tone to psychical causes, neither is adequate to our present knowledge concerning hedonic tone. Of the theories, finally, which relate hedonic tone to physiological processes, one is contrary to fact and the others, however correct any or all may eventually turn out to be, for the present are so lacking in verifiable implications as to be wholly beyond the possibility of proof or disproof, and consequently, at least for the experimentalist, beyond the realm of science.

An Heuristic Hypothesis

The preceding review of theories, with its wholly negative conclusion, indicates some fundamental weakness in current theorizing with respect to hedonic tone. The nature of this weakness becomes evident when we consider that but one of the theories, that of Allport, could be actually tested by means of experimental data. In seeking to cover all possible facts, theories of hedonic tone have lost contact with the facts altogether. The result has been harmful to experimentation and theorizing alike. Experimentation, lacking guidance, has often exhausted itself upon inconsequential problems. Theorizing, lacking factual restraint, has turned into mere speculation. What is needed at present, in the psychology of hedonic tone, is the abandonment of attempts to bring all facts under a single set of fundamental principles and, instead, the formulation of limited working hypotheses capable of experimental verification and development.

The view that there is a relation between hedonic tone and certain specific processes in sense-organs has been seeking recognition for well over a century. In the first part of his "Elemens d'ideologie," published in 1801, Destutt de Tracy maintained that feelings, including joy and sadness, "are true internal sensations," [46] and as recently as 1922, Warren wrote: "A feeling is an experience in which systemic sensations are the main elements." [47]   In the interval, variations upon the same general theme have been proposed by a large number of psychologists, including such eminent men as Stumpf,[48] Brentano[49] and Titchener.[50]

This view has never achieved widespread acceptance.[51] Its detailed development has invariably encountered three major stumbling-blocks. In the first place, the problem of correlating pleasantness with a specific process in sense-organs—a process different from that underlying unpleasantness—has proved a hopeless puzzle.[52] Von Frey, it is true, sought to circumvent this obstacle by identifying pleasantness with the removal of pain,[53] but this expedient conflicted with the phenomenal individuality of pleasantness and with its frequent arousal in the absence of previous pain. In the second place, no processes have until recently been shown to correlate highly with unpleasantness except those underlying pain, and recourse to these has been precluded by the occurrence of pleasant pains.[54] In the third place, experimentation on the "nature" of hedonic tone has led a number of investigators to the conclusion that hedonic tone is phenomenally distinct from the usually accepted sensory qualities.[55]

It is my conviction that all three of these stumbling-blocks have been removed by certain recent developments in experimental psychology. In the first place, investigation has shown that absolute judgments of weight and of hedonic tone are subject to the same general law of contrast. We have seen that if a set of stimuli not involving extremes be presented repeatedly for hedonic judgment, the relatively most pleasant ones will eventually be judged absolutely pleasant, and the relatively least pleasant ones absolutely unpleasant.[56] Likewise, it can be predicted that if any set of stimuli not involving extremes be presented with instructions to give absolute judgments of weight, the observer will eventually call the lightest ones absolutely light and the heaviest ones absolutely heavy.[57] This points unmistakably, it seems to me, to a similarity in the physiological processes underlying experiences of weight and hedonic tone. But in the case of weight, both the experiences absolutely light and absolutely heavy are conceived to correspond to a single type of process in sense-organs, which varies only in respect of the physiological concomitant of stimulus-intensity. Why, then, should a view concerning the relation of hedonic tone to processes in sense-organs be obliged to designate a specific process corresponding solely to pleasantness? Is it not far more probable that pleasantness and unpleasantness both depend upon a single type of process varying only in respect of the physiological concomitant of stimulus-intensity?

The second development to which I wish to refer is the establishment by Nafe and by Hunt of a high correlation between hedonic tone and organic pressure.[58] Nafe's observers, it will be remembered, eventually *identified* pleasantness with bright pressure and unpleasantness with dull pressure. It is clear that this identification cannot be accepted literally. P. T. Young's failure to duplicate Nafe's results with any but a former observer of Nafe,[59] together with Nafe's own statement that in order to experience these pressures an observer ". . . must maintain a psychological, non-perceptive attitude." [60] clearly indicate that identification is contingent upon sensory instructions or their equivalent. On the other hand, this very contingence points to an equally significant alternative interpretation. It suggests, namely, that hedonic tone, though not a mode of pressure, corresponds to processes in sense-organs which, under sensory instructions or their equivalent, mediate modes of pressure. Such an interpretation obviously circumvents the two latter stumbling-blocks mentioned above. It provides as a concomitant of hedonic tone a specific process in sense-organs other than that underlying pain, and at the same time admits of a phenomenal distinction between hedonic tone and sensory qualities.

It is clear that these developments, besides removing certain stumbling-blocks, point to a fairly definite hypothesis concerning the relation of hedonic tone to processes in sense-organs. In the present state of our knowledge I believe that this hypothesis can best be formulated as follows: Hedonic tone depends upon a specific type of process in sense-organs, namely, that which, under sensory instructions or their equivalent, mediates bright and dull pressure. When this type of process occurs under hedonic instructions or their equivalent, it gives rise to relative or absolute hedonic tone. Relative hedonic tone depends directly upon the relative density[61] of the process, greater pleasantness being mediated by a change of density which, under sensory instructions or their equivalent, would mediate greater brightness. Absolute hedonic tone likewise depends upon relative density, but in a less direct way. Absolute pleasantness depends upon a density differing from the average for similar past situations in a manner adequate to occasion greater pleasantness; absolute unpleasantness depends upon such a relative density adequate to occasion lesser pleasantness. The process in question is invariably proprioceptive. It is aroused by external stimuli—e. g., visual stimuli—indirectly through the muscular adjustments which they bring about.

This hypothesis accounts readily for many facts besides those which led to its formulation: for the extreme variability of hedonic judgment, for the long latent time of hedonic tone, for its close relation to locomotor responses, and for its partial dependence upon learning. Its chief merit, however, is that it has already undergone a measure of verification and promises to lend itself to further experimental testing. The hypothesis was first formulated early in 1930,[62] long before the completion of Hunt's experimental work. At that time it was pointed out that the hypothesis involved two definite implications. The first was that, if observers were made to judge stimuli on one occasion with respect to hedonic value and on another with respect to brightness-dullness of concomitant internal pressures, there should result a marked correlation between hedonic value and brightness-dulness. The second implication was based upon Köhler's work on the time-error in judgments of sensory intensity.[63] It was argued that, if pleasantness and unpleasantness be functions of the density of a single process in sense-organs, the time-error for relative hedonic judgments must display a definite asymmetry. It must involve either an excess of judgments "second more pleasant" for short intervals between stimuli and a deficiency of such judgments for long intervals, or a deficiency of such judgments for short intervals and an excess for long. The first of these implications has since been verified by Hunt.[64] The second still remains to be verified, although the few data on the time-error described in Chapter IV already make it probable that it, likewise, will be found to hold.

In its present formulation the hypothesis is relatively indefinite. This fault, however, promises to be but temporary. The hypothesis, for instance, does not specify whether it is an increase in the density of the process in the sense-organs which underlies greater pleasantness or a decrease. Nafe is of the opinion that brightness—and consequently pleasantness—increases with the neural correlate of stimulus-intensity,[65] but a number of facts stand in the way of such a view. Physiological density might well be expected to correlate at least slightly with phenomenal density, yet Nafe writes that, in the case of bright pressure, "The experience, as a whole, is found to be diffuse and volumic, and within the pattern the brightness consists of discreet points, as in tickle and gooseflesh"; whereas ". . . In the experience of dull pressure the quality is . . . volumic and diffuse, but less so than bright pressure." [66] Furthermore, P. T. Young has shown that the bodily reverberations in the case of unpleasantness are more rich and varied than in the case of pleasantness.[67] We have seen in Chapter III, finally, that increase in the intensity of the external stimulus results as a rule in the eventual decrease of the pleasantness of the stimulus. All of these facts, though not absolutely incompatible with Nafe's opinion, suggest the wisdom of withholding judgment in the absence of further evidence. The establishment, however, of a definite asymmetry in the case of the hedonic time-error would provide such evidence. If the time-error should be found to involve a deficiency of judgments "second more pleasant" for short intervals and an excess of such judgments for long intervals, it could be inferred, on the basis of Köhler's physiological hypothesis, that increased pleasantness does indeed depend upon increased density. If, on the other hand, there should be an excess of judgments "second more pleasant" for short intervals, and a deficiency for long, it could be inferred that increase of density mediates increase of unpleasantness. The fragmentary data already available, which were presented in Chapter IV, favor the former alternative. They are too few, however, to warrant a definite decision.

The further indefiniteness of the hypothesis with respect to the locus of the process in sense-organs should likewise yield to experimental attack. As was pointed out in Chapter VIII, Nafe found that the bright pressure correlated with pleasantness is vaguely localized in the upper part of the body, while the dull pressure correlated with unpleasantness is localized in the abdomen or in the lower part of the body,[68] and Hunt confirmed these results.[69] From what we know of cutaneous and organic localization, it seems reasonable to infer that the corresponding processes in sense-organs are somewhat similarly localized. It also seems reasonable to expect that further introspective work, combined with experiments involving selective activation of specific muscular groups, will enable us materially to increase this modicum of knowledge.

The most serious indefiniteness of the hypothesis arises from the phrase "hedonic instructions or their equivalent." Here, again, however, experimentation promises to be of some avail. No instructions appear to be necessary for the arousal of hedonic tone in the case of intense pain stimulation. Is this so of all stimuli having high "general hedonic value"? [70] Early classifications of odors rest largely upon hedonic tone; indeed, Haller's classification was based entirely upon this characteristic.[71] Do olfactory stimuli—and perhaps taste stimuli—arouse hedonic tone in the absence of instructions more readily than do visual and auditory stimuli? It is often said that workers in chemical laboratories are hedonically immune to odors. Is novelty an equivalent of hedonic instructions? Investigation of these questions involves a methodological difficulty, but not an insuperable one. It is generally agreed that for the report of an event to be wholly reliable it is necessary that the instructions determining the report precede the event. This condition is obviously impossible of satisfaction in the investigation of the questions mentioned above. Reliability, however, is not subject to the all-or-none law. Everyday experience and the history of the *Ausfragemethode* show that post-determined reports, though subject to the distorting effects of memory and suggestion, nevertheless yield results of fair reliability. In this case, then, as in the two preceding ones, the relative indefiniteness of the hypothesis is essentially an invitation to further experimental investigation.

The hypothesis formulated above is at present no more than a stepping-stone from experimental facts of the past to experimental facts of the future. Whether it is ultimately to assume theoretical rank will obviously depend upon experimental results. It has not the slightest pretension, however, to the rank of a theory. It covers but one of the many relations essential to a complete theory of hedonic tone, and thus can at best but develop into a single feature of such a theory. As was stated at the beginning of this section, however, it seems likely that the psychology of hedonic tone will derive greater benefit for the present from the formulation of such limited, but verifiable, hypotheses than from more ambitious attempts to provide all-inclusive theoretical structures.

FOOTNOTES AND REFERENCES

[1] W. WUNDT. Grundzüge der physiologischen Psychologie, 4th edit., Leipzig, 1893, I, 555 ff.

[2] H. R. MARSHALL. The Methods of the Naturalist and Psychologist, *Psychol. Rev.*, 15, 1908, 16f.; Pain, Pleasure and Aesthetics, N. Y., 1894, 61.

[3] T. ZIEHEN. Leitfaden der physiologischen Psychologie, 12th edit., Jena, 1924, 290-294 and 355-358.

[4] *Ibid.*, 290.

[5] *Ibid.*, 356.

[6] C. STUMPF. Ueber Gefühlsempfindungen, *Bericht über den II Kongress für experimentelle Psychologie*, Leipzig, 1907, 209; Ueber Gefühlsempfindungen, *Z. f. Psychologie*, 44, 1906, 1 ff. (this article is an expansion of the preceding one); *Cf.* also C. STUMPF, *Z. f. Psychologie*, 28, 1917, 263 ff. An excellent exposition and critical discussion of Stumpf's theory will be found in E. B. TITCHENER, Lectures on the Elementary Psychology of Feeling and Attention, N. Y., 1908, 81-121.

[7] E. B. TITCHENER. A Textbook of Psychology, N. Y., 1919 (1909), 225-236.

[8] W. WUNDT. Grundriss der Psychologie, 14th edit., Stuttgart, 1920, 99; Grundzüge der physiologischen Psychologie, Leipzig, 1902, II, 284-291. An excellent exposition and critical discussion of Wundt's theory will be found in E. B. TITCHENER, Lectures on the Elementary Psychology of Feeling and Attention, N. Y., 1908, 125-168.

[9] H. C. WARREN. Human Psychology, Boston and N. Y., 1920, 279.

[10] J. P. NAFE. The Psychology of Felt Experience, *Amer. J. Psychol.*, 39, 1927, 387.

[11] F. KRUEGER. Das Wasen der Gefühle, Entwurf Einer Systematischen Theorie, *Arch. f. d. ges. Psychol.*, 65, 1928, 91-128. *Cf.* also F. KRUEGER. The Essence of Feeling, Outline of a Systematic Theory, in Feelings and Emotions, The Wittenberg Symposium, Worcester, 1928, 58-86.

[12] *Ibid.*, 108.

[13] *Ibid.*, 103.

[14] "The most fundamental division of conscious experience is into two distinct types. . . . They are termed sensation and ideation, respectively. . . . Sensation is the original and ideation the derivative type of experience. The entire group of sensations furnished by each sort of receptor is called a *sense*. . . . The two *characters* of experience, quality and intensity, are determined primarily by the mode and intensity of the stimulus." (H. C. WARREN, Human Psychology, Boston and N. Y., 1920, 148-149.)

[15] J. F. HERBART. Lehrbuch zur Psychologie, Königsberg und Leipzig, 1816, 120-121.

[16] W. McDOUGALL. Outline of Psychology, N. Y., 1923, 269.

418   THEORY

17 J. W. NAHLOWSKY. Das Gefühlsleben (1862), 2nd edit., Leipzig, 1884, 41-44 and 47-50.

18 J. F. HERBART. A Textbook in Psychology, transl. by M. K. Smith, N. Y., 1891, 28.

19 Ibid., 29. In connection with this theory, cf. W. F. VOLKMANN, RITTER VON VOLKMAR, Lehrbuch der Psychologie, 3rd edit., Vol. 2, Cöthen, 1875, 298 ff.

20 E. v. HARTMANN. Die Moderne Psychologie, Leipzig, 1901, 272-273.

21 W. MCDOUGALL. Outline of Psychology, N. Y., 1923, 269.

22 Ibid., 270.

23 W. MCDOUGALL. Pleasure, Pain and Conation, Brit. J. Psychol., 17, 1927, 178-179.

24 A. LEHMANN. Die Hauptgesetze des Menschlichen Gefühlslebens, Leipzig, 1914, 166-168.

25 H. R. MARSHALL. Consciousness, N. Y., 1909, 242 ff.

26 E. L. THORNDIKE. Educational Psychology, Briefer Course, N. Y., 1914, 53-56.

27 Ibid., 53.

28 Ibid., 55.

29 L. T. TROLAND. A System for Explaining Affective Phenomena, J. of Abnor. Psychol., 14, 1920, 376-387; The Mystery of Mind, N. Y., 1926, 131-145; The Fundamentals of Human Motivation, N. Y., 1928, 284-300.

30 L. T. TROLAND. J. Abnor. Psychol., 14, 1920, 377.

31 C. J. HERRICK. An Introduction to Neurology, 2nd edit., Phila., 1918, 286.

32 F. H. ALLPORT. Social Psychology, Cambridge, Mass., 1924, 84-98.

33 Ibid., 85.

34 Ibid., 89.

35 Ibid., 90.

36 W. M. MARSTON. A Theory of Emotions and Affection Based Upon Systolic Blood Pressure Studies, Amer. J. Psychol., 35, 1924, 469.

37 Ibid., 497.

38 Ibid., 498.

39 Ibid., 499.

40 Ibid., 501-502.

41 Ibid., 505.

42 W. B. CANNON. Bodily Changes in Pain, Hunger, Fear and Rage, N. Y., 1915, 280.

43 If any evidence of this statement be considered necessary, cf. H. C. WARREN, Elements of Human Psychology, Cambridge, Mass., 1922, 215.

44 F. H. ALLPORT. Op. cit., 91.

45 Ibid., 91.

46 A. L. C. DESTUTT DE TRACY. Elemens d'idéologie, première partie, idéologie proprement dite (1801) 1827, 25.

47 H. C. WARREN. Elements of Human Psychology, N. Y., 1922, 203-204.

48 C. STUMPF. Ueber Gefühlsempfindungen, Z. f. Psychol, 1907, 44, 1.

49 F. BRENTANO. Untersuchungen zur Sinnespsychologie, Leipzig, 1907, 112 and 119-125.

50 E. B. TITCHENER. A Textbook of Psychology, N. Y. (1909), 1926, 260 ff.

[51] Even William James dared not include hedonic tone in his theory of Emotions. *Cf.* W. JAMES, What Is an Emotion? *Mind,* 9, 1884, 189 and 201-203; The Physical Basis of Emotion, *Psychol. Rev.,* 1, 1894, 523-524. In the latter article James does not *deny* that hedonic tone may come under his theory of emotions, but he *refuses to assert* it.

[52] "Ob ferner auch besondere Lustnerven anzunehmen sind, wie v. Frey Schmerznerven statuirt, ist . . . eine Frage der Physiologie, nicht der Psychologie." C. STUMPF, *op. cit.,* 22.

[53] M. v. FREY. Die Gefühle und ihr Verhältnis zu den Empfindungen, Leipzig, 1894, 17.

[54] E. B. TITCHENER. *Op. cit.,* 261; A. WOHLGEMUTH, On the Feelings and Their Neural Correlate, with an Examination of the Nature of Pain, *Brit. J. Psychol.,* 1917, 8, 450.

[55] *Cf.* N. ALECHSIEFF. Die Grundformen der Gefühle, *Psychol. Stud.,* 1907, 3, 264; M. YOKOYAMA, The Nature of the Affective Judgment in the Method of Paired Comparison. *Amer. J. Psychol.,* 1921, 32, 369.

[56] *Cf.* A. J. HARRIS. An Experiment on Affective Contrast, *Amer. J. Psychol.,* 1929, 41, 617-624; J. G. BEEBE-CENTER, The Law of Affective Equilibrium, *ibid.,* 1929, 41, 64.

[57] E. G. WEVER and K. E. ZENER. The Method of Absolute Judgment in Psychophysics, *Psychol. Rev.,* 1928, 35, 466.

[58] J. P. NAFE. An Experimental Study of the Affective Qualities, *Amer. J. Psychol.,* 1924, 35, 507; W. A. HUNT, The Relation of Bright and Dull Pressure to Affectivity, *Amer. J. Psychol.,* 43, 1931, 87.

[59] P. T. YOUNG. Studies in Affective Psychology, *Amer. J. Psychol.,* 1927, 38, 175.

[60] J. P. NAFE. *Op. cit.,* 540.

[61] Density is here used to represent the physiological correlate of stimulus-intensity. Should this correlate turn out to be frequency or some other characteristic the hypopthesis could easily be altered accordingly.

[62] J. G. BEEBE-CENTER. The Relation Between Affectivity and Specific Processes in Sense-organs, *Psychol. Rev.,* 37, 1930, 327.

[63] W. KÖHLER. Zur Theorie des Sukzessivvergleichs und der Zeitfehler, *Psychol. Forsch.,* 1923, 4, 115.

[64] W. A. HUNT. The Relation of Bright and Dull Pressure to Affectivity, *Amer. J. Psychol.,* 43, 1931, 87; The Pressure Correlate of Emotion, *Ibid.,* 600.

[65] J. P. NAFE. The Sense of Feeling, in "The Foundations of Experimental Psychology," Worcester, 1929, 399. Nafe considers the neural correlate of stimulus-intensity to be frequency of impulses rather than density.

[66] J. P. NAFE. The Psychology of Felt Experience, *Amer. J. Psychol.,* 1927, 39, 371.

[67] P. T. YOUNG. Pleasantness and Unpleasantness in Relation to Organic Response, *Amer. J. Psychol.,* 1921, 32, 38.

[68] J. P. NAFE. The Sense of Feeling, in "The Foundations of Experimental Psychology," Worcester, 1929, 411.

[69] W. A. HUNT. The Pressure Correlates of Hedonic Tone, Thesis, Harvard University, 1931, 29-42.

[70] *Cf.* J. G. BEEBE-CENTER. General Affective Value, *Psychol. Rev.,* 1929, 36, 472.

[71] *Cf.* H. HENNING. Der Geruch, Leipzig, 1916, 71 ff.

INDEX OF SUBJECTS

INDEX OF NAMES